Basic Keyboarding
for the
Medical Office Assistant
3rd Edition

Edna J. Moss, BA

Grossmount Health Occupations Center
Santee, CA

Southwestern College
Chula Vista, CA

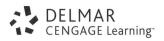
DELMAR
CENGAGE Learning

Australia • Brazil • Japan • Korea • Mexico • Singapore • Spain • United Kingdom • United States

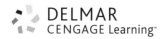
DELMAR
CENGAGE Learning™

Basic Keyboarding for the Medical Office Assistant, Third Edition

Edna J. Moss

Vice President, Health Care Business Unit:
  William Brottmiller

Editorial Director: Cathy L. Esperti

Acquisitions Editor: Rhonda Dearborn

Editorial Assistant: Natalie Wager

Editorial Assistant: Jill Osterhout

Marketing Director: Jennifer McAvey

Channel Manager: Tamara Caruso

Production Editor: Mary Colleen Liburdi

For product information and technology assistance, contact us at
Cengage Learning Customer & Sales Support, 1-800-354-9706

For permission to use material from this text or product,
submit all requests online at **www.cengage.com/permissions**
Further permissions questions can be emailed to
permissionrequest@cengage.com

ExamView® and ExamView Pro® are registered trademarks of FSCreations, Inc. Windows is a registered trademark of the Microsoft Corporation used herein under license. Macintosh and Power Macintosh are registered trademarks of Apple Computer, Inc. Used herein under license.

ISBN-13: 978-1-4018-1189-1

ISBN-10: 1-4018-1189-2

Delmar
Executive Woods
5 Maxwell Drive
Clifton Park, NY 12065
USA

Cengage Learning is a leading provider of customized learning solutions with office locations around the globe, including Singapore, the United Kingdom, Australia, Mexico, Brazil, and Japan. Locate your local office at **www.cengage.com/global**

Cengage Learning products are represented in Canada by Nelson Education, Ltd.

To learn more about Delmar, visit **www.cengage.com/delmar**

Purchase any of our products at your local bookstore or at our preferred online store **www.CengageBrain.com**

Notice to the Reader

Printed in the United States of America
12 13 14 15 16 14 13 12 11 10

Contents

UNIT 5   ALL-PURPOSE DRILLS AND TIMED WRITINGS   83

UNIT 6   NUMBERS AND TOP ROW KEYS   113

Preface

The purpose of *Basic Keyboarding for the Medical Office Assistant, 3rd Edition* is to familiarize the user with beginning medical keyboarding, advanced keyboarding, medical language skills, and grammatical and office skills.

The text is designed to introduce material of increasing difficulty gradually. In this way, experience and proficiency of skill can be gained. Medical keyboarding skill requires the user to concentrate on each assignment and to practice.

NEW TO THIS EDITION

All keyboarding exercises in the third edition have been extensively revised to include more medical terminology with the goal of exposing students to terms and phrases they will encounter in other courses or on the job. Based on the feedback that was received from users of the previous edition, the following information has been added in this edition to help students expand their knowledge of grammar and punctuation and improve their keyboarding speed and accuracy:

- More timed writing exercises in letter and medical reports
- More rules for punctuation and grammar with expanded exercises
- Exercises made up of prefixes, root words, and suffixes
- More instruction on format layout, such as tab settings and margins
- More instruction on word count scales and how they are used in timed writings

The additional timed writing exercises can be easily customized to fit the needs of any user. New icons have been added to the Table of Contents to help readers quickly identify the length of each timed writing exercise. The clock symbol (🕐) indicates a timed writing. The acronym "WAM" has been added next to the lessons that teach users how to compute a timed writing in words a minute. Unit 12 has also been updated to include a greater emphasis on beginning medical transcription. Instructions for formatting a variety of medical reports, such as history and physical examination, operative, consultation, and others, are included in this unit, along with numerous sample reports and practice exercises.

CD-ROM

A CD-ROM containing the majority of medical reports contained in Unit 12 is also available with some texts. The CD-ROM will give students exposure to medical dictation and the opportunity to practice their keyboarding skills while transcribing it. The answers to all of the reports on the CD-ROM are included in Unit 12 of the student text, so students may proofread their work upon completion. CD-ROM exercises may be completed as part of Unit 12, or assigned as extra credit to encourage students to try their hand at transcription when they have gained some confidence in their keyboarding skills.

The text is appropriate for use in high schools, vocational schools, in-service training, and community colleges.

FEATURES

Each lesson identifies learning goals and offers activities to aid in accomplishing those goals. Answers and a keyboarding progress record are included at the end of the text. An instructor's guide is available for use with this text.

Upon completion of these units, the student will meet the following goals.

Unit 1 introduces the user to beginning medical keyboarding and how to compute 1-minute timings.

Unit 2 stresses alphabetic sentences with 1-minute timings; the tab key will be used. How to compute 2-minute timings is also covered.

Unit 3 contains speed paragraphs and exercises for accuracy development. How to compute 3- and 5-minute timings is also covered.

Unit 4 has more speed builders, letter combinations, and medical timed writings.

Unit 5 offers timed writings and shifting drills.

Unit 6 emphasizes language skills such as parts of speech, punctuation, capitalization, the sentence, clauses, phrases, and timed writings.

Unit 7 introduces the number keys, symbols, and timed writings.

Unit 8 introduces additional abbreviations, homonyms, antonyms, eponyms, word division, proofreading, and timed writings.

Unit 9 introduces how capitalization is used and timed writings.

Unit 10 presents memos, minutes, agenda, centering, and timed writings.

Unit 11 introduces formats for keying business letters and timed writings.

Unit 12 covers keying medical reports, such as history and physical reports, operative reports, pathology reports, consultation reports, radiology reports, discharge summaries, discharge instructions, worker's compensation letters, autopsy reports, chart notes, and timed writings.

Unit 13 deals with the job search, marketing skills, and timed writings.

ACKNOWLEDGMENTS

The author would like to thank the following reviewers who assisted in this revision:

Sue Brisky, BPS
College America
Denver, CO

Gina Erio
California College of Technology
Sacramento, CA

Courtney McCash
North Texas Professional Career Institute
Dallas, TX

Linda Pettiogano
Berdan Institute
Totowa, NJ

Mitsy Ballentine, M.Ed.
Greenville Technical School
Greenville, SC

Charlotte Williams, Ph.D.
Stringer-Huff Business Center
Jones County Junior College
Ellisville, MS

The author would also like to thank the following Delmar Cengage Learning staff for their guidance: Cathy Esperti, Rhonda Dearborn, Mary Colleen Liburdi, Natalie Wagner, Mona Caron, and Jill Osterhout.

Beginning Keyboarding

Keyboarding Techniques

Goals

After completing this lesson, you will be able to:

✔ Key by touch, keeping your eyes on the book.
✔ Seat yourself and place your hands correctly on the keyboard.
✔ Arrange your workspace correctly.
✔ Set up your computer for the exercises in this book.

Instructions

1. Keep your feet on the floor for balance (see the illustration on p. 3).
2. Adjust your chair height so that your feet are comfortably on the floor.
3. Place the fingers of your left hand on the a s d f keys, the little finger on a.
4. Place the fingers of your right hand on the j k l ; keys, the little finger on the ;.
5. Key with your fingertips, curving the fingers and keeping them light on the keys.
6. **Be sure to keep your wrists and palms off the keyboard.**
7. **Strike the space bar with the right thumb.**
8. Keep your eyes on the copy as you key.
9. Do not read faster than you key.
10. Tap the space bar, and take your thumb off. The space bar is used to space between words and punctuation.

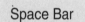

Enter Key:

Use the fourth finger of your right hand. Keep the j finger on the j key. Tap the enter key. Practice using the enter key.

The illustration (on p. 5) shows a typical computer keyboard.

Sitting Diagram

This is the general diagram of the recommended sitting posture for computer users. Keep in mind that fixed postures contribute to the risk of cumulative trauma injury. Variety of posture is crucial, as is the habit of standing up often. The body needs movement. Nothing counts more than comfort, and this illustration is simply a tool to understand what is happening in your body at the computer. Keep these principles in mind as you develop a repertoire of comfortable postures to use throughout the workday, knowing that slumped and leaning postures demand more work from the body leading to early fatigue.

• Top of monitor just below eye level. This supports keeping the head over the shoulders. Comfortable viewing is generally 5 to 30 degrees below horizontal. Place in front of the body to prevent sitting in a twisted posture or turning the head.

• Head over the shoulders to allow the skeleton to carry the weight of the head, relieving overuse of neck, shoulder, and back muscles.

• Monitor distance so that chin doesn't jut forward while the trunk is against the chair back.

• Seat back should support curve in lower (lumbar) spine. Higher seat backs are recommended to relieve spinal pressures. A slight backward angle is preferred to allow the chair to take some load off the spine. Allow the chair to carry a share of the body weight.

• Keyboard height should allow for relaxed shoulders, flat wrists, and at least ninety degrees at the inside of elbow. Sit directly in front, close enough not to have to reach forward. Rest palms on rest only when fingers can remain relaxed.

• Armrests, if used, soft and wide. There should be no contact during keying. Close enough to not force extension of elbows, and low enough for shoulders to be relaxed without slumping or leaning.

• Thighs level with or just above knees to promote a neutral spine.

• Seat pan not so deep that comfortable contact with chair back is prevented. Contact behind the knees must be avoided. Optimal contact with thighs provides greatest degree of effortless support.

• Feet in firm contact with the floor to distribute load through the whole body. Use a footrest only if necessary. Leave space under desk free of any obstruction to legs.

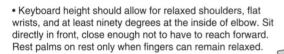

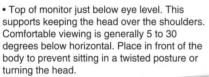
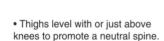
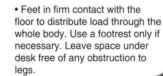

Recommended computer operator position. (Courtesy of Gary Karp, Ergonomics Consultant, Onsight Technology Education Services, San Francisco, CA)

THE COMPUTER KEYBOARD

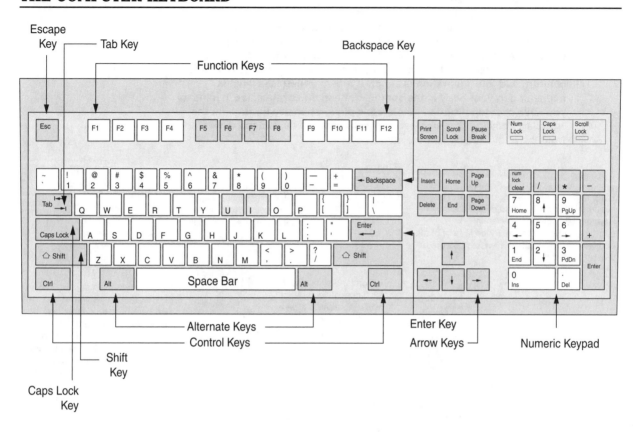

Escape Key

Tab Key

Function Keys

Backspace Key

Alternate Keys

Control Keys

Shift Key

Caps Lock Key

Enter Key

Arrow Keys

Numeric Keypad

Home Row Keys, Space, and Return

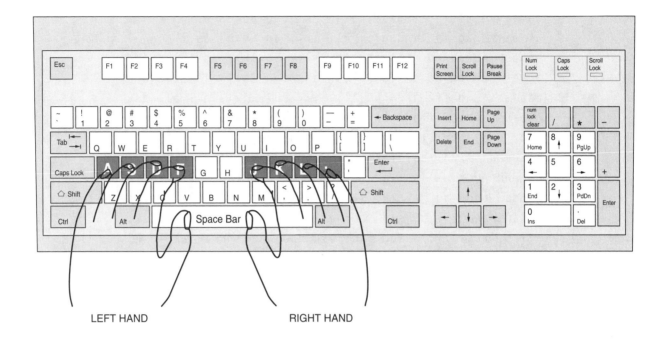

LEFT HAND   RIGHT HAND

HOME ROW KEYS

Goals

After completing this lesson, you will be able to:

✔ Key home row keys.
✔ Use the space bar.
✔ Use the return key.
✔ Key words using the keys learned.

A. Instructions: The Home Row

1. Locate the space bar and strike it with your right thumb.
2. Locate the enter key and strike it with the little finger of your right hand.
3. Use your finger tips to strike keys.
4. Place the fingers of your left hand on the a, s, d, and f keys.
5. Place the fingers of your right hand on the j, k, l, and ; keys.
6. **Keep your eyes on the copy as you key.**
7. After completing two lines, strike the enter key twice.
8. Key each line two times, double space after each group of two.
9. Keep feet on the floor in front of your chair.

HOME ROW KEYS

```
 1   a ss aa ss as as as dd ff dd ff df df df dl
 2   a ss aa ss as as as dd ff dd ff df df df dl
 3   j kk jj kk jk jk jk ll ;; ll ;; ll ;l ;l ;l
 4   j kk jj kk jk jk jk ll ;; ll ;; ll ;l ;l ;l
 5   as as kd kd fj l; asdf; jkl; jkl; ad ad as as
 6   as as kd kd fj l; asdf; jkl; jkl; ad ad as as
 7   as as sad ad ad all ask lad lass fad fall ask alas add
 8   as as sad ad ad all ask lad lass fad fall ask alas add
 9   aaa sss ddd fff jjj kkk lll ;;; asdf; jkl; all all ask
10   aaa sss ddd fff jjj kkk lll ;;; asdf; jkl; all all ask
11   jad; dad; kad; fad; add; lad; dad; kad; fad; flask flask
12   ask a sad lad; all fall; ask a sad dad; all dads; ask dad;
13   as dad adds ad jak lad la all ask lass fad fall kad; a dad;
14   as dad adds ad jak lad la all ask lass fad fall kad; a dad;
15   a lad; ask all; a sad lad; ask dad; jak fall; a flask;
16   a lad; ask all; a sad lad; ask dad; jak fall; a flask;
```

H AND G

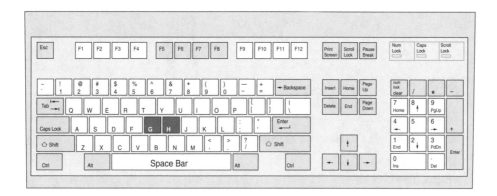

B. Instructions: The H and G Keys

1. **Use your left forefinger for the g key.**
2. **Use your right forefinger for the h key.**
3. Key each line two times; double space after each group of two.

Learn the h key. Use the j finger.

```
17   h hh jj jj ;h ;h lh lh ah ah ha ha ha had
18   h hh jj jj ;h ;h lh lh ah ah ha ha ha had
19   h ha has has had sash sash lash lash half
20   h ha has has had sash sash lash lash half
```

Learn the g key. Use the f finger.

```
21   g gg ff ff gf gf lg lg ag ag kg kg kg kg
22   g gg ff ff gf gf lg lg ag ag kg kg kg kg
23   a ag gas gas gas gash gash glass glass ag
24   a ag gas gas gas gash gash glass glass ag
```

Skillbuilding Warmup

```
25   ask all; a dad has gas; all had a glass; a kaka
26   ask all; a dad has gas; all had a glass; a kaka
27   all has a gall; jak fall; a flask; gag a lad; aa
```

Thirty-Second Timed Writings

Key the following timing. Key line 28 first, start over on line 28 if you complete in 30 seconds.

```
28   ask a dad;  add a lad;  ask ask a kaka;  add jags,        10
```

Key line 29. Start over on line 29 if you complete in 30 seconds.

```
29   ask a lad;  a gall;  lad has gas, gag a lad;               9
```

Instructions

Key the following timing.

Key line 1 first, start over on line 1 if you complete in 30 seconds.

```
1   as dad adds ad jak lad la all ask lass fad fall kad; a dad;   11
```

Key line 2 second, start over on line 2 if you complete in 30 seconds.

```
2   a lad; ask all; a sad lad; ask dad; jak fall; a flask;        11
```

Key line 3 third, start over on line 3 if you complete in 30 seconds.

```
3   ask a sad lad; all fall; ask a sad dad; all dads; ask dad;    11
     □□□□1□□□□2□□□□3□□□□4□□□□5□□□□6□□□□7□□□□8□□□□9□□□□10□□□□11□□□□12
```

Nine New Keys: T, U, E, I, R, and N, Left Shift, Right Shift, Period; and Computing One-Minute Timing

NINE NEW KEYS: T, U, E, I, R, AND N, LEFT SHIFT, RIGHT SHIFT, PERIOD

Goals

After completing this lesson, you will be able to:

✔ Key t, u, e, i, r, and n.
✔ Use the shift key to capitalize letters.

Skillbuilding Warmup

```
jjj fff kkk ddd lll sss ;;; aaa
add a flask; a glad dad; has gas
```

T AND U

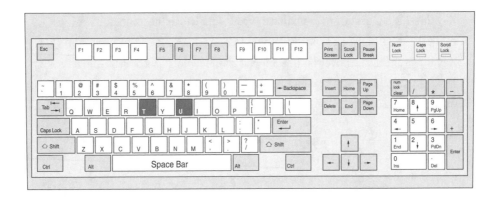

Learn t. Reach with the f finger.

Reminder: Keep at least one finger on the home row at all times to guide back to home position. Key each line two times.

```
1   t tf tf tf ta ta ts ts tl tl at at tag tad hat fat
2   t tf sat gat jat lat tat task flat tag tad tall fast
3   td hat staff data last tag task flat tag tad tall fast
4   td hat tad stat skat stag that slat gast task halt fat
```

Learn u. Reach with the j finger.

Reminder: Keep at least one finger on the home row at all times to guide back to home position. Key each line two times.

1   u uj uj uj ua ua ul ul us uk uk jug lug dug hug ug
2   u uj sud tut auk tut ugh gust tuft dud hug gull tug
3   ud hut aula dust full juj tugg huff dual guff jugs
4   ud hut flu lull luff gull gaud shut dull kudi lust
5   just a gull; lug a jug; sad tut; as a dual; a gust
6   as a hush; suds dull; ugh sulk lad; as a tutu gal;

One-Minute Timed Writing

Take 3 one-minute timed writings. Note: If you finish before time is up, start over again.

7   all glad dads had gas;   5

    ▢▢▢▢1▢▢▢▢2▢▢▢▢3▢▢▢▢4▢▢▢▢5▢▢▢▢6▢▢▢▢7▢▢▢▢8▢▢▢▢9▢▢▢▢10▢▢▢▢11▢▢▢▢12

Skillbuilding Warmup

ttt uuu ddd lll sss ;;; aaa kkk
a fast hug; dust jugs; had flu;

E AND I

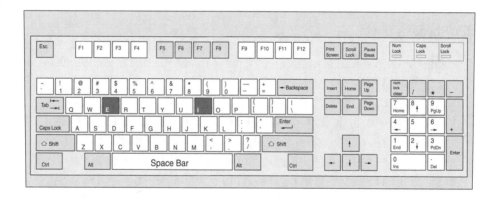

Learn e. Reach with the d finger.

Reminder: Keep at least one finger on the home row at all times to guide back to home position. Key each line two times.

1   e ed ed ed he he ek ek el el ef ef leg she fee see
2   e ed ked sea egg fed let set age deaf heat jet gel
3   es elf leak heal else egg left leak head fell fee
4   es elf hue else left leg jell fade east deka feed
5   heal a leak; eat a egg; as fees; had a seed; a head;
6   ad a suet; test teat; set left leg; as a test tea;

COMPUTING ONE-MINUTE TIMING

A. Instructions: Computing Timed Writing Speed

Note: This edition has provided additional timed writing exercises to better help you teach the rules of grammar, punctuation, speed, and accuracy. It is not necessary, however, to use all of the timed writings provided in this text. Choose the exercises best suited to your class.

Keyboarding speed is measured in words in a minute (WAM). To compute WAM, count every 5 strokes, including spaces.

Example: Computing 1-Minute Timing

1. Keyed 12 words in a 1-minute timing with two errors.
2. Count the errors and multiply by 2.
3. Errors = 2; 2 × 2 = 4.
4. Subtract errors from 12. 12 − 4 = 8.
5. Your net speed: 8/2 errors.

To determine your words per minute, add the number at the end of the last complete line to the number beneath timing of the partially completed line.

Example: 1-Minute Timed Writing

```
Mary returns to the cllinic this morning for follow-up of her    12
herpes encephalitis. He was hospitalized for several days or     24
encephalitis which was diagnosed as herpes.                      33
□□□□1□□□□2□□□□3□□□□4□□□□5□□□□6□□□□7□□□□8□□□□9□□□□10□□□□11□□□□12
```

Learn i. Reach with the k finger.

Reminder: Keep at least one finger on the home row at all times to guide back to home position. Key each line two times.

```
1   i ik ik ik is is it it if if il il aid did kid lik
2   i ik ail aid kik lik ill ilk lit jigs kits kit tie
3   is aid sill silt silk ill like kiss disk dial sill
4   is aid lie fail sail jail dill fill hill diet life
5   kiss a dial; aid a kid; is dill; if a slit; a disk
6   is a sail; kids said; did fall ill; if a lass did;
```

One-Minute Timed Writing

Take 3 one-minute timed writings. Note: If you finish before time is up, start over again.

```
7   he fell; hit head; kids did fall ill;                        8
    □□□□1□□□□2□□□□3□□□□4□□□□5□□□□6□□□□7□□□□8□□□□9□□□□10□□□□11□□□□12
```

Skillbuilding Warmup

```
eee iii ttt uuu ;;; lll aaa kkk
heal a leg; dad is ill; aid kid
```

R

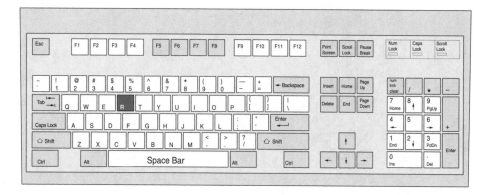

Learn r. Reach with the f finger.

Reminder: Keep at least one finger on the home row at all times to guide back to home position. Key each line two times.

1 r rf rf rf rs rs rd rd rl rl ra ra rid jar sir rat
2 r rf ark art are far red tart risk rad are far fur
3 ra rad jars tear iris tar hard rage hare rash rad
4 ra rad far fret rest fret free area dark sear dart
5 treat a rash; air a jar; is iris; is a rale; a tear
6 is a risk; dark area; sir fret art; as a dart rad;

One-Minute Timed Writing

Take 3 one-minute timed writings. Note: If you finish before time is up, start over again.

7 her rash is hard to treat; rales are heard; is iritis;   11
   □□□□1□□□□2□□□□3□□□□4□□□□5□□□□6□□□□7□□□□8□□□□9□□□□10□□□□11□□□□12

Skillbuilding Warmup

rrr iii ;;; aaa uuu lll kkk t
read test; seal tear; red jar

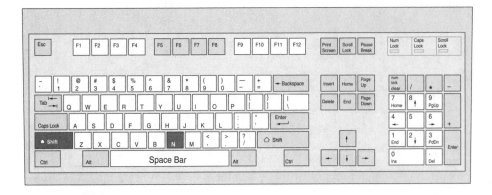

Learn n. Reach with the j finger.

Reminder: Keep at least one finger on home row at all times to guide back to home position. Key each line two times.

1 n nj in in an an ns ns nl nl na na tan den fin kin

2 n nj ant net ink din fen nail fang ink nit nil tin

3 in end near thin and shin skin tine need rain tin

4 in kin inn lung turn near hand then gen nake hang

5 need a tine; nag a kin; is thin; in a fang; a lung

6 in a nail; end near; nit fins net; in a gene hand;

Learn left shift key. Reach with the left little finger.

The left shift key is used to make capital letters for letters keyed with the right hand. Depress the left shift key with the left little finger. Key the capital letter with the appropriate finger of the right hand. Release the left shift key and return to the home row.

1 J J Jan Jan Jana Li Ina Jan Nan Li Ken Hal Nan Ida Jan Lida

2 Jan and Lida; Ken and Hal; Li and Lil; Ida and Nan: Ira and Lil;

3 Jana and Jeff; Jill and Jane Lee; Jill Lake and James King;

4 King and Jain; Jena; Jang; Keen; Ida Lake; Ina King and Jan Lake;

One-Minute Timed Writing

Take 3 one-minute timed writings. Note: If you finish before time is up, start over again.

5 Jan King and Lida King are ill; Ira and Lil had a lung test;   12

   ☐☐☐☐1☐☐☐☐2☐☐☐☐3☐☐☐☐4☐☐☐☐5☐☐☐☐6☐☐☐☐7☐☐☐☐8☐☐☐☐9☐☐☐☐10☐☐☐☐11☐☐☐☐12

Skillbuilding Warmup

nnn ;;; sss ddd ttt aaa eee iiii

Jan Lake; Lida King; Nan and Ida

RIGHT SHIFT

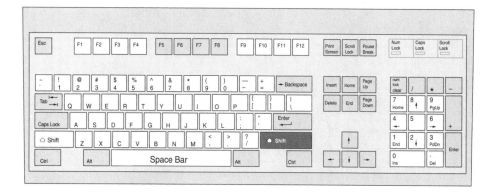

Learn Right Shift Key

The right shift key is used to make capital letters for letters keyed with the left hand. Depress the right shift key with the right little finger. Key the letter with the appropriate finger of the left hand. Release the right shift key and return to the home row. Key each line two times.

1   A A Ada Ada Sara Dan Ann Ted Ann Ed Sid Sal Eli

2   Ada Adair Sara Adell Ed Daen Ann Dale Sal Sales

3   Dan Slade Sali Finn Edna Slade Ali Fin Sid Fend

4   Daas and Adair Adell and Fend Sales and Slade

5   Fran Fend has the flu; a rash on the left leg;

RIGHT SHIFT, SHIFT LOCK, PERIOD

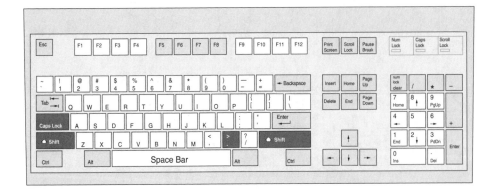

Learn caps lock key. Reach with the fourth finger of the left hand.

Press caps lock key down. If you press it down, it is on until you press it again to turn off; if you press it again, it is on.

When you have words that you want in all capital letters, press the caps lock key down, key them, then release the shift lock key. Key each line two times.

1   AS HA GI GU AD AJ ER HD LH AF KS ER GA FH TA
2   RA RF AU GH DI US DT AA DM HD LE ND NS RA UA
3   EEG GTT HAA ARF DNA UTI TUR FTT HSG ENT RNA URI
4   FHS FHT EGD ARF IUD DRE STD DES ALS TIA EKG LDL

Learn the period. Reach with the l finger.

Instructions

The . key is located below the l key. Move the third finger of your right hand as you reach to the bottom row and tap the . key. Keep at least one finger on the home row at all times to guide back to home position. Key each line two times.

1   11. 1.1. 11 1.1. 1.1. 111 . . .1.1.
2   i.e. lig. gl. rad. Jr. t.i.d. Dr.
3   Dr. Eddie J. Saad has a rash.
4   Alfred G. Read has angina.
5   Fred R. Reid left his snared nail.

Six New Keys: V,O,W,M,C, and Y; and Timed Writings

SIX NEW KEYS

Goals

After completing this lesson, you will be able to:

✔ Key v, o, w, m, c, y.

Instructions: Computing Timed Writing Speed

Keyboarding speed is measured in words a minute (WAM). To compute WAM, count every 5 strokes, including spaces. For timed writings other than a minute, divide the number of words keyed by the number of minutes in the timed writings.

Example: Computing 5-Minute Timing

1. Keyed 115 words in a 5-minute timing with two errors.
2. Count the errors and multiply by 2.
3. Errors = 2; 2 × 2 = 4.
4. Subtract errors from 115. 115 − 4 = 111.
5. Divide by 5 minutes. 111 ÷ 5 = 22. Your net speed: 22/2 errors.

To determine your words per minute, add the number at the end of the last line you completed to the number beneath timing of the partially completed line.

```
Mary returns to the clinic this morning for follow-up of her    12
herpes encephalitis. He was hospitalized for several days or    24
encephalitis which was diagnosed as herpes.                     33
     □□□□1□□□□2□□□□3□□□□4□□□□5□□□□6□□□□7□□□□8□□□□9□□□□10□□□□11□□□□12
```

Skillbuilding Warmup

```
AAA SSS DDD FFF HHH JJJ kKKK LLL ;;;
Dan Slade; Sara Finn; Ann Ali Finn;;
```

V AND O

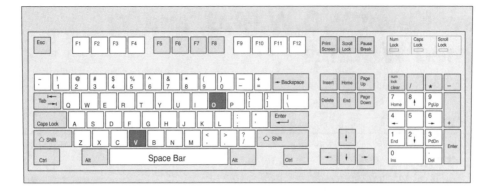

Learn v. Reach with the f finger.

Reminder: Keep at least one finger on home row at all times to guide back to home position. Key each line two times.

```
1  v fv fv fv vj vj vd vd lv vs lv dv vag via vat vig
2  v fv vee vas via vig vat vena vain vig vas veg vag
3  dv via vein vial vagi via vest even kava vela vine
4  ev vas vee vela veal vast vase vest vale hive have
5  even a vase; via veg; is vein; in a vial; a vest
6  in a vena; have veal; vas vast vat; in a hive jar;
```

Learn o. Reach with the l finger.

Reminder: Keep at least one finger on home row at all times to guide back to home position. Key each line two times.

```
1  o ol ol ol oh oh go go so so to no ion rot toe hog
2  o ol old odd fog son ova ossa oral oil dol ego oar
3  on old fork odor soak ion goal loin nose keto sold
4  on old rod oath lose love long rose fold gold gork
5  soak a sole; sod a hod; an ossa, on a nose; a goal
6  to an oath; gold fork; old loin odd; is a long ego;
```

One-Minute Timed Writing

Take 3 one-minute timed writings. Note: If you finish before time is up, start over again.

```
7  She has an ova. Veins are sore.                        7
```
□□□□1□□□□2□□□□3□□□□4□□□□5□□□□6□□□□7□□□□8□□□□9□□□□10□□□□11□□□□12

Skillbuilding Warmup

```
vvv ooo eee ;;; fff ggg aaa sss ttt
had a virus; sore vulva; old ova. v
foot odor; oil in vial a skull oooo
```

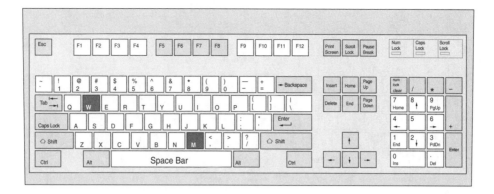

Learn w. Reach with the s finger.

Reminder: Keep at least one finger on the home row at all times to guide back to home position. Key each line two times.

1 w ws ws ws kw kw lw lw aw aw jw wj wet saw new now
2 w ws wit jaw low law wad wean twig new own dew raw
3 wk jaw word swan wash raw ward wait weak fowl twig
4 wk jaw saw wool wing watt writ with wave weak will
5 was a fowl; own a saw; is wool; is a swan; a ward;
6 is a twig; weak hand; new writ law; is a wired jaw;

Learn m. Reach with the j finger.

Reminder: Keep at least one finger on the home row all times to guide back to home position. Key each line two times.

1 m am am am mg mg ml ml km km am dm ram ham med mud
2 m am man fam mid mat mal met mal gram mite mull mint
3 ms mad mesh mast mark elm mall malt male room jams
4 ms mom dams make hams mims must drum stem mild mind
5 mark a mask; met a man; is mesh; if a mass; a gram
6 is a mite; mint milk; mal mind man; is a maim man;

One-Minute Timed Writing

Take 3 one-minute timed writings. Note: If you finish before time is up, start over again.

7 The jaw is wired and mass on mouth is sore.   9

□□□□1□□□□2□□□□3□□□□4□□□□5□□□□6□□□□7□□□□8□□□□9□□□□10□□□□11□□□□12

Skillbuilding Warmup

www mmm aaa lll sss kkk iii jjj ggg
has a wart; had a tumor; no masses;
one wheal; two masks; a mild man; g

C

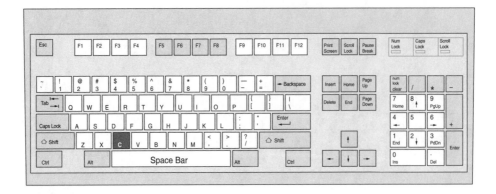

Learn c. Reach with the d finger.

Reminder: Keep at least one finger on the home row at all times to guide back to home position. Key each line two times.

1   c cd cd ca ca hc hc cu ac ac act ice tic cot scan
2   c cd cue cod cut sac ich cone hack race rice scan
3   ce cue neck acne hack cut coma lice face cuff cane
4   cd cue act clot nick tick lice sick inch chin cell
5   nick a tick; cut a fist; is acid; is a clot; a scan
6   is a lice; cold face; has acne now; is a scar ich;

One-Minute Timed Writing

Take 3 one-minute timings. Note: If you finish before time is up, start over again.

7   The tissue showed clots and cells. The CT scan showed an   11
8   enlarged liver; a clot in left leg with edema.   9

    □□□□1□□□□2□□□□3□□□□4□□□□5□□□□6□□□□7□□□□8□□□□9□□□□10□□□□11□□□□12

Skillbuilding Warmup

ccc mmm lll ttt kkk sss aaa eee vv
scan skin; cast a leg; a cecum vvv

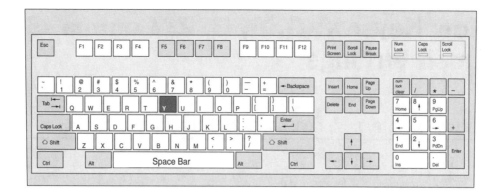

Learn y. Reach with the j finger.

Reminder: Keep at least one finger on the home row at all times to guide back to home position. Key each line two times.

```
1  y jy jy ya ya ys ys ys yd yd yes yes rye gym hay cry
2  y jy ray soy lye sky say yowl yock tyro yet type dyne
3  yd why soya year cyst dry type envy yarn duty jury
4  yd why eye gray clay chevy very clay alk amyl many
5  type a soya; dye a tie; is gray; is a cyst; a yolk
6  is a yolk; blue clay; had wide eye; is a jury type;
```

Skillbuilding Paragraph

One-Minute Timed Writing.

Note: If you finish before time is up, start over again.

```
There is no family history of cancer or heart disease. He does   12
not smoke. He admits to a liter of gin every day; denies         23
allergies. The man had surgery on his right ankle and left       34
knee. He will return to see me at the office in several days.     46
```
□□□□1□□□□2□□□□3□□□□4□□□□5□□□□6□□□□7□□□□8□□□□9□□□□10□□□□11□□□□12

Five New Keys: X, Q, P, B, Z; Comma, Slash, and Timed Writings

FIVE NEW KEYS: X, Q, P, B, Z, COMMA, SLASH, TIMED WRITINGS

Goals

After completing this lesson, you will be able to:

✔ Key x, q, p, b, z, the comma, and the slash.
✔ Key words and sentences.
✔ Key sentences in one-minute timings.

Skillbuilding Warmup

```
yyy www vvv ooo mmm www ddd lll
yaw on leg; had a cyst; a youth
had a cyst; an eyelid; dry eyet
```

X AND Q

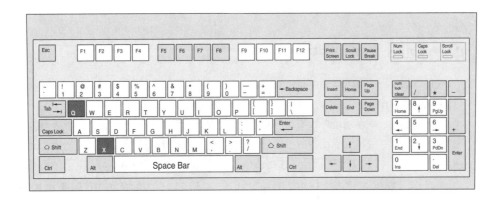

Learn x. Reach with the s finger.

Reminder: Keep at least one finger on the home row at all times to guide back to home position. Key each line two times.

```
1  x xs xs xs ax ax ax xa xa lx lx xy xj fox fax six lax
2  x xs tax sox nix fix pox exam exit axel nix onyx sexy
3  xh axe flex axon waxy axis mixt noxa xero axel exam
4  xh dex mix axon exam mixt axis noxa flex flax waxy
5  flax a seed; fix a pox; is xero; is a noxa; a mixt
6  is a mixt; exam exit; fax exam tax; is a cozy sox;
```

Learn q. Reach with the a finger.

Reminder: Keep at least one finger on the home row at all times to guide back to home position.
Key each line two times.

1 q qz qa qa qt qt qh qh qv qv ql qp qua quo qua qui quat
2 q qa qhr que aqa aqa qqq quen quey quiz quod quid quat
3 ql qns quay quai quat quat quad quid quip quit quiz qu
4 ql qui quo quod equal quod equip quip quale quat quiet
5 quiz a quod; qua qui; is quid; is a quod; a quat; a quay
6 is a quip; quit quit; quo quat qui; is a quad qua; a quay

One-Minute Timed Writing

Take 3 one-minute timings. Note: If you finish before time is up, start over again.

7 There is no evidence of chickenpox or any edema.   10
   □□□□1□□□□2□□□□3□□□□4□□□□5□□□□6□□□□7□□□□8□□□□9□□□□10□□□□11□□□□12

Skillbuilding Warmup

xxx qqq aaa ttt lll sss ddd jj
exit exam; nick onyx, fix soxj
a quad qua; quiet lad; a quat;

P, B, AND Z

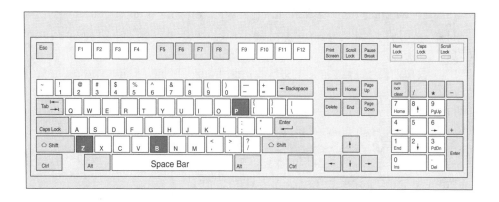

Learn p. Reach with the semicolon finger.

Reminder: Keep at least one finger on the home row at all times to guide back to home position.
Key each line two times.

1 p ;p ;p ;p up pa pa ps ps pd pd pl tip sap pad pen
2 p pl pep ape top gap pia pace pale pain apex palm pons
3 pl pen pill camp pare nap paws spud pulp open pang
4 pl pen pack spur apex pie open deep loop rump span
5 open a pack; sap a paw; in pain; up a pace; a polyp
6 is a polyp; deep loop; has pale lip; is a spur and palm

Learn b. Reach with the f finger.

Reminder: Keep at least one finger on the home row at all times to guide back to home position. Key each line two times.

```
1  b bf bf ba ba bl bl bs bs bk bk bur bud dab lab
2  b bb tab cab jab nab bag bile alba tube back bald
3  ba bed baby band ibex bee bite blue brow base brat
4  ba bay bar beef bath bend bush jobs bask blew bulb
5  bile in bags; bag a bur; is blue; is a tube; a brow
6  is a boil; balm back; bee bite big; is a baby bed;
```

Learn z. Reach with the a finger.

Reminder: Keep at least one finger on the home row at all times to guide back to home position. Key each line two times.

```
1  z za za za oz oz zd zd zl zl zj zj zee zit zit zip
2  z za zap zit zip zoo zed size zero zing zein zest
3  za zea gaze zinc zona zoo quiz daze doze zoom pizza
4  za zip size hazy razz zed zebra zebu zeal tzar maize
5  zest is zeal; zip a zit; is daze; is a zero; a zona
6  is a doze; hazy gaze; zip quiz zap; is a zone a zoo;
```

One-Minute Timed Writing

Take 3 one-minute timings. Note: If you finish before time is up, start over again.

```
7  The patient has diabetes and is in a daze. Valium caused her    12
   to doze.                                                         14
   □□□□1□□□□2□□□□3□□□□4□□□□5□□□□6□□□□7□□□□8□□□□9□□□□10□□□□11□□□□12
```

Skillbuilding Warmup

```
ppp bbb zzz yyy ccc mmm vvv aaa lll
a patient; ankle pain; is a bur; ll
open brow; sore bursa; a colon; ppp
```

TIMED WRITING 1—ONE-MINUTE TIMED WRITING

```
1  The boy had a shot for the flu. He has a cold and sore leg.     12
2  The scan showed a mass on the left leg and a spur on the        11
3  right heel that was causing pain. This was quite a visit        11
4  for the boy with a cyst on the right arm.                        8
   □□□□1□□□□2□□□□3□□□□4□□□□5□□□□6□□□□7□□□□8□□□□9□□□□10□□□□11□□□□12
```

THE COMPUTER KEYBOARD

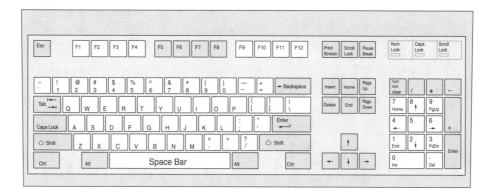

COMMA

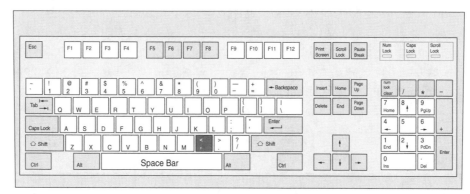

Instructions

Learn the comma. Use the k finger. Key each line two times.

1 k, k, k, leg, ova, ear, sac, pus, ill, mal, eye, toe, red, one,
2 k, k, k, hip, gas, lip, gut, flu, yaw, jaw, gap, fat, rod, rad,
3 bone, cell, bile, nose, clot, knee, cast, pulp, cold, coma, rad,
4 stye, urea, pons, iris, glia, pain, germ, arch, cyst, scan, hip,
5 scan bone, cyst, stye, and knee. Put cast on leg, hand, and hip.

One-Minute Timed Writing

Take 3 one-minute timings on each sentence. Continue to concentrate letter by letter. If you finish before time is up, start over again.

1	Mae was admitted with stomach pain, ascites, fatigue, and	11
	blood in stools.	14
2	The patient had been taking aspirin. She felt dizzy when she	12
	would sit up.	15
3	The patient improved after taking iron pills. She is to	11
	refrain from taking aspirin products.	19
4	The lady has a large lesion over her left breast which looks	12
	like cancer.	15
	Her lungs were clear.	19

☐☐☐☐1☐☐☐☐2☐☐☐☐3☐☐☐☐4☐☐☐☐5☐☐☐☐6☐☐☐☐7☐☐☐☐8☐☐☐☐9☐☐☐☐10☐☐☐☐11☐☐☐☐12

SLASH

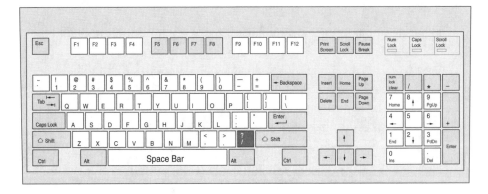

Instructions

Learn the slash. **Reach with the semicolon finger.** Key each line two times.

```
1  /; /; /; /; /; /; /; /; /; /; /; /; /; /; /; /; /; /; /;
2  bi/o my/o ot/o ox/o an/o or/o py/o ur/o ov/o is/o ir/o mi/o zo/o
3  cec/o col/o ile/o ren/o ket/o cry/o gon/o vas/o gli/o ven/o tel/o
4  men/o rhin/o chol/e hem/o lip/o sial/o gluc/o metr/o nat/i lact/o
5  lord/o kyph/o aur/o aer/o tox/o iatr/o dips/o derm/o hydr/o
```

WORD ROOTS

A word root is the main foundation of a word. A combining form is added to a word root. The combining forms are vowels: a, e, i, o, u, or y. The vowels assist in word pronunciation. Use a medical dictionary or medical terminology text for the meaning of word roots.

Examples:

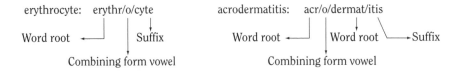

Instructions

Key each line of word roots two times.

Word Roots for the Digestive System

```
1  bucco/o an/o celi/o col/o dent/i
   enter/o lapar/o gloss/o gastr/o hepat/o
```

Word Roots for the Urinary System

```
2  ur/o dips/o ket/o vesic/o urethr/o
   ren/o nephr/o cyst/o meat/o pyel/o
```

Word Roots for the Female Reproductive System

3   colp/o galact/o metr/o mamm/o culd/o
gynec/o cervic/o men/o ov/o salping/o

Word Roots for the Male Reproductive System

4   test/o sperm/o hydr/o andr/o crypt/o
balan/o zo/o prostat/o semin/i orchi/o

Word Roots for the Nervous System

5   dur/o encephal/o my/o thalam/o gli/o
myel/o vag/o pont/o cerebr/o lept/o

Word Roots for the Cardiovascular System

6   ather/o steth/o cardi/o phleb/o atri/o
angi/o thromb/o brachi/o ather/o aort/o

Word Roots for the Respiratory System

7   rhin/o nas/o lob/o cyan/o spir/o
pleur/o capn/o tonsill/o pneum/o sinus/o

Word Roots for the Blood System (Circulatory System)

8   mon/o baso/o kary/o erythr/o hemat/o
poikil/o cyt/o hem/o leuk/o coagul/o

Word Roots for the Lymphatic and Immune Systems

9   splen/o thym/o tox/o myel/o thromb/o
lymph/o immun/o lymphaden/o azot/o ferr/o

Word Roots for the Musculoskeletal System

10   oste/o lord/o kyph/o scoli/o lamin/o
ortho/o calc/o rachi/o sacr/o crani/o

Word Roots for the Skin (Integumentary System)

```
11   seb/o melan/o lip/o caus/o hidr/o
     pil/o phyt/o squam/o xer/o onych/o
```

Word Roots for the Sense Organs

```
12   ocul/o blephar/o corne/o irid/o scler/o
     ot/o cochle/o salping/o myring/o tympan/o
```

Word Roots for the Endocrine System

```
13   gonad/o myx/o estr/o lact/o somat/o
     aden/o thyr/o toc/o crin/o hormon/o
```

Word Roots for Cancer

```
14   carcin/o cac/o onc/o plas/o ple/o
     chem/o mut/o sarc/o polyp/p radi/o
```

Word Roots for Radiology

```
15   leth/o tom/o scint/i mucos/o roentgen/o
     viv/o is/o fluor/o son/o vitr/o
```

Word Roots for Pharmacology

```
16   toxic/o iatr/o alges/o erg/o narc/o
     aer/o cras/o pharmac/o pyret/o hypn/o
```

Word Roots for Psychiatry

```
17   ment/o schiz/o anxi/o hypn/o phil/o
     hallucin/o phren/o neur/o psych/o somat/o
```

Instruction

Take 3 one-minute timed writings. Note: If you finish before time is up, start over again. Circle errors. Compute timing.

1 The patient has had chest pain on exertion for several years.   12
In the past few months, this has been getting worse, with   23
repeated attacks several times a week. He takes Nitrol with   34
minimal relief. The patient has also had wheezing, coughing,   45
and dyspnea usually brought on by exercise. In order to get   56
relief from his chest pain and wheezing, the patient has   67
resorted to taking small sips of alcohol several times a day.   79
He has been in the hospital for pneumonia, myocardial   89
infarction, chronic emphysema, and bronchitis.   98

☐☐☐☐1☐☐☐☐2☐☐☐☐3☐☐☐☐4☐☐☐☐5☐☐☐☐6☐☐☐☐7☐☐☐☐8☐☐☐☐9☐☐☐☐10☐☐☐☐11☐☐☐☐12

2 This young girl was on a scooter when she collided with the   11
trolley. She was lying on the street, covered with a blanket.   23
The paramedics took her to Mobile Hospital where she received   35
treatment and was sent home. She missed school on Friday, but   47
returned Monday and Tuesday. During the past two days, she   58
developed a headache and stomachache. Her right knee is   69
swollen from the accident. She has abrasions on the left arm.   81

☐☐☐☐1☐☐☐☐2☐☐☐☐3☐☐☐☐4☐☐☐☐5☐☐☐☐6☐☐☐☐7☐☐☐☐8☐☐☐☐9☐☐☐☐10☐☐☐☐11☐☐☐☐12

Colon, Question Mark, Apostrophe, Quotation Marks, Hyphen, and Timed Writings

Goals

After completing this lesson, you will be able to:

✔ Key the colon.
✔ Key the question mark.
✔ Key the apostrophe.
✔ Key quotation marks.
✔ Key the hyphen.

COLON AND QUESTION MARK

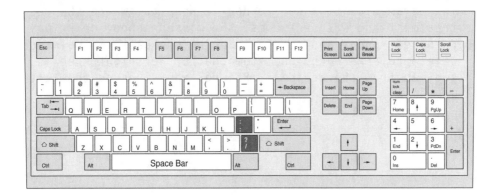

Instructions

Key each line two times, double-spacing between groups of two.

Learn the colon. **Reach with the shift of the semicolon finger and use the left shift to type a colon.** Headings and subheadings in medical reports are capitalized (e.g., Preoperative Diagnosis, Family History, etc.).

1   : : : : : ; ; ; ; :; :; :: :; :; :: :;
2   PATIENT: Jeffery Sampson
3   DATE: 09/09/2005
4   SURGEON: Parry D. Moss, MD
5   ANESTHESIOLOGIST: Anita L. Young, MD
6   ANESTHESIA: General.
7   PREOPERATIVE DIAGNOSIS: Brain tumor.
8   POSTOPERATIVE DIAGNOSIS: Brain tumor.
9   LUNGS: No rales.
10 HEART: No murmurs.

Learn the question mark. **Hold down the left shift key and press the slash key.**

1 ? ? ? ; ? ; ? ; ? ; ? ; ? ; ??? ?;? ?;? ?;? ?;?
2 Have you any pain? What is your address?
3 How do you feel? What is your telephone number?
4 What is your name? Who is your doctor?
5 Do you have insurance? Are you tired?

APOSTROPHE/QUOTATION MARKS

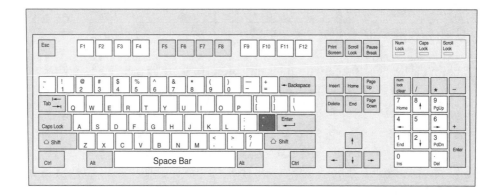

Instructions

Learn the apostrophe. **Reach with the semicolon finger.** Key each line two times.

1 ' ; ; ; ' ; ' ; ' ; ; ' ' ' ; ' ; ; ' ; ' ; ' ;
2 Jane's chart is missing.
3 Who's chairing the radiology conference?
4 It's an excellent CT scan.
5 Is this Bob's MRI report?

Instructions

Learn quotation marks. **Hold down the left shift key and press the apostrophe key.** Key each line two times.

1 " " ; " " ; " ; " ; " ; " ; " ; " ; " ; " ; " ; "
2 "I don't know," said Dr. Jones. "When did he go?"
3 "Where is it?" she asked. "Please tell me."
4 "What time is it?" "Where is the chart?"
5 "I have to perform a CT scan today."

HYPHEN

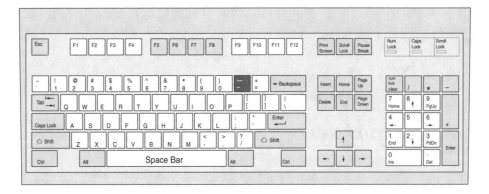

Instructions

Learn the hyphen. **Reach with the semicolon finger.** Key each line two times.

```
1  -a -p ad- ab- -;- -;- af- -al an- p- p- p- p- p- -;- ;-; ;-; -
2  -gram -itis -genic -logy -ical -opsy -osis -cyte -cele -emia -
3  -mania -lysis -ptysis ante- endo- auto- anti- cata- hemi---
4  hypo- macro- retro- meta- micro- supra- para- epi- dys- intra-
5  X-rays showed the lumbar spine to be normal. X-rays showed left
   arm to be broken.
```

PREFIXES

A prefix is a word part added to the beginning of a word root.

Example:

dia- diarrhea

Instructions

Key each line of prefixes two times. Dashes are not used in medical typing

```
 1  uni-     bi-      tri-      poly-     di-        hemi-
 2  an-      de-      un-       contra-   dia-       eu-
 3  iso-     neo-     trans-    per-      sym-       pre-
 4  pros-    pan-     peri-     mega-     kern-      ir-
 5  ex-      en-      epi-      con-      pseudo-    cata-
 6  homo-    dys-     echo-     ecto-     ante-      post-
 7  pro-     tetra-   dorsi-    exo-      extra-     hyper-
 8  in-      intra-   ipsi-     inter-    macro-     mal-
 9  meta-    micro-   meso-     pachy-    nulli-     oxy-
10  peri-    para-    per-      supra-    primi-     tachy-
```

SUFFIXES

A suffix is a word ending that describes a noun or adjective. See the meaning of suffixes in a medical dictionary or medical terminology text.

Example:

anesthesia -ia

Instructions

Key each line of suffixes two times.

```
 1   -ia       -ism     -sis      -ac       -al        -ic
 2   -logy     -ist     -iatrics  -algia    -gram      -ia
 3   -scope    -tomy    -y        -ion      -ar        -itis
 4   -oma      -cyte    -genic    -ac       -al        -ile
 5   -opsy     -osis    -scopy    -opia     -ous       -oid
 6   -dynia    -emesis  -eal      -clast    -centesis  -blast
 7   -lepsy    -lexia   -hexia    -pathy    -philia    -tresia
 8   -uria     -tocia   -tome     -spasm    -rrhea     -phyte
 9   -poiesis  -ptosis  -ptysis   -tripsy   -plasty    -desis
10   -schisis  -pexy    -stomy    -ectomy   -graph     -meter
```

Skillbuilding Practice

Take 3 One-Minute Timed Writings. Note: If you finish before time is up, start over.

Top Row

```
 6   I saw the patient after hand surgery.        8
 7   Write to their doctor to inform them.        8
 8   She is having some fatigue and apnea.        8
```

Home Row

```
 9   Alex had a sharp pain in the right arm.      8
10   Louis was seen for asthma and ataxia.        8
11   Al has dyspnea, heartburn, and cysts.        8
```

Bottom Row

```
12   The man fell and fractured his elbow.        8
13   She had a one vessel bypass surgery.         8
14   Bobbie has had chest pains for weeks.        8
```

     □□□□1□□□□2□□□□3□□□□4□□□□5□□□□6□□□□7□□□□8□□□□9□□□□10□□□□11□□□□12

Instructions

Key each line two times, double-spacing after each group of two. Rekey each error two times.

3-Letter Words

1 cut red ear eye rib fat ova rub hip rod flu add dry tic age
2 eat ego bug gag ice gut net sac toe mal mat mad gum oil lip
3 jaw pus egg pin arm zip oat low sex gas ice old leg air dye

4-Letter Words

1 ovum duct bile skin pain gall cold vein pulp oral cell sore
2 urea scan cyst pons axon coma gait lung cure uric acid drug
3 cord aura disk head body cuff apex iron heme clot ulna cyst
4 hard shin pore back cast foot loss bind disc tick weak tube
5 gout sole pore odor hive slit burn corn nevi anus acne wart
6 pain iris lens mall womb lobe neck male stye vivo uvea mold

5-Letter Words

1 feces rugae uvula liver villi colon cecum colic ulcer virus
2 enema polyp urine renin renal edema fetus sperm ovary fluid
3 tumor organ nerve brain mania palsy aorta atria septa liver
4 pulse piles lipid nasal hilum cilia sinus rales croup axial
5 serum acute lymph toxin joint fossa cleft vomer thumb tibia
6 sinus pubis ilium bursa sebum wheal basal tinea pinna fugue

6-Letter Words

1 enzyme tongue buccal enamel dentin tissue fundus mucosa cheeks
   lipase iritis stress eyelid cornea vagina costal muscle
2 saliva rectum lipase palate nausea cancer hernia meatus tubule
   ureter senile mitral coccyx pelvis septal mental nipple coryza
3 turbid ketone pyuria embryo uterus gonads gamete adnexa cervix
   areola cyesis axilla breast thorax kidney tendon comedo larynx
4 testes stroma plexus neuron glioma severe septum murmur atrium
   patent injury throat septic fascia penile cortex labile serous
5 asthma lavage plasma globin immune fibrin anemia spongy thymus
   spleen ocular dermal lesion aortic cardia visual lumbar lipoid
6 palate fibula bursae bunion retina sclera goiter tetany benign
   macula stupor meatus melena nausea lupoid nodule plaque

7-Letter Words

1 glucose lingual pharynx jejunum condyle
2 sigmoid amylase insulin ascites urinary
3 kidneys ureters albumin protein ovaries
4 puberty ovarian toxemia gravida scrotum
5 seizure embolus venules carotid systole
6 hypoxia bronchi trachea anosmia calcium

```
 7   purpura myeloma allergy antigen foramen
 8   carpals sternum xiphoid patella mastoid
 9   pyrexia abscess melanin rubella vesicle
10   measles neuroma vertigo gastric osteoma
```

8-Letter Words

```
 1   thoracic cervical surgical leukemia pancreas
 2   duodenum appendix glycogen anorexia diarrhea
 3   jaundice pyorrhea bacteria hepatoma oncogene
 4   catheter enuresis polyuria syndrome ischemia
 5   diabetes mellitus fimbriae menarche estrogen
 6   prostate duodenum cerebrum meninges comatose
 7   epilepsy dyslexia shingles thrombus aneurysm
 8   diastole cyanosis effusion temporal clavicle
 9   vertebra osteitis lipocyte glaucoma macrotia
10   oxytocin estrogen incision myxedema sarcomas
```

9-Letter Words

```
 1   digestive esophagus dysphagia polyposis dysentery
 2   cirrhosis hemoccult nephritis bilirubin hematuria
 3   pregnancy ovulation carcinoma dysplasia curettage
 4   eclampsia vasectomy hydrocele gonorrhea analgesia
 5   neuralgia contusion occlusion pacemaker radiology
 6   isoenzyme orthopnea granuloma pathology emphysema
 7   pulmonary angiogram phlebitis digitalis diaphragm
 8   sinusitis epistaxis pertussis tomograms phalanges
 9   arthritis sebaceous causalgia seborrhea psoriasis
10   tonometry retinitis endocrine potassium thyroxine
```

10-Letter Words

```
 1   gynecology obstetrics podiatrist pharmacist infectious
 2   melanocyte homosexual chromosome metabolism morphology
 3   adiposuria laparotomy metastasis adenodynia gastrocele
 4   cellulitis septicemia percussion cardiogram palliative
 5   arrhythmia hemothorax defecation creatinine mastectomy
 6   leukorrhea congential hemophilia thyropathy glycosuria
 7   cerebellum ventricles vestibular refraction strabismus
 8   osteopenia dermatitis ecchymosis stomatitis urethritis
 9   myometrium episiotomy varicocele epididymis polydipsia
10   urinometer lithotrite polycystic antiemetic hemoptysis
```

Take 3 one-minute timed writings. Note: If you finish before time is up, start over again.

```
Jean is well oriented and in acute distress due to injury to    12
the right hip. The patient has had eye surgery and shows        23
irregular pupils. The mucous membranes of the nose and throat   35
appear to be intact. However, tha patient has complaints of     46
tenderness of her gums and tongue. There are no rales. The      57
abdomen is soft and nontender. The patient has arthritis in     69
both feet. She has a fracture of the right hip with a turning    81
out of the right ankle.                                         86
```

□□□□1□□□□2□□□□3□□□□4□□□□5□□□□6□□□□7□□□□8□□□□9□□□□10□□□□11□□□□12

Alphabetic Concentration Sentences and the Tab Keys

Alphabetic Concentration Sentences

SPECIFIC FINGER DRILLS

Goals

After completing this lesson, you will be able to:

✔ Better control the index finger.
✔ Become aware of when errors occur.

Instructions

Unit Two lessons are for alphabetic practice to diagnose where errors occur.
1. Practice units that are suited for the individual.
2. Key the pretest and posttest one time. Rekey each error two times.

PRETEST AND POSTTEST—THREE-MINUTE TIMING

```
1        The patient is up-to-date on her immunization status.      11
2   She has had a breast exam, pelvic, and Pap smear performed by    23
3   Dr. Joe Quick who discussed hormonal replacement therapy         34
4   with the patient. She is to have a mammogram performed this      45
5   month.  She had a normal thyroid function test in September      56
6   She was encouraged to perform monthly breast self-exams and     67
7   report any changes to me or Dr. Joe Quick. She was encouraged   79
8   to continue exercising on a regular routine basis. She was      90
9   counseled on seat belt use and sun exposure.                    99
    □□□□1□□□□2□□□□3□□□□4□□□□5□□□□6□□□□7□□□□8□□□□9□□□□10□□□□11□□□□12
```

LEFT HAND, FIRST FINGER STROKES

Instructions

Key each line one time. Rekey each error two times. Double-space between each group of two lines. Complete before alphabetic concentration sentences.

Drill 1: R

```
1   rachigraph radiator radiocarpal radioparency rash
2   rate rat radialis react reactant reactivate reagin
3   reagent reamer receptor recall rectal reposition
4   reserve reservoir residency residual resilient
5   resorb rhinitis rhizome rhizotomy rhizomelic
```

Drill 2: F

1 fiat fiber fibra fibril fibrillation fibrin
2 fibroid fibroma fibromyitis flaccid flagella flank
3 flange flap flare flak flatfoot flatulent fracture
4 fragment frambesia francium fratricide fraternal
5 free freezing ferment fern ferrin fertile fester

Drill 3: V

1 varicosis varicosity varicula variola variolar vas
2 variolic varus variolate ventro venom venin vent
3 ventrad ventral ventrose verbomania vergence vital
4 vitalist vitamer vitamin vitium vitriol vitellus
5 vitiligo vivisect voice vocal voces vole volley

Drill 4: T

1 triorchidism triolism triose triotus tripara
2 triplet triploid triplopia trismic trabecula trabs
3 trace trachea tragal tragus train tractus transfer
4 tissue tissular titer titrate titre titrimetry
5 titubation tip tingle tendon tenia teniasis tense

Drill 5: G

1 germ germicide germinal genesis generic geroderma
2 gerontopia gestalt gestation giga giantism gingiva
3 gingivitis gingivosis ginglyform gingivalgia gate
4 ginseng gastrolith gate gait gatism gauge gauss
5 gauze gavage gauntlet glimmer googolplex give

Drill 6: B

1 bacillus bacteriemia bacteremia bacterioid bag bake
2 ball ballistics balm bias bibasic bibulous biceps
3 biduous bifacial bifid bifocal bifurcate bucardia
4 buccula bud bulbous budding buffer bulb bulbar
5 bulboid beat bed bedbug bedfast bedlam bedsore

RIGHT HAND, FIRST FINGER STROKES

Goals

After completing this lesson, you will be able to:

✔ Better control the forefinger.
✔ Become aware of when errors occur.

Key each line one time. Rekey each error two times. Double-space between each group of two lines.

Drill 1: U

1 ulcera ulcus ulectomy ulegyria ulerythema uletic
2 uletomy uletic urachal urachus uracil uracrasia
3 uranium unranoplasty uranoplegia uranoschisis uten
4 uratoma uteralgia uterine uterolith uterus utilize
5 utricle uvea uva unstriated univalence unofficial

Drill 2: J

1 jargon jaundice jugum jugulum jumentous junctura
2 juvenile juxtangina jigger jitters jaw jimson jog
3 joint jugular jugum juxtaposition juxtapyloric
4 juxtaspinal juxta-articular juxtaglomerular justo
5 major jacket jusculum juvantia jellyfish japes

Drill 3: M

1 mold mole molecular molecule molilalia molimen
2 mollin mollusc mollusk maidism maidismus maieutic
3 maim main maise maisin make maizenate miana mica
4 micella micelle micron micrergy microbe microbion
5 mucase mucidin mucigen mucilage mucin mucoclasis

Drill 4: Y

1 yard yatobyo yaw yawey yawning yaws yeast yerba
2 yerli ylang-ylang-ylene yochubio yodoxin yoke yolk
3 yogurt yperite yttrium yerk yesterday ypsiliod yet
4 ypsiliform yukon yttrium yare yellowy yews yamen
5 yammer yarrow yare yauld yodoxin yakking yurt

Drill 5: H

1 habit habitat habitus hair halide halitosis hiant
2 halituous halitus hallux hiatopexia hibernoma
3 hidradenitis hidroa hidropoiesis hidrosis hiccup
4 holotonia holotopy holozole holophytic hologynic
5 holoacardius holotetanus holothurin holotopy hum

Drill 6: N

1 nalline narcotic nardil nares nasal narry nasion
2 nasitis natremia negatol necrectomy necrosis

```
3   necrencephalus necrobiotic nematosis nelavan nema
4   nodose nodulous nomotopic nona nonelectrolyte
5   nonigravida nonmetal normal nosophilia nitron
```

LEFT HAND, SECOND FINGER STROKES

Goals

After completing this lesson, you will be able to:

✔ Better control the second finger.
✔ Become aware of when errors occur.

Instructions

Key each line one time, double-spacing after each group of two lines. Rekey each error two times.

Drill 1: E

```
1   ear earth earwax ear-minded earache eardrops eat
2   eardrum earplug edema edentia edematous edible
3   edulcorant edematogenic edetate edrophonium ergo
4   exacerbation exaltation examination exangia exam
5   exanthema excision excerebration exarticulation
```

Drill 2: D

```
1   dacryon dacryolin danazol dacryocyte dactylogram
2   dactylology dactylus dapsone dartoid deaf death
3   dearticulation deaquation decay debilitate
4   decapsulation debridement dracontiasis drain dram
5   denature diplopia disequilibrium diplocardia
```

Drill 3: C

```
1   capsitis captopril carbamide carbidopa Carbocaine
2   canthus canthitis caput capsulitis cradle cramp
3   craniectomy creatinine creatinemia crematorium
4   creosote crevicular cretin cuirass culicifuge
5   culicide cult cultivation cuneate cupruresis cissa
```

RIGHT HAND, SECOND FINGER STROKES

Goals

After completing this lesson, you will be able to:

✔ Better control the second finger.
✔ Become aware of when errors occur.

Key each line one time, double-spacing after each group of two lines. Rekey each error two times.

Drill 1: I

1   ileac ileocecal ileus ileum iliocostal iliospinal
2   ilium ileorrhaphy ileectomy imagination imbalance
3   imbrication imidazole imbecile imbed imbibition
4   imbecility imide incus incurvation incudostapedial
5   indentation indigestion incyclotropia incisor

Drill 2: K

1   kakidrosis kakke kakosmia kakotrophy kallidin
2   kalium kaliopenia kaolin keratinase keratinous
3   keratitis kenotoxin kerasin keloid keloidosis kelp
4   kibe kidney kneading kilounit kineplasty kinesia
5   kinase kinesodic kinin knee kneecap kneippism

Drill 3: E and I

1   eidetic eicosanoids eikonometry eiloid einsteinium
2   eisodic eleidin enceinte erythropoietic ileitis
3   erythropoiesis erythropoietic iniencephalus apneic
4   ambient abortient absorbefacient acetylcysteine
5   achievement acheiria acheiropodia acleistocardia

LEFT HAND, THIRD FINGER STROKES

Goals

After completing this lesson, you will be able to:

✔ Better control the third finger.
✔ Emphasize the reaches where errors occur.

Instructions

Key each line one time. Rekey each error word two times. Double-space between each group of two lines.

Drill 1: W

1   wafer wakeful walk walker walking wall walleye
2   ward wart wash wasp waste wasting water wattage
3   wave weak wean weanling web weeping welding welt
4   wetbrain wen weight weismannism wrist wryneck writ
5   wreath wrinkle wrongful wristdrop wrightine

Drill 2: S

1 strain strap strangury stratum streak stress sap
2 streptococcemia stressor sphincter spherule spider
3 spheroplast sphygmoid spiculum spica spicule sac
4 sclerous scolecoid scolex scorpion scrofula suffer
5 scrotitis scotoma sacculation sacrectomy sacral

Drill 3: X

1 excochleation exclusion exclave excoriation excite
2 excitation excise excision excitoglandular axes
3 excreta exenteration excystation excurvation expel
4 exenteration exencephalia exeresis exergonic axe
5 exfetation exflagellation exfoliation exhalation

RIGHT HAND, THIRD FINGER STROKES

Goals

After completing this lesson, you will be able to:

✔ Better control the third finger.
✔ Become aware of when errors occur.

Instructions

Key each line one time. Rekey each error word two times. Double-space between each group of two lines.

Drill 1: O

1 oakum oasis obcecation obduction obsessive oblique
2 occipitomastoid obtund oneirology oncogene opiate
3 oulitis osmidrosis osmiophilic optic orbit opioid
4 opisthotic opsoclonus opsogen opsonic opsonin obit
5 occlusion ochlesis oospore ootheca ooplasm oocyte

Drill 2: L

1 laparoenterotomy laparoscope lobe labrocyte labrum
2 lactorrhea lacuna labium lazaretto lax laxative
3 levator levodopa leukorrhea leukoplasia licorice
4 lippitude liquor fall lienitis lattice lochial
5 lochia lymphemia lupus lubricant lyssa lupus luxus

LEFT HAND, FOURTH FINGER STROKES

Goals

After completing this lesson, you will be able to:

✔ Better control the fourth finger.
✔ Become aware of when errors occur.

Instructions

Key each line one time. Rekey each error two times. Double-space between each group of two lines.

Drill 1: Q

1 quack quadrangular quadrant quadrate quadribasic
2 quadriceps quadrantanopia quadrantanopsia quale
3 quart quartile quartipara quantity quadripolar
4 quadrisect quadrivalent quadruped quadruple quip
5 qualimeter qualitative quinone quotient quotidian

Drill 2: A

1 attitude attention attachment atticotomy attolens
2 attractions attrition aquaphobia aquapuncture
3 aqueductus arcate arcanum arboviruses asiderosis
4 ascites ascorbic ascospore asphyxiation asphyxiant
5 acetone acetate acetic achromatic achromatin

Drill 3: Z

1 zirconium zazen zelotypia zero zooblast zeitgeist
2 zonesthesia zonulysis zoobiology zooblast zoom
3 zoodermic zoodynamic zooerast zoescope zone zonal
4 zonae zonary zonula zonipetal zygomycosis razz
5 zygomaticum zygomatic fizzle zygomatic zygocyte

RIGHT HAND, FOURTH FINGER STROKES

Goals

After completing this lesson, you will be able to:

✔ Better control the fourth finger.
✔ Emphasize the reaches where errors occur.

Instructions

Key each line one time. Rekey each error two times. Double-space between each group of two lines.

Drill 1: P

```
1  polyps pachyderma pap priapus palpate palpebra pip
2  palpebral palsy pheochrome pheromone phenomelanins
3  phenytoin phenothiazine phenomenology phenotype
4  pup pimelosis piniform pinocyte piarachnoid pauper
5  piceous pica pop poikilonymy poikiloblast podiatry
```

ALPHABETIC CONCENTRATION DRILLS

Goals

After completing this lesson, you will be able to:

✔ Concentrate when keying long words.

Instructions

Key each line one time. Rekey each error two times. Double-space between groups of two words.

Drill 1: A

```
1  abarticulation abdominocentesis
2  abdominohysterectomy abdominohysterotomy
3  abdominouterotomy abdominovesical
4  abetalipoproteinemia abrachiocephalia
5  acanthamebiasis acanthocephaliasis
6  akidogalvanocautery acephalothoracia
7  acetazolamide acetylcholinesterase
8  achondrogenesis azoxybenzene
```

Drill 2: B

```
1  bulbocavernosus bacterioagglutinin
2  bacteriological bacterioprecipitin
3  balanopreputial ballistocardiograph
4  balneotherapeutics baresthesiometer
5  bartonellosis basiarachnoiditis
6  bathyhyperesthesia bendroflumethiazide
7  benzodiazepine betamethasone
8  biochemorphology biodegradation
```

Drill 3: C

1 calcaneoapophysitis calcaneonavicular
2 calcaneoscaphiod calcaneotibial
3 callosomarginal cystometrography
4 capillaropathy capsulolenticular
5 carbamazepine carbaminohemoglobin
6 carcinomatophobia cardiocatheterization
7 cardiohepatomegaly cardiopneumograph
8 carpometacarpal cartilaginification

Drill 4: D

1 dacryocystorhinostenosis dacryocystosyringotomy
2 dacrocystoblennorrhea decarboxylization
3 deciduosarcoma decisuomatosis
4 dehydrocorticosterone dehydroandrosterone
5 dehydroepiandrosterone dehydroisoandrosterone
6 deinstitutionalization dendrophagocytosis
7 deoxyribonucleoside deoxyribonuclease
8 depolymerization dermatoheteroplasty

Drill 5: E

1 eccentro-osteochondrodysplasia
2 erythroblastemia echinococcotomy
3 echoencephalogram electrocochleography
4 electrocorticography electrocardiophonograph
5 electroencephalography electrohysterography
6 electronystagmography electrothermotherapy
7 encephalomeningitis encephalomeningocele
8 encephalomyelitis encephalocystocele

Drill 6: F

1 faciocephalalgia facioscapulohumeral
2 fibrillogenesis fibercolonoscope
3 fibrinogenopenia fibroepithelioma
4 fibroenchondroma fibromyomectomy
5 fibromyxosarcoma fludrocortisone
6 fluoxymesterone fluprednisolone
7 flurandrenolide fusostreptococcicosis
8 frenuloplasty frontomaxillary

Drill 7: G

1 galactophagous galvanocontractility
2 gynandromorphous galvanotherapeutics
3 ganglioglioneuroma gastroenterocolostomy
4 gastroenteroanastomosis gastroduodenostomy
5 gastroduodenoscopy gastroesophagostomy
6 gastropancreatitis gingivostomatitis
7 ginglymoarthrodial glomerulonephritis
8 glomerulosclerosis gynandroblastoma

Drill 8: H

1 hallucinogenesis halmatogenesis
2 hamartomatosis helminthagogue
3 helminthemesis helminthophobia
4 hemodynamometer hemagglutination
5 hemangioendothelioblastoma hematoperitoneum
6 hematoporphyrinuria hematolymphangioma
7 hematospectroscope hematospectroscopy
8 hematospermatocele hemiachromatopsia

Drill 9: I

1 ichthyoacanthotoxism ichthyohemotoxin
2 ichthyotoxicology iliothoracopagus
3 ilioxiphopagus ileosigmoidostomy
4 immunoelectrophoresis immunochemotherapy
5 immunocompromised infundibulectomy
6 infusodecoction intellectualization
7 intercricothyrotomy intraligamentary
8 iridectomesodialysis iridocyclochorioditis

Drill 10: J

1 jejunocolostomy jejunojejunostomy
2 juxtaglomerular jejunocecostomy
3 jejunectomy jejunorrhaphy
4 jejunoileostomy jejunoileitis
5 jugomaxillary juxtangina juxta-articular
6 juxtaposition juxtapyloric juxtaspinal
7 jugulation juncturae jujitsu jackscrew
8 jactation jactitation jaculiferous jalap

Drill 11: K

1 kallikreinogen karyomicrosome kyphoscoliosis
2 karyomorphism katathermometer kratometer
3 keratoacanthoma keratoconjunctivitis
4 keratoleukoma kupramite krypton
5 kinetocardiography kynophobia kyphoscoliosis
6 kynurenine kymocyclograph kocherization
7 kymography keto-tetrahydrophenanthrene
8 ketohydroxestratriene ketogenic

Drill 12: L

1 labioglossolaryngeal labioglossopharyngeal
2 lactobutyrometer lacto-ovovegetarian
3 lagophthalmos laparocolostomy
4 laparocystidotomy laparogastroscopy
5 laparohysterosalpingo-oophorectomy
6 laparogastronomy laparotrachelotomy
7 laminagraphy lanceolate laryngotome
8 laryngotracheobronchoscopy lull

Drill 13: M

1 macrencephalia macroamylasemia
2 macroglobulinemia macromyeloblast
3 macropromyelocyte macrostereognosis
4 malassimilation mandibulopharyngeal
5 manudynamometer masculinovoblastoma
6 maxillomandibular mediastinopericarditis
7 medicomechanical medicopsychology
8 medulloadrenal myxochondrosarcoma

Drill 14: N

1 narcoanesthesia nasopharyngography
2 nemathelminth nephrohypertrophy
3 nephrocapsectomy nephrocystanastomosis
4 nephropyelography neuroencephalomyelopathy
5 neurofibrosarcoma neurochorioretinitis
6 neuroanastomosis neuroastrocytoma
7 neutralization neuro-ophthalmology
8 nyctalbuminuria nudomania nudophobia

Drill 15: O

1. occipitobregmatic oesophagostomiasis
2. olecranarthropathy oligodendroblastoma
3. oligoleukocythemia oligozoospermatism
4. osteopoikilosis omentumectomy
5. omphaloangiopagus onychoheterotopia
6. onycho-osteodysplasia oophorohysterectomy
7. oophorosalpingectomy ophthalmencephalon
8. oxydoreductase oxyetheroptherapy

Drill 16: P

1. panhysterosalpingo-oophorectomy
2. papilloadenocystoma papillocarcinoma
3. pappillomaviruses paramyxoviruses
4. paraosteoarthropathy pachypelviperitonitis
5. parathyroidectomy pancreatemphraxis
6. parisitophobic pedodynamometer
7. pericardiosymphysis peniaphobia
8. perioophorosalpingitis pachyleptomenigitis

Drill 17: Q

1. quadrantanopia quadrantanopsia
2. quadrangular quadricepsplasty
3. quadritubercular quadrigeminus
4. quenuthoracoplasty quadrigeminum
5. quadriparesis quadrigemina
6. quadridigitate quadricuspid
7. querulent quickening quinestrol
8. quinethazone quinoline quinone

Drill 18: R

1. rachialbuminimeter rachialbuminimetry
2. rachianesthesia radiculoneuropathy
3. radiculomeningomyelitis radiculomyelopathy
4. radioanaphylaxis radiocardiography
5. radiocinematograph radioelectrocardiogram
6. radiopharmaceuticals radioimmunodiffusion
7. ramollissement rectococcypexia
8. rhytidoplasty rhodogenesis rhinosporidiosis

Drill 19: S

```
1  saccharification saccharogalactorrhea
2  sacrococcygenus salpingemphraxis
3  salpingo-oophorectomy salpingo-ureterostomy
4  saturnotherapy sassafrass sarsaparilla
5  salpingo-ovariectomy salpingoperitonitis
6  salpingostomy salpingocatheterism
7  sanguinopoietic sclerectoiridodialysis
8  semisupination semenologist semicanalis
```

Drill 20: T

```
1  tachyrhythmia tachycardia
2  tachyphylaxis tachytrophism tapeinocephalic
3  tarsocheiloplasty tarsophalangeal
4  tarsometatarsal tarsomegaly tautomerase
5  taurodontism telecardiogram telecardiophone
6  telecurietherapy telelectrocardiogram
7  thalassemia thrombocytopathy thrill
8  thryemphraxis tic thyrophyma tokodynagraph
```

Drill 21: U

```
1  ulceromembranous ululate uvula uvulotome
2  ultracentrifugation uranostaphyloschisis
3  uranostaphylorrhaphy uranostaphyloplasty
4  ureteroheminephrectomy ureteroneocystostomy
5  ureterosigmoidostomy ureterotrigonoenterostomy
6  ureterovesicostomy urethroperineoscrotal
7  urohematonephrosis utriculosaccular uvulitis
8  uvalaptosis utriculoplasty uzara
```

Drill 22: V

```
1  vaccinogenous vaccinotherapeutics
2  vaginoabdominal vaginomycosis
3  vaginoperineorrhaphy vaginoperineotomy
4  vaginolabial vaginography vaginoperitoneal
5  vaginoplasty vagosympathetic valvuloplasty
6  vascularization vasoconstriction
7  vasoepididymostomy vaso-orchidostomy
8  vacciniculturist valetudinarianism
```

Drill 23: W

1. waterhammer wavelength weanling
2. weightlessness wheal wheat wheeze whisper
3. whistle windchill whooping whitlow white
4. winking wisdom work-up wound W-plasty
5. wreath wrinkly wrist wrist writing wryneck
6. wrongful Winstrol Winslow Wirsung
7. wolffian woolgather word Wohlfahrtia
8. waw whiteleg whoop wink whack wart wydase

Drill 24: X

1. xanchromatic xanthochromatic
2. xanthocyanopsia xanthocyanopsia
3. xanthogranuloma xanthokyanopy
4. xeromammography xiphisternum
5. xeroradiography xerophthalmus
6. xenogenesis xenophthalmia xenoparasite
7. xanthoprotein xanthuria xiphocostal
8. xiphopagotomy xiphopagus

Drill 25: Y

1. yellow yttrium yushi youth ypsiliform
2. yogurt yohimbine yin-yang yersiniosis
3. yerba yawning yeast yell yohimbine
4. Y. pseudotuberculosis Y. enterocolitica
5. Yutobar Yersin's serum ylang-ylang
6. Youngs operation ypsiliform ytterbium
7. Yzquierdo's bacillus yahoo yochubio
8. yerbine yeki saying yes

Drill 26: Z

1. zeaxanthin zenkerize zestocautery
2. zoacanthosis zootechnics zoogeography
3. zooacanthosis zoo therapeutics
4. zootrophotoxism zuckergussdarm
5. zuckergussleber zwischenscheibe
6. zygapophyseal zygomaticofacial
7. zygomaticofrontal zygomaticomaxillary
8. zygomaticosphenoid pizzazz

VERTICAL STROKES

Goals

After completing this lesson, you will be able to:

✔ Concentrate on vertical-stroke words.
✔ Notice when errors are made.
✔ Key when one finger has to strike two or more consecutive keys on different rows of the keyboard.

Instructions

Key each drill one time. Rekey each error two times. Double-space between each group of three lines.

Drill 1: A Finger

1   azygos azymia azotemia pizza azygography
2   azathioprine azoospermia azoturia azymic
3   azotenesis azotification azurophilia azoic
4   Azolid Azotobacter pizzazz Azulfidine aqueductus

Drill 2: S Finger

1   swallow swab swage swoon switch swimmer
2   swelling sweet Swedish swarming Swan paws
3   flaws brews slows swaged swan Swiss
4   swath sway swathe brews slows laws
5   veins grows flows news

Drill 3: D Finger

1   decay desmitis demeed dear deciduitis decoction
2   dementia decrement demulcent dextrinuria cedar
3   cellulitis centrum cephalea centesis centiliter
4   cecopexy celiopathy cerebripetal edematous

Drill 4: F Finger

1   fragiform frangipani fraise framboesia
2   fremitus freer frottage frenzy fragilocyte
3   fratricide fructosan fruit fructosuria frugivorous
4   frustration frenectomy frenetic friction fretum

Drill 5: F Finger

1   graft grain gram grammole grandiosity
2   grahamellosis grease gregaloid gregarinosis
3   grippe grattage grave grass gravel gravedo
4   graviditas griffin grippal groin groove grog

Drill 6: J Finger

1   juvenile juvantia jute jusculum jurisprudence
2   juniper junk juncturae junctional junctura
3   junction jumentous jumping julep juice jugum
4   jugular jugulation juglone Juglans jugate jugged

Drill 7: J Finger

1   hum hump Humatin humeral humectant humectation
2   humeri humeral humeroradial humeroscapular
3   humerus human humidity humidifier humor humoral
4   humus husk hunchback hunger hyaline humulon

Drill 8: J Finger

1   mummified muciferous muciform mucigen mucilago
2   mucigenous mucin mucilaginous mucinase mutism
3   mute mutilate musk musculus mutagen mustard
4   mussel mutilation mucinase mucinogen mulatto

Drill 9: J Finger

1   nubile nubility nucha nuchal nuclear nuclease
2   nucleoid nucleolonema nucleolus nucleus nuclide
3   nude nudism nudophobia nudomania nulligravida
4   nullipara nulliparous numb number numeral nurse

Drill 10: J Finger

1   unit unigravida ungual unguicular uncus uncal
2   unciform uncinate uncinatum inanimate succubus
3   incisura incisure incubus incudal incus umbo
4   umbra umbilical umbrella umbilicate umbilicus

Drill 11: K Finger

1   kibe kidney kilocycle kilogram kinase kinematics
2   kinetosis kinin kink kinesitherapy
3   kininases kininogen kinocilium kinomometer kilo
4   kineplasty kineplastic kinematograph kinescope

Drill 12: L Finger

1   load lobar lobate lobelia lobotomy lobular lobule
2   lochia lochiocolpos lockjaw loco locus logaditis
3   logaphasia logasthenia logoklony logoplegia
4   logomania logamnesia logorrhea logopathy logopedia

ALPHABETIC CONCENTRATION SENTENCES

Goals

After completing this lesson, you will be able to:

✔ Keep eyes and fingers working together.
✔ Read no faster than you key.

Instructions

Key each sentence twice, double-spacing after each group of two. Proofread right to left for errors. Strive for accuracy. (Practice sentences with highest errors.)

a A patient was at Addiston Clinic for an acute cardiac arrest.

b The broken bloody bones are in the limb bones, collarbone, and shoulder blade.

c Carol had a cough, a cold, chills, and chest pain for three days.

d The diseased nose contained different odors, dust, and had nosebleeds.

e Ears are comprised of the external ear, the middle ear, and the internal ear.

f Fred had fluid in the left ear, and this afflicted ear became deaf.

g The guy gargles and gnaws gum.

h The healthy male was afraid he was headed for another heart attack.

i Iron is in a pigment called bilirubin.

j Janet had a jejunojejunostomy at Justice Clinic.

k Keratin, on the skin of nails, has a protective blanket so the nail will not flake.

l The liver secretes fluid called bile, produces blood proteins, and destroys red blood cells.

m Myxedema is mucous material under the dermis that has become puffy.

n Nervous Niles had necrosis of the nose, and now has rhinitis and a painful nail.

o Organs produce ova, which provide a place for growth of the embryo.

p The physician examined a patient and saw pruritus, papules, and polyps.

q The quick quiet quack was quaffing quinine.

r The retina is a sensitive nerve of the eye having receptor cells called rods.

s She had symptoms of pleurisy and several episodes of bronchitis lasting for six days.

t Thomas saw two tumors located in the mouth on the tongue.

u Urine that has a cloudy appearance might be turbid with pyuria.

v Verruca is a growth caused by a virus, and juvenile verrucae are on the hands of children.

w Wheal is a swollen, wide area of the skin.

x   Xeroderma is dry skin, xanthoma is a tumor, and a xanthocyte is a cell.

y   Yellow bone marrow is composed of fat cells of the yellow bone.

z   Dr. Zanz prescribed Zantac and zinc.

More Alphabetic Concentration Sentences

a   Eating an apple gave Marissa a stomachache and diarrhea.

b   Bob, Billy, Benita, and Barbara went to the Brown Clinic.

c   Chocolate candy can cause Carl to have caries.

d   Dorothy's dad drove to the dentist at the Douglas Medical Center.

e   The rewards were presented at Shelley's Eye Center.

f   Filipe had flavorful, fresh fruits at the Fischer's Health Clinic in Fairfax.

g   George was unable to chew sugarless gum because of his glossitis.

h   Harry had heard that Henrietta had hallux and halitosis.

i   Inquiries were made about Inman's innutrition, inoccipitia, iniencephaly, and infrapsychic.

j   John Jackson discussed his jejunitis and jejunojejunostomy at the Jewett Clinic.

k   Dr. Kelly's studies confirmed the following diagnoses: karyogenesis and karyokinesis.

l   Lovely Lula has laryngitis and lalophobia.

m   Dr. MacMunn is presenting a manuscript about mononucleosis, mountain fever, and myxedema.

n   The Nairobi center, on Nairobi Street, is researching nanoid and nanomelia.

o   On Monday, the patient will be examined for organotropia.

p   The patient lay supine upon the table and was prepared for a Pfannenstiel incision.

q   Dr. Quilla performed quadricepsplasty on the quadriplegic.

r   Dr. Raman recommended radicotomy and radiotropic.

s   Saenger's case contains saccharephidrosis.

t   The patient is taking tablets for tachycardia and tachytrophism.

u   The patient is listed in fair condition with ulalgia, ulatrophy, and urorubin.

v   The patient went to surgery for a vaginovulvar repair.

w   The water was washed from the patient's wound.

x   Xylanthrax and xylenin are used for the assay.

y   Dr. Yound did research on yawning and ylang-ylang.

z   Zenkerize rented space for the Zander apparatus.

LESSON 8

Tab Key, Computing Two-Minute Timing

TAB KEY

Goals

After completing this lesson, you will be able to:

✔ Use the tab key.

Instructions

For paragraph indentation, use the tab. The first line of a paragraph should be indented 5 spaces or 0.5 inch. Follow the software's instructions for setting tabs.

Use the A finger to tab. Practice using the tab key.

There were some rales in the lower right base of her chest.

The patient has a history of arthritis, anemia, asthma, and diabetes.

Skillbuilding Paragraph

Tab. One-minute timed writing.

1	The patient was seen at Mobile Clinic. She had injured	11
2	her right knee while dancing. The pain developed over the	22
3	right knee. The examination revealed fluid in the right knee.	34

Skillbuilding Paragraphs

Instructions

See page 55 on how to compute two-minute timing.

Take 3 two-minute timings. Try to make no more than two errors in 2 minutes. Rekey each error twice. Key for accuracy and then speed. Concentrate on each letter of each word. Key the timing to establish your goal.

29 WAM

Bob was born with a cleft lip and palate. He will undergo	12
surgery of his nose.	16
He has had multiple surgeries to revise his nose and upper	28
lip.	29

□□□□1□□□□2□□□□3□□□□4□□□□5□□□□6□□□□7□□□□8□□□□9□□□□10□□□□11□□□□12

COMPUTING TWO-MINUTE TIMING

A. Instructions: Computing Timed Writing Speed

Keyboarding speed is measured in words in a minute (WAM). To compute WAM, count every 5 strokes, including spaces. For timed writing other than a minute, divide the number of words keyed by the number of minutes in the timed writings.

Example: Computing 2-Minute Timing

1. Keyed 110 words in a 2-minute timing.
2. Count errors and multiply by 2.
3. Errors = 3; $2 \times 3 = 6$.
4. Subtract errors from 110. $110 - 6 = 104$.
5. Divide by two minutes. $104 \div 2 = 52$. Your net speed: 52/3 errors.

To determine your words per minute add the number at the end of the last complete line to the number beneath timing of the partially completed line.

Example: 2-Minute Timed Writing

The timed writing was completed two times for a total of 66. The number beneath the timing of the part completed is 8. $66 + 8 = 74$. See the following example:

Mary returns to the clinic this morning for follow-up of her	12
herpes encephalitis. He was hospitalized for several days or	24
encephalitis which was diagnosed at herpes.	33

☐☐☐☐1☐☐☐☐2☐☐☐☐3☐☐☐☐4☐☐☐☐5☐☐☐☐6☐☐☐☐7☐☐☐☐8☐☐☐☐9☐☐☐☐10☐☐☐☐11☐☐☐☐12

31 WAM

Some headaches are due to changes in blood flow of the	11
brain. This causes pain, with nausea and vomiting.	21
A tension headache may be triggered by stress, certain	32
foods, eye strain, or lack of sleep.	39

33 WAM

Back pain is caused by strain of the muscles that support	12
the spine. This is a common injury.	18
Back strains cause pain and muscle spasms. The back	29
injury often takes weeks to heal.	36

36 WAM

This child has had a runny nose and symptoms of a mild	11
cold with a slight cough for about three or four weeks.	22
There has been a marked change with difficulty in	33
breathing for the past hour.	39

43 WAM

The patient was tearful and demanding. She spoke of	11
feeling depressed and having difficulty coping.	20
This patient increased her somatic complaints when her	32
medication needs were not met. The patient had low self-esteem	46
and pushed a tray over the edge of the table.	54

☐☐☐☐1☐☐☐☐2☐☐☐☐3☐☐☐☐4☐☐☐☐5☐☐☐☐6☐☐☐☐7☐☐☐☐8☐☐☐☐9☐☐☐☐10☐☐☐☐11☐☐☐☐12

49 WAM

      She was well and sitting in her wheelchair reading the   11
daily news. She became restless but was alert. She is a   22
cooperative lady.   25

      There were coarse rales in the lower right chest. Her   36
diagnosis was acute pneumonia. The patient became lethargic and 48
hypertensive. No anemia or diabetes mellitus.   57

52 WAM

      This patient was admitted because of dizziness, nausea,   11
weakness, and shortness of breath. He had been treated for   22
angina and emphysema.   26

      On the morning of admission, he developed nausea,   37
shortness of breath, dizziness, weakness and was unable to   48
stand and take care of himself. He had hypertension, chest   59
pain, and vertigo for several days.   63

55 WAM

      This lady was transferred from a nursing home to the   74
Mobile Hospital for dehydration, cystitis, and vomiting. She   85
became febrile on the day of admission.   93

      The lady had been living alone prior to nursing home   11
admission and had become severely dehydrated due to an   22
inadequate fluid intake. The patient was unresponsive and   33
dyspenic with shallow, rapid respiraions. She is frail   44
and undernourished.   48

61 WAM

      This man was seen by the doctor with complaints of   11
increasing symptoms of bladder neck obstruction. He complained 23
of the urinary stream requiring a longer time to initiate.   34

      There was no history of urinary tract infections or   45
hematuria. Also, there was no past history of diabetes or   56
urethritis. The examination showed enlargement of the prostate 68
gland.   69

65 WAM

      The patient today presented with lower quadrant pain,   11
diarrhea, and nausea. The patient was worked up for possible   23
appendicitis but all tests were negative. Hemoglobin and   34
hematocrit were less than normal and found to be very low.   45

      The patient was started on iron therapy with ferrous   56
sulfate and bed rest. The nausea, diarrhea, and pain subsided. 68
Her diagnoses are iron deficiency anemia with hepatomegaly and 80
probable gastroenteritis.   85

□□□□1□□□□2□□□□3□□□□4□□□□5□□□□6□□□□7□□□□8□□□□9□□□□10□□□□11□□□□12

---

70 WAM

       The patient has arteriosclerotic heart disease, having   11
suffered a heart attack in December. On the day of admission,   23
he had the sudden onset of dyspnea at rest. There was no chest   35
pain, weakness or other symptoms. Nitroglycerin afforded some   47
relief, but the dyspnea persisted and he presented to the   58
emergency room.   61

       An examination there revealed evidence for signs of   72
moderate congestive heart failure. His electrocardiogram was   84
unchanged from previous records. His only medication is   95
digoxin.   96

73 WAM

       Other medical problems include stable diabetes mellitus,   12
treated with insulin each day. He also has significant manic   24
depressive disease for which he has been hospitalized twice   35
recently. He has been in a hypomanic state lately and has   46
discontinued his psychotropic medications. He has been under   58
the care of Dr. Sykes.   62

       Recently, he reported attacks of falling asleep while   73
driving his car or watching television. He made an appointment   85
to see a neurologist.   89

85 WAM

       His physical examination revealed tachypnea and   10
orthopnea, but no acute respiratory distress. He was alert and   22
cooperative. The dermatophytosis and tinea pedis seemed to be   34
clearing compared with previous exams. Acute conjunctivitis   45
was present in the eyes. He has full dentures.   54

       The neck veins were not distended. There were increased   66
anterior and posterior diameters of the thorax. Fine rales and   78
expiratory wheezes were heard in all lung fields. No gallop or   90
murmur was heard. There was a trace of pretibial edema.   101
Neurological exam was grossly intact.   108

□□□□1□□□□2□□□□3□□□□4□□□□5□□□□6□□□□7□□□□8□□□□9□□□□10□□□□11□□□□12

LESSON 8 ■ Tab Key, Computing Two-Minute Timing   57

    The patient was hypomanic during his hospital stay with   12
restlessness and exerted considerable pressure on the nursing   24
staff to be discharged. He refused follow-up by his   34
psychiatrist, and I felt that he should not restart lithium or   46
psychotropic medications.   51

    He suffers from neurosis. Dr. Sykes is aware of his   62
status. His seizures occurred while he was taking lithium. The   74
patient refused a CAT scan and EEG.   81

    The patient was discharged to home. He goes to the Brown   93
House, which is a half-way house. He will be seen for a   104
follow-up visit in my office.   110

□□□□1□□□□2□□□□3□□□□4□□□□5□□□□6□□□□7□□□□8□□□□9□□□□10□□□□11□□□□12

Skillbuilding Paragraphs—Timed Writings

Lesson 9 Three- and Five-Minute Timed Writings: 🕐 Three- and Five-Minute Timed Writings WAM   Page 60
Computing Three-Minute Timing,
Computing Five-Minute Timing

COMPUTING THREE-MINUTE TIMING

Instructions: Computing Timed Writing Speed

Keyboarding speed is measured in words a minute (WAM). To compute WAM, count every five strokes, including spaces. For timed writing other than a minute, divide the number of words keyed by the number of minutes in the timed writings.

Example: Computing 3-Minute Timing

1. Keyed 142 words in a 3-minute timing with four errors.
2. Count errors and multiply by 2.
3. Errors = 4; $2 \times 4 = 8$.
4. Subtract errors from 142. $142 - 8 = 134$.
5. Divide by three minutes. $134 \div 3 = 44$. Your net speed: 44/4 errors.

To determine your words per minute, add the number at the end of the last complete line to the number beneath timing of the partially completed line.

Example: 3-Minute Timed Writing

The timed writing was completed four times for a total of 132. The number beneath timing of the completed is 10. $132 + 10 = 142$. See the following example:

```
Mary returns to the clinic this morning for follow-up of he      12
herpes encephalitis. He was hospitalized for several days or     24
encephalitis which was diagnosed a herpes.                       32
□□□□1□□□□2□□□□3□□□□4□□□□5□□□□6□□□□7□□□□8□□□□9□□□□10□□□□11□□□□12
```

Three- and Five-Minute Timed Writings: Computing Three-Minute Timing, Computing Five-Minute Timing

Goals

After completing this lesson, you will be able to:

✔ Take a timing for speed and accuracy.
✔ Key with control to improve accuracy.

Instructions

See page 59 on how to compute three-minute timing.

Indent five spaces or 0.5 inches for the paragraph. Double space.

Practice long words individually.

TIMED WRITING 1—THREE-MINUTE TIMING—DOUBLE SPACE

1	The patient was admitted to Mobile Desert Hos-	10	10
2	pital. We discussed her past history of gallblad-	20	20
3	der problems. A CT scan showed cholelithiasis and	30	30
4	choledocholithiasis. Her medical history revealed	40	40
5	that she had passed a kidney stone and was thought	50	50
6	to have some psychological stress-related problem.	10	60
7	Upon physical examination, she was discovered	20	70
8	to be febrile. She had generalized abdominal ten-	30	80
9	derness. Her urine, which was quite dark, was the	40	90
10	color of brown sugar, and she had very dark stool.	50	100
11	The day after she was admitted, she underwent	10	110
12	a laparoscopic cholecystectomy. At the time of	20	120
13	surgery, an excision was made, and pus and stones	30	130
14	squirted. The patient's condition improved quickly	40	140
15	post surgery.	43	143
16	The nurse gave the patient instructions as to	10	153
17	how to care for herself, then discharged her from this	20	163
18	hospital. The patient was to call for an appoint-	30	173
19	ment in two weeks for a postoperative assessment.	40	183
20	The patient was asymptomatic at discharge. I	50	193
21	am confident that she is recovered from illness.	10	203

□□□□1□□□□2□□□□3□□□□4□□□□5□□□□6□□□□7□□□□8□□□□9□□□□10

TIMED WRITING 2—THREE-MINUTE TIMING—DOUBLE SPACE

1	Mr. Eduard Corona came to this emergency room	10	10
2	disoriented. His daughter brought him in, telling	20	20
3	the doctor that for the past few weeks Mr. Coro-	30	30
4	na has been "going downhill." Mr. Corona has been	40	40
5	found to have organic brain syndrome. Due to this	50	50
6	syndrome, he has experienced many problems. He has	10	60
7	increasing problems with memory and has committed	20	70
8	antisocial acts such as concealing his food in his	30	80
9	pants and hiding his clothing in odd places in the	40	90
10	house. This has caused his daughter much anxiety.	50	100
11	He has organic brain syndrome and feels depressed.	10	110
12	He was placed in a well-run convalescent hos-	20	120
13	pital for nine months, gradually improved, and re-	30	130
14	turned home. The day before he was brought in he	40	140
15	exhibited no symptom other than that he was unable	50	150
16	to respond to his family. He has hypertension and	10	160
17	takes medication that controls it adequately.	20	170
18	Several years ago, he had a hemicolectomy for	30	180
19	a large number of polyps in the colon and a trans-	40	190
20	urethral resection of the prostate. His weight is	50	200
21	stable. No report of headaches or visual anomaly.	10	210
22	The patient exhibits no cough, chest pain, or	20	220
23	shortness of breath. There is no known history of	30	230
24	myocardial infarction or ankle swelling. No prob-	40	240
25	lem with bowel movements.	45	245

TIMED WRITING 3—THREE-MINUTE TIMING—DOUBLE SPACE

1	This patient complains of severe pain, mainly	10	10
2	in her right hip, for the past two days. She also	20	20
3	complains of one week of uncontrollable diarrhea.	30	30
4	She sustained a gunshot wound many months ago	40	40
5	that has left her with paraplegia and loss of sen-	50	50
6	sation. She does have chronic back pain; however,	10	60
7	she takes medication for this pain. Additionally,	20	70
8	she had an infection of her right foot requiring a	30	80
9	below-knee amputation. She is being treated (with	40	90
10	Paxil) for chronic depression, which is currently	50	100
11	stable. She has a Foley catheter, suffers chronic	10	110
12	urinary tract infections, and so takes medication.	20	120

□□□□1□□□□2□□□□3□□□□4□□□□5□□□□6□□□□7□□□□8□□□□9□□□□10

13	First, the doctor performed an examination of	30	130
14	her head, eyes, ears, neck, and throat. She lacks	40	140
15	headaches and has no difficulty swallowing. There	50	150
16	has been no shortness of breath; no chest pain; no	10	160
17	leg swelling; and no history of heart problems. In	20	170
18	the past she had pneumonia but got well quickly.	30	180
19	She has had no recent nausea or vomiting nor	40	190
20	any abdominal pain. She has no pyuria and no rec-	50	200
21	tal pain. A right hip x-ray revealed fractures of	10	210
22	that hip with displacements of fracture fragments.	20	220
23	This patient is being admitted to the hospital.	30	230

TIMED WRITING 4—THREE-MINUTE TIMING—DOUBLE SPACE

1	The patient presented to the office with epi-	10	10
2	gastric pain. He has had intermittent right upper	20	20
3	quadrant and back pain for the past several weeks.	30	30
4	This pain has been unusually intermittent and when	40	40
5	I saw the patient at an office visit, the physical	50	50
6	findings were negative. He has been taking Zantac	10	60
7	for peptic ulcer disease and has it under control.	20	70
8	Prior to admission, the patient noted that he	30	80
9	started turning yellow and his urine turned brown.	40	90
10	He underwent a CT scan of his abdomen. A calculus	50	100
11	was found in the neck of the gallbladder, and addi-	10	110
12	tional calculi were found in the common bile duct.	20	120
13	Although the patient denies diarrhea and vomiting,	30	130
14	he has been anorexic and has recently lost several	40	140
15	pounds. He previously had removal of a cyst and a	50	150
16	hemorrhoidectomy. He recovered well from surgery.	10	160
17	He has no known allergies. He does not smoke	20	170
18	or drink alcohol. He has had shortness of breath.	30	180
19	He has no known heart problems. He has experienced	40	190
20	extreme work-related stress during the past year	50	200
21	This patient was married and has four sons.	9	209
22	This patient was admitted to the hospital for	19	219
23	further evaluation and treatment.	26	226

□□□□1□□□□2□□□□3□□□□4□□□□5□□□□6□□□□7□□□□8□□□□9□□□□10

TIMED WRITING 5—THREE-MINUTE TIMING—DOUBLE SPACE

1	The patient is alert, cooperative, well nour-	10	10
2	ished, and well developed but is pale and possi-	20	20
3	bly anemic. She coughs but reports no congestion.	30	30
4	She was admitted to Mobile Hospital for upper	40	40
5	gastrointestinal series. It showed something sus-	50	50
6	picious in her upper throat near the pharynx. She	10	60
7	underwent upper gastrointestinal esophagoscopy and	20	70
8	gastroscopy in November; when the doctor was doing	30	80
9	the esophagoscopy, she noticed that the patient had	40	90
10	a polypoid mass behind her larynx. This doctor	50	100
11	sent her here for more detailed evaluation.	9	109
12	The patient was alert and pleasant. Laryngo-	19	119
13	scopy was somewhat difficult but did reveal a pol-	29	129
14	ypoid mass in the larynx appearing to be benign.	39	139
15	She has had a hacking cough for the past week	49	149
16	and apparently has intermittent upper gastrointes-	10	159
17	tinal-type bleeding but reports no other problem.	20	169
18	A CT scan will be done because of the finding	30	179
19	of the benign mass in the larynx. No evidence of	40	189
20	paralysis, nodule, cyst, or other abnormalities in	50	199
21	the larynx were found. CT scan is scheduled today.	10	209
22	The patient is in good general health. She's	20	219
23	been told about the operative procedure and poten-	30	229
24	tial complications, including bleeding, poor heal-	40	239
25	ing, infections, hematoma, and reaction to the an-	50	249
26	esthesia. She accepted the risks. Her only prior	10	259
27	surgery was a tonsillectomy and adenoidectomy as a	20	269
28	child. She has had no allergies. She is on medi-	30	279
29	cation for hypertension.	35	284

TIMED WRITING 6—THREE-MINUTE TIMING—DOUBLE SPACE

1	Mr. Jeff Lee Ptosis was seen in my office for	10	10
2	injuries he sustained in an accident two days ago.	20	20
3	He was very concerned about the possible effect of	30	30
4	the accident. He was driving a small truck; near-	40	40
5	ing a stop sign, he braked and was struck from the	50	50
6	rear by a speeding auto that did not try to brake.	10	60
7	He wasn't wearing his seat belt. He felt his	20	70
8	neck snap back and then forward, then his forehead	30	80

□□□□1□□□□2□□□□3□□□□4□□□□5□□□□6□□□□7□□□□8□□□□9□□□□10

9	hit the steering wheel. He felt dazed at the time	40	90
10	but did not lose consciousness and remained lucid.	50	100
11	He was taken to the Mobile Hospital Emergency	10	110
12	Center. X-rays of his cervical and thoracic spine	20	120
13	were taken, which showed a change in his chest. No	30	130
14	other acute injury manifested. He felt a severe	40	140
15	headache for two days after the accident, but this	50	150
16	resolved spontaneously. He took aspirin for pain.	10	160
17	Positive findings after my examination of the	20	170
18	patient included pronounced tenderness of the neck	30	180
19	muscles. Diagnosis included head trauma with con-	40	190
20	cussion, cervical strain, and soft tissue injuries.	50	200
21	Ultrasound stimulation was continued for four	10	210
22	weeks, after which he was switched to electrostim-	20	220
23	ulation therapy. He still felt mild tenderness of	30	230
24	his muscles but was almost symptom-free. As long	40	240
25	as he continues with the exercise program designed	50	250
26	for him and does not sustain further injuries, he	10	260
27	should do well.	13	263

TIMED WRITING 7—THREE-MINUTE TIMING—DOUBLE SPACE

1	The patient has a history of pain in his left	10	10
2	groin. He has been diagnosed as having a left in-	20	20
3	guinal hernia. However, in the past several days,	30	30
4	this area has gotten more painful and has bothered	40	40
5	him. Receiving a specialist's agreement with this	50	50
6	diagnosis, the patient is being admitted for elec-	10	60
7	tive surgery. Surgery is scheduled for this week.	20	70
8	The patient's other significant history is of	30	80
9	having degenerative arthritis. This arthritis in-	40	90
10	volves symptomatically most of his joints. He has	50	100
11	recently been prescribed nonsteroidal anti-inflam-	10	110
12	matory drugs. He also has gastritis. The patient	20	120
13	also recently has complained of palpitations. The	30	130
14	palpitations are thought to stem from anxiety. He	40	140
15	has had an EKG exercise test that he was unable to	50	150
16	complete because of foot pain; however, there were	10	160
17	no indications of ischemia; no further complaints.	20	170
18	He is allergic to PENICILLIN and SULFA DRUGS.	30	180
19	Twelve years ago, the patient had surgery for	40	190
20	rhinoplasty. He also has had a right hip replace-	50	200

□□□□1□□□□2□□□□3□□□□4□□□□5□□□□6□□□□7□□□□8□□□□9□□□□10

21	ment. He has a history of polio, but there are no	10	210
22	known sequelae. He has complained of a feeling of	20	220
23	bloating and of abdominal pain. The patient is	30	230
24	to be admitted to Mobile Hospital for elective	40	240
25	repair of the inguinal hernia.	46	246

TIMED WRITING 8—THREE-MINUTE TIMING—DOUBLE SPACE

1	This patient was admitted to the hospital for	10	10
2	pneumonia and urinary tract infection. During his	20	20
3	stay, it was thought he had urinary sepsis and was	30	30
4	treated for this condition. His urine culture was	40	40
5	negative, and no blood cultures were obtained when	50	50
6	he was hospitalized. The medication taken by this	10	60
7	patient initially caused serious lethargy. By his	20	70
8	final day in the hospital, this had quite improved.	30	80
9	Still, he was not ambulatory and had no appe-	40	90
10	tite so was kept on intravenous fluids and intra-	50	100
11	venous antibiotics. He has had no abdominal pain,	10	110
12	no vomiting, no diarrhea, and no other complaints.	20	120
13	The past medical history revealed that he had	30	130
14	a history of hypertension, which is not active at	40	140
15	the present time. When young, he underwent an ap-	50	150
16	pendectomy, had pneumonia, and broke his left arm.	10	160
17	There are no audible wheezes in his chest. The	20	170
18	patient is a lethargic male who is sometimes alert	30	180
19	and responsive; he moves all his extremities well.	40	190
20	This patient will be transferred to a skilled	50	200
21	nursing facility for antibiotic treatment for this	10	210
22	infection and also for physical therapy to aid him	20	220
23	in becoming ambulatory.	25	225

TIMED WRITING 9—THREE-MINUTE TIMING—DOUBLE SPACE

1	This is one of many prior admissions for this	10	10
2	pleasant female; she has a history of lung cancer.	20	20
3	The patient presented with abdominal pain, nausea,	30	30
4	vomiting, and severe hemorrhaging. She denies fe-	40	40
5	ver and chills. In the emergency room, the doctor	50	50
6	found her to have abdominal pain and hemorrhaging.	10	60
7	She was treated for her pain and given intravenous	20	70
8	fluids. The patient is allergic to CODEINE, which	30	80

□□□□1□□□□2□□□□3□□□□4□□□□5□□□□6□□□□7□□□□8□□□□9□□□□10

9	she claims causes an itch, and EMPIRIN. Her blood	40	90
10	pressure is within normal limits and she is lucid.	50	100
11	Her past surgical history includes two opera-	10	110
12	tions for lung cancer and a hysterectomy. She now	20	120
13	lives with her mother. Her father also had cancer	30	130
14	and died several weeks ago. The patient's brother	40	140
15	and sisters are healthy and lack unusual symptoms.	50	150
16	While her appetite has been poor for the last	10	160
17	few days; her condition is stable. She is encour-	20	170
18	aged to eat regularly, with which she does comply.	30	180
19	She smokes one pack of cigarettes a day. She	40	190
20	is alert, oriented, and cooperative. Today she is	50	200
21	being discharged to go home. She is a teacher.	10	210

TIMED WRITING 10—THREE-MINUTE TIMING—DOUBLE SPACE

1	Mrs. Evie Serum was a passenger in a cab when	10	10
2	a second car struck the cab from behind. Her neck	20	20
3	and head were snapped forward and backward on	30	30
4	impact. Her back and neck were injured because of	40	40
5	the accident. The patient's neck pain is confined	50	50
6	to the mid-cervical spine, the sides, and the base	10	60
7	of the neck. The pain is recurrent, aggravated by	20	70
8	the turning of the head. Occasionally, pain comes	30	80
9	on spontaneously, with no obvious causative agent.	40	90
10	My examination of the cervical spine revealed	50	100
11	a normal range of movement; this includes flexion,	10	110
12	extension, sideward bending, and rotation. Palpa-	20	120
13	tion shows tenderness in the cervical spine and in	30	130
14	the spine. Paravertebrae and muscles were tender.	40	140
15	My examination of the lumbar spine shows this	50	150
16	patient's gait to be normal. Heel and toe walking	10	160
17	are normal. Extension and sideward bending to the	20	170
18	right bring pain that is referred to the low back,	30	180
19	with tenderness to palpation of the lumbar spine.	40	190
20	This patient is responding well to her treat-	50	200
21	ment. This treatment consists of physical therapy	10	210
22	and an anti-inflammatory agent. She attends phys-	20	220
23	ical therapy three times a week and will return to	30	230
24	work in six weeks.	34	234

□□□□1□□□□2□□□□3□□□□4□□□□5□□□□6□□□□7□□□□8□□□□9□□□□10

COMPUTING FIVE-MINUTE TIMING

Instructions: *Computing Timed Writing Speed*

Keyboarding speed is measured in words a minute (WAM). To compute WAM, count every 5 strokes, including spaces. For timed writings other than a minute, divide the number of words keyed by the number of minutes in the timed writings.

Example: *Computing 5-Minute Timing*

1. Keyed 172 words in a 5-minute timing with two errors.
2. Count errors and multiply by 2.
3. Errors = 2; 2 × 2 = 4.
4. Subtract errors from 272. 272 − 4 = 268.
5. Divide by 5 minutes. 268 ÷ 5 = 53. Your net speed: 53/2 errors.

To determine your words per minute, add the number at the end of the last complete line to the number beneath timing of the partially completed line.

Example: *5-Minute Timed Writing*

The timed writing was completed five times for a total of 165. The number beneath timing of the part completed is 7. 165 + 7 = 172. See the following example:

```
Mary returns to the clinic this morning for follow-up of her    12
herpes encephalitis. He was hospitalized for several days or     24
encephalitis which was diagnosed as herpes.                      33
    □□□□1□□□□2□□□□3□□□□4□□□□5□□□□6□□□□7□□□□8□□□□9□□□□10□□□□11□□□□12
```

TIMED WRITING 11—FIVE-MINUTE TIMING—DOUBLE SPACE

```
        This elderly lady was brought to the emergency room in a    12
confused state. She had had a chronic productive cough with         23
yellow purulent sputum. A chest x-ray revealed a density at         34
the left lung base, and she was admitted for treatment of           45
pneumonia. The patient is not a very good historian. She was        57
seen in June and August of this year. At that time, she had         68
pneumonia and was hospitalized at Mobile Hospital. At that          79
time, there was a history of urinary incontinence and slurred       91
speech. She has continued to smoke cigarettes. She has a           102
history of hypertension and has been on various medications        113
for this in the past. When I saw her in August, she was not        124
aware of having any lung disease. The home situation was quite     136
difficult in that she was living with a daughter who was           147
separated from her husband. The patient's husband died several     159
years ago.                                                         161
        The patient denies any cephalgia. She is aware of some     172
nasal congestion and nasal discharge. She denies any               182
difficulty swallowing but readily admits that she is eating        193
little more than liquids. She denies being aware of any fever      205
or chills. She states that she has chest pain but is unable to     217
adequately describe this or point to its location. She denies      129
dysuria; indeed, she denies having any significant symptoms        140
other than mild dyspnea and a cough productive of sputum.          151
    □□□□1□□□□2□□□□3□□□□4□□□□5□□□□6□□□□7□□□□8□□□□9□□□□10□□□□11□□□□12
```

This is a well-developed elderly, poorly nourished and   162
chronically ill-appearing confused lady. She seems to realize   174
she is in the hospital but is not oriented to time. She is   185
afebrile. There is no evidence of cervical adenopathy or   196
thyromegaly.   198

She probably needs placement outside her daughter's home.   210
It seems unlikely that the daughter is able to care for her   221
adequately.   223

TIMED WRITING 12—FIVE-MINUTE TIMING—DOUBLE SPACE

The patient is a male who was admitted because of chest   12
pain, cough, and sputum who was subsequently found to have   23
pneumonia. Patient has a previous history of coronary artery   35
disease with a previous myocardial infarction and has been   46
seen for these two problems by Dr. Sampson and Dr. Burns. In   58
addition, patient has a long drinking history and a very   70
distended abdomen. I have been asked to see him in realtion   81
to evaluation of ascites.   86

Patient claims that he drinks alcohol every day. He has   98
been previously told he had cirrhosis but has never had a   109
liver biopsy. He claims that his abdomen has been distended   120
for several years. On previous admissions, he has been   131
described as having ascites, but as far as I can tell has   142
never had a paracentesis. He has no history of known   152
hepatitis, no history of jaundice, and no history of any   163
neoplastic disease. On previous evaluations, he has been found   175
to have minimally elevated liver enzymes. On this admission,   187
his SGOT is slightly elevated.   193

Physical exam shows this male to be in no acute distress.   205
He is afebrile. Fundi show flat disks with no hemorrhage or   216
mild arteriolar narrowing. Oropharynx is benign. Neck is   227
supple. Carotid upstroke is normal; no carotid bruits. Thyroid   239
is normal. There are rhonchi throughout both lungs with some   250
rales. Abdomen is markedly distended. There is no definite   261
fluid wave. Spleen is not palpable. Bowel sounds are normal.   272
The rectal exam showed no masses or tenderness. Also,   282
extremities showed no clubbing, cyanosis, or edema. Central   293
nervous system screening neurologic exam is within normal   304
limits.   305

If the patient has ascites in light of his normal liver   316
function tests, further evaluation will be required, including   328
a paracentesis, a liver biopsy, and an abdominal   338
ultrasonography. Hypothyroidism might be another cause for his   350
ascites.   352

▫▫▫▫1▫▫▫▫2▫▫▫▫3▫▫▫▫4▫▫▫▫5▫▫▫▫6▫▫▫▫7▫▫▫▫8▫▫▫▫9▫▫▫▫10▫▫▫▫11▫▫▫▫12

TIMED WRITING 13—FIVE-MINUTE TIMING—DOUBLE SPACE

This male was in a moped versus motor vehicle accident	11
in which he sustained a left humerus fracture and a right	22
femur fracture.	25
The patient was taken to the main operating room where	36
he received general endotracheal anesthetic. The injured leg	47
was placed into the boot holder and into position, with	58
padding to his heel and his foot. The left arm was placed	69
onto an arm holder, and the right arm was placed up over the	81
patient's chest and well padded. All extremity pressure	92
points were well padded.	97
Image was obtained to demonstrate good image of the	108
fracture and good reduction with traction of the fracture on	120
the fracture table. Reduction was satisfactory; therefore,	131
the leg was prepped and draped in a sterile fashion.	141
An incision was made over the greater trochanter. The	152
subcutaneous fat was divided down to the muscle fascia. The	163
muscle fascia was incised. The fossa was then located on the	174
greater trochanter. The guide rod was then placed across the	185
fracture site; this was done with minimal difficulty. The nail	197
was passed under fluoroscopic control across the fracture	208
site and from the hip to the knee. With this process	218
completed, all other instrumentation was removed from the	229
nail; and the femur was scanned from proximal to distal;	240
and it demonstrated excellent alignment and fixation of the	251
fracture.	253
The wound was irrigated with sterile saline, and a layer	265
closure was performed ending with skin staples. A sterile	276
dressing was applied to the wound, and the patient was taken	287
off the fracture table and placed onto his bed. The knee had	298
a full range of motion.	302

TIMED WRITING 14—FIVE-MINUTE TIMING—DOUBLE SPACE

This Caucasian male with multiple recent admissions to	11
this hospital returned to the emergency room the evening of	22
admission complaining of severe back pain, and his family was	34
quite concerned over his intermittent severe confusion. He was	46
most recently hospitalized from February to March with fever	58
and dehydration associated with confusion. At that time, the	70
patient improved on IV hydration and treatment with adicillin.	82
He was seen by Dr. Sykes who felt that he had subacute	93
delirium. The patient was exhibiting evidence of	103
hallucinations. It was felt that he had considerably impaired	115
judgment. The patient became alert, oriented, and seemingly	126
competent. He was discharged at his insistence to his home in	138
Mobile with a prescription for Anspor, in addition to his	149
usual prednisone, aminophylline, and digoxin. He returned to	161
home where, I would gather from his family, he did not	172
maintain an intake of food and fluid. For reasons that are	183

☐☐☐☐1☐☐☐☐2☐☐☐☐3☐☐☐☐4☐☐☐☐5☐☐☐☐6☐☐☐☐7☐☐☐☐8☐☐☐☐9☐☐☐☐10☐☐☐☐11☐☐☐☐12

---

not clear to me, his prescription for the antibiotic was not   195
filled; and the patient apparently became dehydrated.   205
Although he has multiple family members living in his   215
immediate environment, it is certainly questionable as to   226
whether they are able to adequately provide for this man's   237
considerable supportive needs. At any rate, he returned to   248
the emergency room with a fever. His abdomen is tender and   259
his liver now appears to be enlarged.   266

    Chest x-ray failed to demonstrate any major change.   277
Basically, he has a bronchogenic carcinoma, primary in the   288
right upper lung, discovered last summer. He had radiation   299
therapy to this area due to a determination by CAT scan of   310
noresectability. Radiation did not seem to relieve the pain.   322
The patient had a number of hospitalizations for pain,   333
culminating in an anterior vertebral body surgical procedure.   345
Since then the patient has had considerable relief of his   356
left shoulder and neck pain, but he has remained quite   367
agitated and intermittently confused.   374

TIMED WRITING 15—FIVE-MINUTE TIMING—DOUBLE SPACE

    The patient was admitted with chief complaints of   11
depression, intense anxiety, and many fears concerning her   22
ability to function and to maintain herself at home. The   33
patient had been recently discharged from Mobile Hospital   44
after being evaluated for abdominal and chest pain. She also   56
had urinary retention secondary to anticholinergic effects of   68
her medication. She had been evaluated for depression during   80
her hospitalization, and it was felt that the patient was very 92
anxious and depressed and reacting to her symptoms. She was   103
not able to be treated with antidepressant medication due to   115
her urinary retention.   119

    The patient complained of abdominal pain. Her abdomen   130
was soft and nontender. There was no organomegaly, no masses,   142
no rebound tenderness. Her bowel sounds were normoactive.   153

    It is recommended that the patient be hospitalized   164
because she apparently is unable to function and has had   175
noted neurogenic bladder with urinary retention. She stated   186
that she cannot handle herself on an outpatient basis and   197
that she becomes extremely depressed and despondent to the   208
point she is unable to function. It is felt that she be given   220
immediate crisis-oriented, reality-focused therapy to help   231
clarify her environmental stresses and help her increase her   242
self-esteem. During her hospitalization, she should be   253
treated with medications to relieve her anxiety and to be   264
seen in reality-oriented psychotherapy to clarify her present   276
life situation and any environmental problems that she may be   288
experiencing. Since she is having urinary retention, it is   299
recommended that her medications be decreased and that she be   311
maintained on psychotherapy alone. She is a very difficult,   322
demanding patient with marked somatic complaints and has   333
noted feelings of isolation and abandonment. She will need to   345

□□□□1□□□□2□□□□3□□□□4□□□□5□□□□6□□□□7□□□□8□□□□9□□□□10□□□□11□□□□12

be supported and gently confronted to help her recognize her   356
somatization complaints are to gain attention and are products   368
of her anxiety and depression. It is also necessary that she   379
be followed by her primary care physician and urologist during   391
her hospitalization.   395

TIMED WRITING 16—FIVE-MINUTE TIMING—DOUBLE SPACE

Helen is a right-handed black female patient who reports   12
feeling a dull, sharp and burning pain involving the bilateral   24
wrists with numbness and a tingling extending into the elbow.   36
She is presently employed as an assembler. She was evaluated   48
by an orthopedic surgeon. The patient was advised that she was   60
suffering from bilateral carpal tunnel syndrome. Wrist splints   72
were recommended. The patient wore splints while sleeping and   84
noted her condition did not worsen. She received no   94
injections. She began experiencing numbness and tingling in   105
her hands while working. The pain became more frequent and she   117
was having more pain at night.   123

The patient was referred to another physician for an EMG   135
and nerve conduction velocity testing. She went for a surgical   147
evaluation. Dr. Hudson recommended surgery. In February, Dr.   158
Hudson administered cortisone injections to her wrists and   169
provided splints to be used at night.   176

Helen underwent a left carpal tunnel surgery in May and   188
two weeks later underwent a right carpal tunnel surgery.   199
Physical therapy was provided for her at the orthopedic clinic   211
for four months. There was some improvement of her condition   223
but symptoms gradually returned. The patient was evaluated by   235
Dr. Hudson, and her condition is permanent and stationary.   246

However, when she returned to repetitive assembling she   258
became somewhat more symptomatic. The patient continued   269
working and changed employers for one year with persistent   280
symptoms. She does have degenerative disc disease in the   291
cervical spine. The work that she was performing over the   302
years has caused aggravation of her disc disease.   312

Helen fell down a flight of stairs at work resulting in   324
neck pain. She has experienced a gradual increasing in neck   336
pain. The physician ordered a MRI. The MRI of the cervical   347
spine revealed degenerative disc disease and spondylosis in   359
the cervical spine. The physician prescribed exercises and   370
anti-inflammatory medications for her neck. Her condition has   382
improved.   384

TIMED WRITING 17—FIVE-MINUTE TIMING—DOUBLE SPACE

Morgan is a white male who was in a fight with his friend   12
where he was kicked in the face and back. On examination, at   24
that time, it was noted there was pain over the lumbar spine   36
with generalized contusions and abrasions. There was pain with   48
marked radiculopathy. Because of that, he was sent to Mobile   60

□□□□1 □□□□2 □□□□3 □□□□4 □□□□5 □□□□6 □□□□7 □□□□8 □□□□9 □□□□10 □□□□11 □□□□12

Outpatient Medical Group, where a possible chip fracture of   71
the lumbar spine was diagnosed. Because of the marked pain   82
this patient was having without nerve root compression and   93
spinal cord compression, he was sent home on pain medication, 105
bedrest, and a heating pad. Over the next several hours, the   117
patient had severe pain, uncontrolled with outpatient therapy. 129
I have been called multiple times today by his mother, father, 141
and the patient himself asking for more relief. Because of   152
this continued pain, he is being admitted to Mobile Hospital   164
for observation and treatment. He was hospitalized several   175
years ago for surgical removal of a superficial tumor. No   186
other hospitalizations are reported.   193

    Presently he lives with his parents. He takes drugs to   204
excess, alcohol to excess, and has in the past been   214
hyperkinetic, and had taken Ritalin for many years.   224

    His family has a positive history of cancer, diabetes,   235
heart disease, kidney problems, hypertension, and asthma. No   247
family history of tuberculosis, epilepsy, myasthenia gravis,   259
or glaucoma has been reported.   265

    He has had measles, chickenpox, and rubeola with no   276
history of mumps, polio, rheumatic fever, diphtheria, malaria, 288
or encephalitis.   291

    There is cephalgia with frontal facial swelling and pain   303
with no history of syncope, convulsions, or seizures. Prior   314
to this problem, there has been no major musculoskeletal   325
abnormality.   327

TIMED WRITING 18—FIVE-MINUTE TIMING—DOUBLE SPACE

    Joan, a right-handed widow, was referred because of   11
epilepsy. The patient apparently has been in the hospital for 23
about a week because of pulmonary infection which seems not   34
to have cleared. She has a history of previous alcoholism.   45
There is no suggestion that she has recently been abusing   56
medication in any way. No details of prior neurologic history 68
are available, but it does not appear that she had had prior   80
major problems.   83

    This afternoon the patient began to twitch and then had a 95
major motor seizure. She was seen by Dr. Jones who gave her   106
parenteral phenobarbital. However, she remained stuporus; and 118
a second seizure occurred about an hour later at which time   129
she was transferred to the intensive care unit. At that time, 141
I was contacted and suggested that she be given phenobarbital   153
intramuscularly. She was intubated, but within an hour,   164
seizures began and have continued to the present.   154

    A spinal fluid exam done by Dr. Jones revealed clear   165
fluid under normal pressure with a normal protein and no   176
cells. The patient had been receiving theophylline, but this   188
has not been in the toxic range. While electrolytes are a   199
little on the low side, they are certainly not in a range that 211
seizures would result, and other blood chemistries are   222
noncontributory.   225

☐☐☐☐1☐☐☐☐2☐☐☐☐3☐☐☐☐4☐☐☐☐5☐☐☐☐6☐☐☐☐7☐☐☐☐8☐☐☐☐9☐☐☐☐10☐☐☐☐11☐☐☐☐12

When the patient was initially seen, she had a   235
generalized convulsion and was breathing rapidly, and blood   247
pressure was palpable. There were a variety of sounds over   258
the chest. General exam did not reveal congestive heart   269
failure. Color was poor, and there may have been a little   280
pallor. The neck was supple. Pupils were slightly reactive.   291
The eyes tended to be forced downward and occasionally   302
jerking. The convulsive movements were generalized, and it was 314
impossible to assess focal changes.   321

The patient was given Valium, phenobarbital, and   332
Dilantin. Blood pressure dropped gradually over the next hour. 344
However, within several minutes, all convulsive activity   355
stopped, and the patient seemed more relaxed. She seemed to   366
have stabilized.   369

TIMED WRITING 19—FIVE-MINUTE TIMING—DOUBLE SPACE

Debra has been known to have hypertension for several   11
years. On the day prior to admission, she was feeling well.   22
Since early morning on the day of admission, she has not felt 34
well and has experienced chills during the day. As the day   45
progressed, she became more and more dyspneic. Prior to   56
admission, she was barely able to carry on a conversation   67
because of dyspnea. There has been some coughing but no   78
significant production of sputum. There has been generalized 90
muscle pain and especially pain in the chest with deep   101
inspiration. She denies any nausea or vomiting.   110

Her father was a diabetic and died from a heart attack;   121
mother was known to have had tuberculosis and died as a   132
result of a self-inflicted gunshot wound. She has brothers   143
and sisters who are living and in good health and two   154
daughters who are living and well.   161

The patient is married and lives in a rural community   172
with her husband who is employed as an attorney. She denies   183
the use of tobacco and alcohol.   189

There has been progressive hearing loss in the left ear,   201
and recent examination by an otolaryngologist diagnosed the   212
problem as neurosensory loss. She denies any exertional   223
dyspnea or pain prior to the onset of this illness. She has   234
been taking blood pressure medication for several years. She 246
has frequent episodes of arthritis involving mostly the feet, 258
attributed to hyperuricemia. She has been taking thyroid   269
supplements for approximately two months with good response. 280
Aside from obesity, she has never shown any overt symptoms of 292
hypothyroidism.   295

The patient is a markedly obese white woman who appears   307
to be dyspneic at rest. Respirations are rapid and shallow.   318
She is alert and oriented, no cyanosis nor icterus apparent. 329

□□□□1□□□□2□□□□3□□□□4□□□□5□□□□6□□□□7□□□□8□□□□9□□□□10□□□□11□□□□12

The patient is a black male child who was apparently well   12
until about a week prior to admission when he developed   23
recurrent tarry stools, not associated with pain or vomiting   35
or any evidence of distress. Prior to this admission, this   46
kept recurring for approximately a week. The child developed   58
some recurrent vomiting associated with grossly bloody stools.   70
The child also had some episodes in the last several hours   81
prior to admission of the urine being slightly blood-tinged.   92

There is no history of toxins, or drug ingestion. The   103
mother has been giving the child some medication for the last   115
week which are known as bleeding tablets containing lime   126
phosphate.   128

There is no history of hemolytic disease in the family or   138
any other possible ingestion related to insecticides. The   149
child was admitted to Mobile Hospital for work-up including a   161
barium enema which showed questionable liver enlargement.   172

The child was a full-term baby born to this mother at   183
Mobile Hospital, the product of a normal spontaneous delivery.   195
The child did well during the neonatal, antenatal, and   206
postnatal period and went home with the mother from the   217
hospital without problems. The only anemia was associated with   229
this pregnancy.   232

The mother had been on Tofranil approximately a week   243
prior to delivery and did breast feed for a short period of   254
time, but this was discontinued after a couple of weeks. Since   266
that time, the mother has been on Tofranil and tranquilizers,   278
type unknown.   281

The child has had a normal course up until this time and   293
no other problems. He has had a DPT and oral polio   303
vaccination. The growth and development has been essentially   315
normal. There is a female sibling at home who is well. The   326
parents are both living and well. There is a strong family   337
history of cancer, primarily involving the lungs and female   348
organs, that is, the breast and the genitourinary tract.   359

□□□□1□□□□2□□□□3□□□□4□□□□5□□□□6□□□□7□□□□8□□□□9□□□□10□□□□11□□□□12

Double Letters, Speed Builders, and Timed Writings

Double Letters and Longer Words, Three- and Five-Minute Timed Writings

Goals

After completing this lesson, you will be able to:

✔ Key double letters.
✔ Key longer words.

Instructions

Key each line one time, double-spacing after each. Strive for accuracy and then speed.

1 cuff cocci flaccid siccus buccula vaccine coccyx
2 feed sleep spleen need effuse odditis attack attic
3 fatty canna skull tubba fissure needle gross
4 dizzy affect fussy nipple billion stiff pitting
5 The druggist struggled with the medication.
6 The mammoplasty resulted in mammalgia.
7 Oocytase destroyed the oocyte and oopore.
8 It seemed she suffered from appendicitis.
9 Appropriate dressings were applied to the verruca.
10 The patient came in with hemorrhaging hemorrhoids.

LONGER WORDS

1 neoplasia varicella anesthesia infection chemical
2 cirrhosis hematuria hemostasis auditory scoliosis
3 This patient has polyuria and polydipsia.
4 tonsillar tinnitus esophagus dysphagia diarrhea
5 chickenpox keratitis pneumonia metacarpal larynx
6 The patient is suffering from depression.
7 sinusitis operation orthopnea comfort occipital
8 dyscrasia allergies digitalis abdominal prosthesis
9 coccygeal headaches dizziness prognosis lethargic
10 Arthroscopy is used for diagnosis of the knee.

SPEED BUILDERS—LETTER COMBINATIONS

```
 1   ch chafe chain chart charta chest chief child chin
 2   pu pus purge pulvis puna pupil pure pump pupa
 3   The chief complaint is pus in the chest.
 4   ac acute acid acardia acyanotic acinitis action
 5   fl flu fluid fluke flux flush flutter flora flow
 6   Drink fluids and fresh fruit juice for the flu.
 7   te tea tear teat teeth tela tenia tense tent
 8   sp spa space spared spasm sperm spica spill splint
 9   The splint on the arm is causing a spasm.
10   mi mix mica milk mind mitral mite morror mitosis
11   di die dila digit diffuse disc distress disk
12   She is being treated for a diffused disc.
13   en end energy enteric ental entrain entity enema
14   gr groin groove group growth grief gross ground
15   The girl grieves about the tumor on the groin.
```

THREE- AND FIVE-MINUTE TIMING—DOUBLE SPACE

```
 1        Mary has been transferred from Laveen to          9
 2   Mobile Hospital for treatment of gross hematuria.     19
 3   Her history is unobtainable from the patient and      29
 4   most of the information is from the patient's         38
 5   daughter.  The daughter went to Laveen to settle      47
 6   the patient's estate and found her mother barri-      56
 7   caded in her home.  Gross hematuria was noted on      65
 8   examination in the emergency department.  Also,       74
 9   bloody clothing was found scattered around the        83
10   home.  The patient is incompetent mentally and has    93
11   been declared so by the psychiatrist.  She was       102
12   brought here for treatment.  An adequate history     111
13   is unobtainable.  The patient denies any urologic    121
14   problems.  She is healthy with a good hemoglobin     130
15   and hematocrit, but an irregular mass was noted      139
16   on the IVP.                                          141
17        Brief examination of the patient shows no       150
18   marked evidence of cerebrovascular accident,         159
19   tenderness, or abdominal masses.  The patient is     168
20   uncooperative.  Pelvic examination was deferred to   178
21   the time of cytoscopy.  The situation was discussed  188
22   with the patient's daughter, and we will proceed     197
23   with a cytoscopy and biopsy of this lesion.          205
```

        □□□□1□□□□2□□□□3□□□□4□□□□5□□□□6□□□□7□□□□8□□□□9□□□□10

Three- and Five-Minute Timed Writings

Goals

After completing this lesson, you will be able to:

✔ Key for speed and accuracy.

Instructions

Continue to concentrate letter by letter for accuracy and speed.

TIMED WRITING 1—STROKE—FIVE-MINUTE TIMING—DOUBLE SPACE

1	A stroke, affecting the cardiovascular system	10
2	and arteries, stops or reduces the blood supply to	20
3	the brain. When an artery in the brain is clogged	30
4	with a blood clot, a stroke occurs; neither oxygen	40
5	nor blood reaches part of the brain's nerve cells.	50
6	A stroke can also occur when a vessel in the brain	10
7	bursts. There are several kinds of strokes: cere-	20
8	bral thrombosis stroke occurs when blood clots in-	30
9	side an artery that ferries blood to the brain, so	40
10	blocking the blood flow; atherosclerosis stroke is	50
11	likely to occur when blood clots form in a vessel.	10
12	Embolism is the other kind of stroke in which	20
13	a blood clot blocks the blood vessels. The hemor-	30
14	rhage stroke occurs when blood bursts in the cere-	40
15	bral artery. The vessel wall widens, bulges, then	50
16	bursts. This is called an aneurysm.	8

TIMED WRITING 2—CONGESTIVE HEART FAILURE—FIVE-MINUTE TIMING—DOUBLE SPACE

1	Damage to, or strain of, the heart muscle can	10
2	cause congestive heart failure. The flow of blood	20
3	to and from the heart slows and brings swelling in	30
4	the legs, ankles, liver, and spleen. Also, fluids	40
5	collect in the lungs and cause shortness of breath	50
6	when the person is lying down. Digitalis is given	10
7	to strengthen the heart; diuretics are often taken	20
8	to help the body eliminate excess water.	28

□□□□1□□□□2□□□□3□□□□4□□□□5□□□□6□□□□7□□□□8□□□□9□□□□10

TIMED WRITING 3—ASTHMA—FIVE-MINUTE TIMING—DOUBLE SPACE

1	Asthma is a disease of the respiratory system	10
2	that includes the lungs. Some symptoms are wheez-	20
3	ing, coughing, and rapid breathing. Asthma can be	30
4	controlled, but it is not curable. With good med-	40
5	ical care, asthma patients usually live productive	50
6	lives. Asthma is common, restricting activity for	10
7	only some sufferers. An inhaler is commonly used.	20
8	In an asthma attack, bronchial tubes restrict;	30
9	muscle spasms constrict the tubes, which clog with	40
10	mucus. Air becomes trapped in the alveoli and new	50
11	air cannot enter. This condition can be severe or	10
12	mild. Asthma attacks may be caused by stress, ex-	20
13	ercise, or allergic reactions to dust, pollen, and	30
14	pollutants in the environment.	36

TIMED WRITING 4—ANGINA PECTORIS—FIVE-MINUTE TIMING—DOUBLE SPACE

1	Angina pectoris is pain in the chest. Angina	10
2	condition is myocardial when the heart muscle does	20
3	not get enough blood; this lack of blood supply is	30
4	called "ischemia." Angina medications alter blood	40
5	supply to the heart muscle and thus supplement the	50
6	oxygen supply. Vasodilators--drugs that relax the	10
7	blood vessels--improve the flow of blood, allowing	20
8	more oxygen to reach the heart. Nitroglycerin may	30
9	also be used.	33

TIMED WRITING 5—HEART ATTACK—FIVE-MINUTE TIMING—DOUBLE SPACE

1	Coronary heart disease is called coronary ar-	10
2	tery disease. If the blood supply to a portion of	20
3	the heart muscle becomes minimal or stops, a heart	30
4	attack occurs. The build up of lipid in the lining	40
5	of coronary arteries is called atherosclerosis and	50
6	can cause abnormal clotting of blood. This abnor-	10
7	mal clotting leads to thrombosis. Thrombosis is a	20
8	clot in the artery.	24

     □□□□1□□□□2□□□□3□□□□4□□□□5□□□□6□□□□7□□□□8□□□□9□□□□10

TIMED WRITING 6—BONE—FIVE-MINUTE TIMING—DOUBLE SPACE

1	Bones are made of phosphorus, potassium, cal-	10
2	cium, and sodium. Bone is living tissue, and for-	20
3	mation of new bone is needed for growth and repair	30
4	of everyday wear. Calcium gives bone strength and	40
5	protein. Bones are held together by ligaments and	50
6	protect and support internal organs. Blood marrow	10
7	is contained in bones; this marrow produces eryth-	20
8	rocytes, yellow bone marrow, and other blood cells	30
9	as well. The cavities of bone, lined with marrow,	40
10	contain red and white blood cells.	47

TIMED WRITING 7—POLYPS—FIVE-MINUTE TIMING—DOUBLE SPACE

1	Polyps are abnormal growths that are the size	10
2	of a pinhead to considerably larger. They grow as	20
3	a flower grows on a stem. Polyps found in the co-	30
4	lon lining are unhealthy growths. They may result	40
5	from a high-fat, low-fiber diet, heredity, or even	50
6	exposure to cancer-causing substances. Polyps are	10
7	also found in the bladder, uterus, and nose. Pol-	20
8	yps can be benign, noncancerous growths, or malig-	30
9	nant, cancerous growths. After removal, the polyp	40
10	tissue is sent to a pathology lab for analysis.	50

TIMED WRITING 8—BLOOD PRESSURE—FIVE-MINUTE TIMING—DOUBLE SPACE

1	Everyone has blood pressure. The measurement	10
2	of the force with which blood pushes against arte-	20
3	rial walls gives the blood pressure reading. When	30
4	arterioles become narrow, blood pressure rises; it	40
5	is harder for the blood to pass through, making	50
6	the heart muscle work harder. High blood pressure	10
7	can be caused by aging, high dietary sodium, undue	20
8	stress, and heredity. High blood pressure can de-	30
9	velop into stroke, coronary heart disease, or con-	40
10	gestive heart failure, and can damage the kidneys.	50
11	Diet, medication, exercise, weight loss, and heed-	10
12	ing a doctor's advice can all drop blood pressure.	20
13	Lifestyle changes and working with the health pro-	30
14	fessionals can reward the high blood pressure vic-	40
15	tim with a long life.	44

□□□□1□□□□2□□□□3□□□□4□□□□5□□□□6□□□□7□□□□8□□□□9□□□□10

TIMED WRITING 9—HERNIAS—THREE-MINUTE TIMING—DOUBLE SPACE

```
 1       A hernia is caused by a weak area in the mus-        10
 2  cle of the stomach.  An umbilical hernia is caused        20
 3  by abdominal pressures including pregnancy, obesi-        30
 4  ty, a bulging navel, and excessive coughing.  Most        40
 5  hernias occur in the abdominal wall.  A hernia can        50
 6  cause pain.  Most hernias do not go away, and sur-        10
 7  gery may be the sole recourse.  A hernia may cause        20
 8  intestinal problems, digestive problems, vomiting,       30
 9  high fever, and bloody stools. Infants can be born        40
10  with hernias, umbilical and inguinal hernias.  The       50
11  hernia occurs in the abdominal wall.  The inguinal       10
12  hernia is a weakness in the intestine--this is the       20
13  most common type.                                        24
```

TIMED WRITING 10—GALLBLADDER—THREE-MINUTE TIMING—DOUBLE SPACE

```
 1       The gallbladder, an organ under the liver, is       10
 2  found in the abdomen.  It stores bile, which helps       20
 3  with digestion by breaking down the fats in foods.       30
 4       Gallstones are formed from liquid and bile in       40
 5  the gallbladder.  Bilirubin, cholesterol, and cal-       50
 6  cium can also form gallstones.  These stones some-       10
 7  times move and get stuck in the bile duct, causing       20
 8  pain.  Gallstones can also block the duct, causing       30
 9  nausea, vomiting, heartburn, back pain, and abdom-       40
10  inal pain.  Doctors test to find the stones' size.       50
11       The ultrasound test uses high-frequency sound       10
12  waves to scan the abdomen.  A doctor can determine       20
13  the appropriate treatment if gallstones are found.       30
14  A cholecystectomy is a surgical procedure that re-       40
15  moves the gallbladder.  Blood tests show stones in       50
16  the bile duct.  Medication can dissolve gallstones       10
17  but sometimes works very slowly.  Lithotripsy is a       20
18  shock wave that crumbles some kinds of gallstones.       30
        □□□□1□□□□2□□□□3□□□□4□□□□5□□□□6□□□□7□□□□8□□□□9□□□□10
```

All-Purpose Drills and Timed Writings

Medical Words, Five-Minute Timed Writing

Goals

After completing this lesson, you will be able to:

✔ Key concentration drills to increase accuracy.
✔ Key medical words.

Instructions

Key each line two times. Rekey each error word two times. Double-space between groups of two lines.

Drill 1

1 situ cells vivo vitro
2 body birth gene tumor
3 gait blood dose myoma

Drill 2

1 skin hymen head shunt
2 acne organ hair palsy
3 pain apnea boil lobar

Drill 3

1 lobe nails uric sebum
2 vein horny urea sweat
3 pons death void x-ray

Drill 4

1 duct tinea para basal
2 anus labor node wheal
3 dead nevus scan mucus

The bronchoscopy risk was explained to the patient. The   11
patient was in the operative suite being monitored continuously 23
on a cardiac monitor. Oxygen was running with a mask, and a   34
nasal cannula was placed in the nose. Preoperative anesthesia 46
included Xylocaine to both nares. The flexible bronchoscope   58
was passed via the left naris and over the vocal cords. The   70
vocal cords appeared normal. There was no bleeding. The   81
bronchoscope was placed into the trachea, and the carina   92
had a normal appearance.   97

Copious yellow secretions were present in the left   108
bronchus. The right and left bronchial trees were lavaged   119
with normal saline and aspirated until clear. Examination   130
of the bronchial tree revealed no lesions. Following lavage   141
and cleaning of the bronchial trees, bronchial brushings   152
were obtained and submitted to cytology. No complications   163
occurred during the procedure. The bronchoscopy revealed   174
bilateral bronchopneumonia.   179

□□□□1□□□□2□□□□3□□□□4□□□□5□□□□6□□□□7□□□□8□□□□9□□□□10□□□□11□□□□12

Key Alternate Hand Words, Five-Minute Timed Writing

Goals

After completing this lesson, you will be able to:

✔ Key concentration drills to increase accuracy in keying alternate hand words.

Instructions

Key each line two times. Rekey each error word two times. Double-space between groups of three lines.

Drill 1

1 abortio adenitis anorexia appendix bile
2 cecum colicky cranial dyspnea focal
3 heparin hernia hiatus hemi macro gloss
4 guaiac macula gait melena ocular pedal

Drill 2

1 band basophil diaphragm gallop ileum
2 jaundice nocturia orally phenol renal
3 serum sinus suture thrill tissue boggy
4 coma benign anal acetone febrile femoral

Drill 3

1 psoas rhonchi sinus trophic venous angina
2 basal codeine contusion cyanosis cutaneous
3 tibia thyroid sputum penicillin scan vital
4 apical axilla cystitis emesis fimbria dilate

Drill 4

1 liter mitral nodes mucosa oral ovary
2 pelvic saline tonsils tubal visual femur
3 fundus medulla flap aural chronic naris
4 sublingual squamous purulent duodenal

This pleasant lady was seen in my office with a history	11
of postural hypotension and syncope. The patient denies other	23
recent postural hypotension and syncope, although she had	34
fallen in the past, incurring several fractures. Her	44
gastrointestinal history revolves around intermittent	55
dysphagia. She has had no peptic ulcer disease or reflux	66
esophagitis symptoms. No hematochezia. However, her stools	77
are black because of iron therapy. She does not drink tea or	89
coffee. She has a history of rheumatoid arthritis and has	100
been on numerous medications, including prednisone. There is	112
no known history of coronary artery disease, kidney stones,	123
or diabetes. Because of her arthritis, exercise is limited.	134
She also has a history of mucous colitis. She had mild	145
anterior cervical lymphadenopathy and significant dental	156
caries. Urinalysis was within normal limits. Chest x-ray	167
was normal. Physical examination was essentially	177
unremarkable.	180

□□□□1□□□□2□□□□3□□□□4□□□□5□□□□6□□□□7□□□□8□□□□9□□□□10□□□□11□□□□12

Double Letters, Five-Minute Timed Writing

Goals

After completing this lesson, you will be able to:

✔ Stroke evenly to help you key accurately.
✔ Key multiple double letters.

Instructions

Key each line two times, double-spacing between groups of two.

```
 1   aa bazaar aardwolf quaalude aamus amaas aardvark
 2   bb Abbott bubbling cobbler rabbit-fever clubbed
 3   cc cocci occipital buccula saccharose sicchasia
 4   dd bedridden bladder sudden adductus addiction add
 5   ee bleeder spleen spondee pedigree sneeze teeth
 6   ff stiff suffusion suffocate caffeine paraffin
 7   gg agglutination tagging Riggs plugger aggregate
 8   ii Hawaii carinii skiing Hawaiian mesenterii
 9   ll lolling pulling yell polling llama calling lull
10   mm mummy mammary mammalian glimmer yammer simmer
11   nn spanner linnet tonnage dinner bunny tanned
12   oo oozoid zoo fool soon moon zoology zoom tool
13   pp hopper Lapp tipper zipper napping yipping
14   rr starred sparring tarred warring hemorrhage
15   ss sussed passed tussive tussis tussiculation
16   tt fatty pitting stutter squatting sagittal
17   uu continuum vacuum
18   vv flivver savvy
19   zz nozzle puzzle sizzle embezzling pizza dazzle
```

MULTIPLE DOUBLE LETTERS

```
 1   aggressive oozooid bookkeeper possession cesspool
 2   woolly appellate orrhorrhea coolly unnecessary
 3   accommodated arrowroot accessible sleeplessly
 4   misspelling commandeer arrowroot balloon
 5   orrho-immunity offshoot foolproof commissary
 6   para-appendicitis para-aminohippurate
 7   rabbetting oophorrhagia pyoblennorrhea buffoon
 8   cassette footstool squirrelly
```

Mrs. Pear, a black female, was admitted to the hospital	12
because of passing blood in her stools, weakness, and	22
inability to get out of bed. She states that she has not	33
had control of her bowels due to diarrhea and has crampy	44
abdominal pains. She denies indigestion or poor appetite.	55
She also states that she has had gout for many years, but	66
no other ongoing illnesses.	72
Her mother died of a cerebral hemorrhage; her father,	83
of carcinoma of the stomach; and a brother died of	93
tuberculosis. She was born in Africa and came to Mobile	104
last summer. She has been married twice. She had the usual	116
childhood diseases. No history of rheumatic fever or scarlet	128
fever. She had diphtheria as a child with no sequelae. She	140
does not smoke or drink alcoholic beverages. She developed	151
asthma and hay fever after moving to Arizona. She has had	162
a tonsillectomy and adenoidectomy. Her only medication is	173
Metamucil as needed. Her hobbies are reading and playing	184
the piano. Ten years ago, she went through early menopause	195
and decided not to take hormone replacement therapy.	205

□□□□1□□□□2□□□□3□□□□4□□□□5□□□□6□□□□7□□□□8□□□□9□□□□10□□□□11□□□□12

Spacing, Five-Minute Timed Writing

Goals

After completing this lesson, you will be able to:

✔ Achieve accuracy in spacing between words and individual letters.
✔ Space after left and right strokes.
✔ Space quickly after each word in a sentence.

Instructions

Use your right thumb for spacing. Key each line two times, double-spacing after each group of two.

Drill 1: Alphabet and Punctuation

```
1  a u d n y t e q . f b ; j c p w i , x r h s k m z
2  t o l ? g v r u w i r o f v x m n e q - ' " i p a
3  e b z , e i y g l h b e w i u y d l h c n p a u s
4  r c n b e i h w h j e w o p a h w q x z / n o u s
5  v b w q ; : y e r z a l h g i u o n b c x . y r l
```

Drill 2: Right Hand

```
1  loin lymph nylon hypo lip lipoid ilium ill phylum
2  oil poly pupil pump kink kinin hip joy lop moon
3  jump pop nip pun loon pool jimmy mini pill hop
4  hump ninny kill look limp lump pull poly him you
5  hymn mink link homo pomp yip look kink puppy poi
```

Drill 3: Left Hand

```
1  face sac sad scar sera dead fear feces saw gage
2  gavage gate cadaver tag fever feeder dead dear
3  deed tear gear garage tar war gave rage face
4  fax faze raze sax sex sever tag bag gab barred
5  wax cadaver vex read reed deer gab cab seceded
```

Drill 4: Sentences

```
1  How old are you?
2  Return to the clinic.
```

3 Schedule your appointment.
 4 A repeat CT scan will be done.
 5 It is difficult to measure its length.
 6 There is no history of depression.
 7 The patient is allergic to penicillin and codeine.
 8 The child was given general anesthesia.
 9 This is a greenstick fracture.
10 The gallbladder is a small sac under the liver.
11 The ice in the box is to put on the left arm.
12 It is up to you to go to the doctor for your foot.
13 She was ill with the flu but now seems to be well.
14 The man has a sore foot and arm veins are flat.
15 She was seen by the doctor for back pain.
16 The clot in the left leg is to be observed.
17 The patient was admitted in the early afternoon.
18 Her cold is in the chest, and her throat is sore.
19 The child was given a mask to put on his face.
20 Dave has rattling in the throat and had a dry cough.

FIVE-MINUTE TIMING—DOUBLE SPACE

Recently, he has apparently been getting incontinent.	11
He has been unable to sleep and has been agitated for several	22
months. His legs are very weak, and it is a struggle for him	33
to walk. He has to walk with help and is only able to do so	44
with a walker. He has no weakness on either side, and no	55
specific neurological defects. The patient has been losing	66
weight and has had no appetite. For the last few days, he	77
has been losing urine, and his stomach has felt firm. The	88
patient was examined and found to have markedly distended	99
bladder above the umbilicus. A Foley catheter was inserted	110
with difficulty in the prostatic area as if there was an	121
obstruction. The Foley catheter was left in, and his bladder	133
was slowly decompressed in the office. His prostate was	144
enlarged and quite high and firm. There were no feces present	156
in the rectum. The patient has now been admitted to the	167
hospital for further evaluation of his urinary retention.	178

□□□□1□□□□2□□□□3□□□□4□□□□5□□□□6□□□□7□□□□8□□□□9□□□□10□□□□11□□□□12

Shifting, Five-Minute Timed Writing

Goals

After completing this lesson, you will be able to:

✔ Use the shifting keys comfortably to capitalize words.

Skillbuilding Warmup—One-Minute Timing—Double Space

Under general anesthesia, two large chronically infected	12
tonsils were removed by Sluder tonsillotome. There was slight	24
bleeding during the tonsillectomy. Large masses of adenoid	35
tissue were removed from the nasopharynx with adenotome and	46
curette.	48

□□□□1□□□□2□□□□3□□□□4□□□□5□□□□6□□□□7□□□□8□□□□9□□□□10□□□□11□□□□12

Instructions

Key each line two times for accuracy. Double-space between each group of two sentences.

1 Amniocentesis may be used to detect Down syndrome and other birth defects.

2 A radiologist will evaluate Mrs. Eva Brown's mammogram.

3 At Mobile Emergency Clinic, myelograms are used to diagnose spinal tumors, disk problems, and the spinal cord.

4 An arthroscope is an instrument that was taken to Perlman Clinic on Girard Avenue in Phoenix, Arizona.

5 MRI and CT are used in diagnosing brain and spinal cord lesions.

6 The physician ordered a PET scan for the patient with Alzheimer's disease.

7 The EEG showed that the patient has a brain tumor.

8 The 39-year-old male patient is being admitted today for an EKG, possible coronary artery bypass graft (CABG), and a percutaneous transluminal coronary angioplasty (PTCA).

9 His cardiac MRI showed lesions of large blood vessels at the Mobile Clinic.

10 The Western blot test showed that the patient has HIV.

Sara noted blood in her urine recently and came to the   11
office. At that time, a urine culture was done, which showed   23
the presence of *Escherichia coli* of the urine. She was   34
started on tetracycline and the urinary symptoms cleared,   45
but she continued having chills. Pelvic examination was   56
performed at that time, which revealed anterior fixation   67
of the cervix and some hemorrhage from the cervical os. She   78
was referred for gynecological consultation, and it was   89
recommended that she have a dilation and curettage. She   100
denies any dysuria or any vaginal bleeding. There has been   111
no recent weight loss and no significant abdominal pain.   122
Until two years ago, the patient has had no serious illnesses   133
except hospitalization for treatment of an eye injury.   143
During the last four years, she has had several respiratory   154
infections and anxiety reactions with paranoid ideation.   165
Last year, she developed septicemia and severe cystitis.   176
Two years ago, she was treated for bronchial pneumonia,   187
hypertension, and chronic fatigue. No known familial   197
illnesses. Several of her offspring are in excellent   207
health.   208

The patient is a widow. She is not known to use   218
tobacco or alcohol and is not employed outside the home.   229
She is allergic to penicillin. Occasional episodes of   240
dysequilibrium. She denies exertional chest pain, cough,   251
or dyspnea. The patient ia a well-developed, well nourished   263
white woman who appears to be in no general distress. No   274
apparent dyspnea, cyanosis, or icterus.   282

☐☐☐☐1☐☐☐☐2☐☐☐☐3☐☐☐☐4☐☐☐☐5☐☐☐☐6☐☐☐☐7☐☐☐☐8☐☐☐☐9☐☐☐☐10☐☐☐☐11☐☐☐☐12

Timed Writings and Sentences, Timed Writings

Goals

After completing this lesson, you will be able to:

✔ Key longer paragraphs.
✔ Key for speed and accuracy.
✔ Key sentences.

Instructions

Five-minute timing—double space.

TIMED WRITING 1

1	This patient sustained an injury to his right	10
2	knee. Since then, he has had pain and swelling in	20
3	this knee. He has had diminished range of motion.	30
4	He has felt the knee lock and give way. Conserva-	40
5	tive physical therapy for this patient has consis-	50
6	ted of anti-inflammatory medication, crutches, and	10
7	rest. This therapy does not seem to be making his	20
8	symptoms improve. He is presenting to the Surgery	30
9	Center for diagnostic arthroscopy. He still walks	40
10	with a crutch and an antalgic gait. Mild swelling	50
11	exists above the right lower extremity; he will be	10
12	admitted soon for diagnostic and operative arthro-	20
13	scopy of the right knee. He understands there are	30
14	risks, including bleeding, infection, stiffness in	40
15	the knee, and other problems; he accepts the risks	50
16	and wishes to proceed with the surgery.	8

Sentences: One-Minute Timings

1	The patient is taking Naprosyn as needed for pain.	10
2	The patient is married and employed as a mechanic.	10
3	He is a healthy man and has normal blood pressure.	10
4	He denies having cardiorespiratory symptomatology.	10
5	She complained of cough but the lungs were clear.	10

▯▯▯▯1▯▯▯▯2▯▯▯▯3▯▯▯▯4▯▯▯▯5▯▯▯▯6▯▯▯▯7▯▯▯▯8▯▯▯▯9▯▯▯▯10

6	His heart rate is regular and the rhythm is usual.	10
7	Ligamentous exam of the man's left knee is normal.	10
8	The neurovascular exam of the left knee is normal.	10
9	She reports tenderness over the lateral joint line.	10
10	His right leg suffers intermittent ankle swelling.	10

TIMED WRITING 2—THREE-MINUTE TIMING—DOUBLE SPACE

1	The patient's chief complaint is right shoul-	10
2	der pain from a car accident two months ago. This	20
3	apparently was a rear-end accident, the car moving	30
4	at relatively high speed. She had immediate onset	40
5	of headaches and neck pain. Her shoulder pain de-	50
6	veloped after the accident. This shoulder pain is	10
7	located across the top of the right shoulder. She	20
8	has been going to physical therapy at Laven Clinic,	30
9	and her neck pain is almost gone. This shoulder	40
10	pain comes on intermittently with various shoulder	50
11	movements. Reaching type movement and behind-the-	10
12	back movements aggravate this pain. She does have	20
13	crepitus in this shoulder. She feels that rubbing	30
14	the muscles alleviates the pain and that the pain	40
15	is intermittent in nature. She feels that she has	50
16	been aggravating this pain and that it is just not	10
17	going away. She had had a shoulder problem before	20
18	the accident. She lacks symptoms down the arm and	30
19	is otherwise apparently healthy.	36

Sentences: One-Minute Timings

1	No deformity or atrophy of either shoulder exists.	10
2	The range of motion, passive and active, is usual.	10
3	On palpation, there is really no tenderness found.	10
4	The biceps provocative test proved to be negative.	10
5	Neurovascular exam of the right upper extremity is	10
	normal and neck range of motion is full.	18
6	The residual soft tissue inflammation is caused by	10
	cervical hyperextension injury.	16
7	The physicians are injecting lidocaine and Kenalog	10
	into the subacromial space.	15
8	The patient's rotator cuff strength is quite good.	10

☐☐☐☐1☐☐☐☐2☐☐☐☐3☐☐☐☐4☐☐☐☐5☐☐☐☐6☐☐☐☐7☐☐☐☐8☐☐☐☐9☐☐☐☐10

9	This pain is atypical and probably comes from sub-	10
	acromial pathology.	14
10	It was post-traumatic impingement of the shoulder.	10

FIVE-MINUTE TIMED WRITING—DOUBLE SPACE

This child was admitted to the hospital with a history	1
of hepatitis, severe abnormality of the electrolytes, and	22
subsequently, sepsis. The state of consciousness was	33
worsening, and this prompted the placement of an endotracheal	45
tube, placement of the child on a respirator, and the use of	56
barbiturates intravenously. These medications, of course,	67
ruled out the observation of consciousness and neurologic	78
function. The other problem is poor blood clotting.	88
Studies here showed that the child is clotting well, even	99
though the past studies are abnormal. The indications for	110
intracranial monitoring appear to be present, and it appears	122
she will clot.	125

□□□□1□□□□2□□□□3□□□□4□□□□5□□□□6□□□□7□□□□8□□□□9□□□□10□□□□11□□□□12

Speed Sentences, Five-Minute Timed Writing

Goals

After completing this lesson, you will be able to:

✔ Key sentences with simple words quickly.

Instructions

Key each line accurately two times, double-spacing between groups of two. Begin keying very slowly and increase your rate of speed.

1   Her symptoms are pain, discharge, and sore throat.
2   The fungal disease has spread to the patient's bones and brain.
3   There are red spots on the face and pain in the joints.
4   Spores are growing in the lungs, and the disease is spreading throughout the body.
5   The air sacs in your inflamed lungs are filled with pus, mucus, and bacteria.
6   The patient has night sweats, vomiting, diarrhea, and difficulty breathing.
7   This patient has a cold, congestion in the lungs and sinuses, and a sore throat.
8   The symptoms were bleeding, chest pain, and lack of oxygen.
9   This patient is complaining of dyspnea, nocturia, headaches, vomiting, and lack of energy.
10 She has a benign tumor of the bile duct, and this condition has left her depressed.
11 He has no history of dyspnea, angina, or problems with polyuria.
12 Abnormal cells were found and another exam will be performed.
13 Pyuria and glycosuria appeared in the urine.
14 Those adults and children are allergic to dust, pollen, and animals.
15 Her vision is poor at night but good in the day.

The patient is a well-developed, dehydrated, chronically	11
ill female lying quietly in bed complaining of lower abdominal	23
pains. Nasal mucosa is clear. Auditory canals are clear.	34
Her pharynx is not injected. Her mouth is edentulous. Her	45
tongue and pharynx are quite dehydrated. Carotids are	56
palpable equally bilaterally. Thyroid is not enlarged.	67
Lungs are fairly clear to percussion and auscultation.	77
Breasts are quite atrophied. There are no masses, tenderness,	89
or discharge in the breasts. The heart sounds are quite	100
distant. Rectal examination showed no masses to the	110
examining finger, but there is a large amount of stool	120
present, which makes examination difficult. Pelvic	130
examination shows blood in the vagina. Extremities are warm,	142
dry, and dehydrated. Cranial nerves II-XII appear intact.	153
Deep tendon reflexes are equal bilaterally. She does not	164
have a positive Babinski reflex.	170

□□□□1□□□□2□□□□3□□□□4□□□□5□□□□6□□□□7□□□□8□□□□9□□□□10□□□□11□□□□12

Sentences with Longer Words, Five-Minute Timed Writing

Goals

After completing this lesson, you will be able to:

✔ Key sentences with long words.
✔ Read no faster than you key.

Instructions

Key each line accurately one time, double-spacing between groups of two. Begin keying each sentence slowly, then increase your speed.

1 The patient underwent a tonsillectomy and adenoidectomy at Mobile Medical Clinic.

2 She was advised to have an appendectomy to correct
  the condition but refused at the time.

3 Pelvic inflammatory disease is an infection of the
  uterus, ovaries, and fallopian tubes.

4 She was diagnosed with carcinoma of the breast, so
  a radical mastectomy was done.

5 The patient had a cholecystectomy and resection of
  the prostate. He is recovering well.

6 The doctor diagnosed a Wilms tumor in the patient,
  surgery was done, and chemotherapy was introduced.

7 This patient was evaluated with myelography, which
  showed a neoplasm of the spinal cord.

8 The physician ordered cerebrospinal fluid analysis
  to diagnose the disease of the brain.

9 The patient is suffering from bradycardia and car-
  diomyopathy disease.

10 Electroencephalography was performed on this child
   to locate and evaluate the brain tumor.

11 Doctors use the stethoscope to listen to and diagnose conditions of the lungs, heart, and abdomen.

12 Blood pressure is measured with sphygmomanometers.

13 Systemic lupus erythematosus is a disease of one's
   musculoskeletal system affecting the skin, nervous
   system, heart, lungs, kidneys, and joints.

14 This patient was brought to the operating room. A
   bunionectomy was performed.
15 The young woman suffered from menometrorrhagia and
   dysmenorrhea.

FIVE-MINUTE TIMING—DOUBLE SPACE

     Maria had an acute onset of extensive weakness on the   11
right side. The patient was noted to have chest x-ray   22
findings of congestive heart failure but had no evidence of   33
hypertension or arrhythmias. The patient diuresed and was   44
given supportive medical care and did well. The patient did   55
develop a urinary tract infection and was placed on Macrobid   66
with good results. Her electrocardiogram showed a previous   77
myocardial infarction. The patient did have cardiac enzymes,   88
which showed no evidence of a recent myocardial infarction,   99
and a thyroid test showed a normal thyroid function. She did   111
develop hypokalemia and was placed on supplemental potassium;   123
also a CT scan showed a thrombotic stroke.   131
     The patient remained hemiplegic on the right side with   142
extreme weakness. The patient was given physical therapy   153
with range of motion. She was initially scheduled to be   164
transferred to Mobile Rehabilitation Program; however, she   175
was not strong enough to tolerate chair activities. The   186
patient was transferred to Mobile Hospital where she will be   198
followed by Dr. Cart.   202

□□□□1□□□□2□□□□3□□□□4□□□□5□□□□6□□□□7□□□□8□□□□9□□□□10□□□□11□□□□12

Paragraphs—Three- and Five-Minute Timed Writings

Goals

After completing this lesson, you will be able to:

✔ Key paragraphs with longer words.

Instructions

Key the following paragraphs twice; first for practice, second for timing.

TIMED WRITING 1—THREE-MINUTE TIMING—DOUBLE SPACE

1	Emphysema is an illness caused by swollen air	10
2	sacs in the lungs. The loss of elasticity and the	20
3	breakdown of the alveoli walls result in decreased	30
4	air movement in the air sacs. Emphysema is a very	40
5	serious disease. As the air sacs thin, holes form	50
6	in the tissues of the lungs, and the lungs pass on	10
7	less oxygen to the bloodstream. The patient feels	20
8	shortness of breath and cannot exhale fully. This	30
9	disease seriously damages the heart and lungs and	40
10	is commonly found in adults who smoke.	48

TIMED WRITING 2—THREE-MINUTE TIMING—DOUBLE SPACE

1	Bronchitis, which is sometimes chronic, is an	10
2	inflammation of the bronchial tubes. These tubes,	20
3	connected to the windpipe, become infected, so air-	30
4	flow is decreased to and from the lungs. The per-	40
5	son afflicted with the condition will cough up	50
6	purulence from the lungs. Bacterial infection, ciga-	10
7	rette smoking, air pollution, industrial dust, and	20
8	irritating fumes are causes of chronic bronchitis.	30
9	The patient develops a rapid heartbeat, coughs up	40
10	more yellow mucus, and feels shortness of breath.	50

◻◻◻◻1◻◻◻◻2◻◻◻◻3◻◻◻◻4◻◻◻◻5◻◻◻◻6◻◻◻◻7◻◻◻◻8◻◻◻◻9◻◻◻◻10

TIMED WRITING 3—THREE-MINUTE TIMING—DOUBLE SPACE

1	Certain occupational diseases cause pneumoco-	10
2	niosis, an abnormal lung condition. Asbestosis is	20
3	caused by inhaling minute asbestos particles. As-	30
4	bestos is used in insulation for buildings. Tachy-	40
5	pnea, chest pain, and upper respiratory infections	50
6	are some of the symptoms. Silicosis, another dis-	10
7	ease, is caused by inhaling silica dust. Symptoms	20
8	include dyspnea, pulmonary hypertension, and a dry	30
9	cough. Silicosis is known as "grinders' disease."	40
10	People at risk are those working with china and	50
11	granite carving and stone grinding. Lastly, black	10
12	lung disease is a coal miner's disease. Coal dust	20
13	is inhaled into the lungs. Some symptoms are dys-	30
14	pnea and coughing up black sputum.	37

FIVE-MINUTE TIMING—DOUBLE SPACE

This is one of several Casa Grande Hospital admissions	11
for this Caucasian female with a past medical history of	22
arteriosclerotic heart disease, hypertension, diabetes,	33
organic brain syndrome, and hypothyroidism with chief	43
complaint of rectal bleeding. The patient was recently	54
discharged from this hospital after having suffered an	65
episode of rectal bleeding complicated by inability to locate	77
the exact source, thought to be secondary to diverticulosis.	88
Repeat sigmoidoscopies failed to visualize the exact	98
etiology.	100
The patient was doing well post barium enema, which	111
seemed to have stopped the bleeding, and was sent back home.	122
The lhysician was called for a similar problem of her rectal	133
bleeding, which had started the morning of admission. She	144
had another large bowel movement with bright red blood and	155
was found to have a low hematocrit and hemoglobin. The	166
patient was admitted to the ICU where she will be stabilized	178
through the use of intravenous blood transfusions.	188

□□□□1□□□□2□□□□3□□□□4□□□□5□□□□6□□□□7□□□□8□□□□9□□□□10□□□□11□□□□12

Paragraphs—Five-Minute Timed Writing

FIVE-MINUTE TIMING—DOUBLE SPACE

```
        Charlie, who is a carpenter, was admitted after complaining 12
of intermittent episodes of shortness of breath for about          23
several months' duration. He states that during the past           34
couple of months he has had difficulty breathing when he lies      46
down. Also he has had some episodes that strongly suggest           57
paroxysmal nocturnal dyspnea. His chest x-ray since admission       69
has shown minimal pneumonic changes, generalized pulmonary          80
emphysema, normal sized heart. He had a chest x-ray in              90
November, which revealed minor changes. An electrocardiogram at    102
that time revealed nonspecific ST segment and T wave changes       113
of minor degree. He had another electrocardiogram following        124
his present admission that revealed deeper inversion of T          135
waves in the anteroseptal region. There are small Q waves in       146
the inferior leads, which may very well have been due to septal    158
activation. There is no definite evidence of an inferior wall      170
injury.                                                            172
        Another electrocardiogram today revealed fewer T wave      183
changes, which may have been due to electrode placement in the     195
medial precordial area. The patient's blood test showed some       207
nonspecific change, which may well be due to liver dysfunction.    219
His LDH and SGOT were slightly elevated. Since he has been         230
hospitalized here, he has been extremely shaky, and it is          241
apparent that this shakiness is due to nervousness.                251
        I would recommend the patient be placed on a tranquilizer  263
such as Valium. If this fails to control his nervousness, then     275
a more potent tranquilizer should be used.                         283
        The past medical history of significance reveals that the  295
patient was hospitalized here in September with right upper        306
quadrant pain, which was at first thought to be muscle strain      318
of the abdominal wall. Later, the patient was readmitted in        329
November for an exploratory laparotomy, excisional biopsy, and     341
an appendectomy. It was concluded that the patient had chronic     353
periappendicitis. The remainder of the past medical history       364
reveals that the patient has been treated for hypertension.        375
Recently he has taken Inderal LA. He also has diverticulosis.      387
```

□□□□1□□□□2□□□□3□□□□4□□□□5□□□□6□□□□7□□□□8□□□□9□□□□10□□□□11□□□□12

Paragraphs—Five-Minute Timed Writing

FIVE-MINUTE TIMING—DOUBLE SPACE

Maria is a black female patient whose last menstrual	11
period began a week ago. Her most recent Pap smear was	21
performed today, the results of which are pending. The patient	33
is using an intrauterine device for contraception. She was	44
seen at the Brown Gynecology Clinic this morning for treatment	56
of probable pelvic inflammatory disease.	64
The patient awoke yesterday morning with severe bilateral	76
lower quadrant pelvic pain. The pain has remained constant	87
since that time and has been increasing in severity. In	98
association with the pain, she complains of nausea and	109
vomiting but has no other gastrointestinal complaint. Her last	121
bowel movement was yesterday. She has no urinary tract	132
complaints; but voiding increases her discomfort, as does	143
activity. Also, she complains of chills and fever. Due to the	155
pain she was seen at Brown Gynecology Clinic yesterday; the	166
diagnosis is unknown. She was treated with Demerol and was	177
sent home. Today she was evaluated by Dr. Good who referred	188
her to me to rule out pelvic inflammatory disease versus acute	200
appendicitis.	203
The patient has no gynecologic complaints, specifically	215
no history of metrorrhagia, dyspareunia, dysmenorrhea, or	226
recent abnormal vaginal discharge or pruritus. She has no	237
history of pelvic inflammatory disease and has no history of	249
prior pelvic surgery. She has no breast complaints. She has no	261
gonorrhea or chlamydia infection.	268
The patient had a tonsillectomy and adenoidectomy several	280
years ago. Her only other hospitalization was for back	291
problems. She denies any drug allergies and currently is	302
taking Demerol for pain. She has no past history of any	313
serious medical diseases or illnesses, including hypertension,	325
heart disease, diabetes, rheumatic fever, or sexually	336
transmitted disease. The patient does not smoke, and drinks	337
alcohol socially.	340
This patient is a physical education instructor by	351
profession who has been very active and teaching aerobic	362
exercises. Maria, the patient, has been placed on bedrest,	373
fluids, and medication.	378

□□□□1□□□□2□□□□3□□□□4□□□□5□□□□6□□□□7□□□□8□□□□9□□□□10□□□□11□□□□12

Paragraphs—Five-Minute Timed Writing

FIVE-MINUTE TIMING—DOUBLE SPACE

Mary is a single female whose last menstrual period was 11
approximately several weeks ago. She has been on Ovrette for 22
contraception during the past year. I was asked to consult 33
because her semiannual examination required a Pap test. For 44
the past several weeks, she has a history of increasing breast 56
tenderness and was advised by a physician to come off birth 67
control pills and to obtain another gynecology consultation. 78

Approximately two weeks ago, the patient noted increased 90
breast swelling unlike any she had before, particularly on 101
the right side, right upper quadrant. She was advised to 112
discontinue birth control pills for several months and to 123
resume them in the event that the pill could be causing an 134
inappropriate stimulation of the breast duct and alveoli. She 146
decided, however, not to go off birth control pills because 157
she had late-onset menarche and was having irregular cycles. 168
Therefore, she was put on the pill for regulation of menses 179
and also for severe dysmenorrhea. In addition, she claimed to 191
have had yeast infections for which she received Mycostatin. 202

She has a sister with a poor contraceptive history, 113
failure with an intrauterine device, and a diaphragm-producing 124
pain. The patient has had numerous surgeries; an appendectomy 136
and a rectovaginal fistula. She had a right salpingo- 147
oophorectomy and resection of an adnexal cyst. She has 158
received a blood transfusion in the past. She has had several 170
recurrent urinary tract infections. 177

Patient, in addition, claims to have had late-onset of 188
menses. In March she had menorrhea and salpingitis. 198

Her mother is living and well with known diabetes 209
requiring insulin. Father is living and well. Grandmother died 221
of carcinoma of the bladder. 227

The patient claims to have had chronic asthma and 238
bronchitis the last few months. 244

▢▢▢▢1▢▢▢▢2▢▢▢▢3▢▢▢▢4▢▢▢▢5▢▢▢▢6▢▢▢▢7▢▢▢▢8▢▢▢▢9▢▢▢▢10▢▢▢▢11▢▢▢▢12

Paragraphs—Five-Minute Timed Writing

FIVE-MINUTE TIMING—DOUBLE SPACE

The patient was admitted to Mobile Hospital with the	11
chief complaint of marked depression, intense anxiety, and	22
multiple fears. The patient could not function at home. She	33
began to feel withdrawn and unable to care for herself. She	44
had a physical examination on admission, which was essentially	56
within normal limits, except for noted colostomy in the left	68
lower quadrant of the abdomen and eruption of lesions on her	80
forearms and fingers on both hands.	87
The patient was very tense and anxious. She was very	98
despondent. She complained of racing thoughts, marked	108
confusion, and inability to think. She had no insight except	119
that she needed help, and her judgment was intact. She had	130
marked inability to goal direct her thoughts. Her	140
concentration and attention were markedly impaired. She had	151
noted feelings of loneliness, isolation, and withdrawal, and	162
marked loss of self-esteem and self-confidence. The patient	173
was completely unable to function by history and unable to	184
manage on her own.	188
The patient was treated with Valium, Tylenol, Mycostatin,	200
Metamucil, Kenalog cream, and vitamins. At first, the patient	212
was very depressed, anxious, and withdrawn. She had noted	223
difficulties in controlling her behavior and her emotions. She	235
had numerous consultations by Dr. Russ for her skin, diagnosed	247
as eczema of hands by Dr. Sampson and Dr. Burns for urinary	258
retention, by Dr. Brown for medical complaints, by Dr. Walker	270
for hemorrhoids, and by Dr. Hubbard for endometriosis.	280
She continued to be very anxious and depressed and	291
avoided any one-to-one contact and avoiding interacting with	302
the staff or the group. The patient was instructed to	312
participate in group therapy and to ventilate her feelings.	323
She participated in assertiveness training through individual	335
psychotherapy, which was on an intense daily basis. She became	347
less depressed. She was able to tolerate frustration and	358
demands and environmental stresses and wished to be discharged.	370
The patient was discharged and told to attend outpatient	381
psychotherapy.	383

□□□□1□□□□2□□□□3□□□□4□□□□5□□□□6□□□□7□□□□8□□□□9□□□□10□□□□11□□□□12

Paragraphs—Five-Minute Timed Writing

FIVE-MINUTE TIMING—DOUBLE SPACE

This is a young man with a history of extensive scarring	12
secondary to burns sustained in a gas explosion. Among his	23
residual problems has been a tight band-like scar around the	34
right ankle. Two weeks ago, the patient sustained a sprain of	46
the right ankle. The patient noted progressive swelling in the	58
ankle, which was treated with an Ace bandage. The patient noted	70
the appearance of blisters. He started running a fever about	81
a week ago. Four days prior to admission, the patient became	92
aware of drainage from some of the blisters that had ruptured	104
on the right leg. The patient had massive cellulitis involving	116
the right lower extremity below the knee. The patient was	127
taken to the operating room, and a fasciotomy was performed.	139
There was evidence of infection involving the ankle joint.	150
Urinalysis was normal. The patient was treated with	161
Keflex. Postoperatively, the patient was started on an	171
intravenous cephalosporin. Bacteriologic examination of	182
specimens obtained at surgery had revealed gram-positive cocci	194
in pairs and chains. White blood cells were also present on	205
Gram stain.	207
General physical examination after surgery reveals	218
multiple areas of scarring on the face, upper extremities,	229
and lower extremities. The patient has had an amputation of	240
his left index finger. The thumb is contracted and minimally	251
functional. There is a decrease in the right femoral pulse at	263
the groin. No audible bruit. The lungs are clear; there were	275
no heart murmurs heard, and the abdomen is soft with no masses.	287
The bacteriologic evidence revealed streptococcal and	298
staphylococcal infection as the major pathogens. The treatment	310
of choice at this time will be the use of both penicillin and	322
Oxacillin to provide best coverage for both streptococcal and	334
staphylococcal bacteria. The local infection on the joint and	346
leg seems to be under good control. There was scant purulent	357
material.	359

□□□□1 □□□□2 □□□□3 □□□□4 □□□□5 □□□□6 □□□□7 □□□□8 □□□□9 □□□□10 □□□□11 □□□□12

Paragraphs—Five-Minute Timed Writing

FIVE-MINUTE TIMING—DOUBLE SPACE

This little girl continued to have symptoms of an upper	11
respiratory infection with rhinorrhea and a fever until two	22
days prior to presenting to the Mobile Clinic when her fever	33
became more severe and her symptoms grew worse. She began to	45
complain of sores in her mouth. Sores covered most of her	56
mouth and made it quite difficult for the patient to eat. For	68
the past several days, she has had very little to eat or	79
drink. She was brought to the clinic by her mother because of	91
a fever and mouth sores.	96
Generally, the patient appeared well developed and well	107
nourished. She is irritable and somewhat lethargic although	118
not in a great deal of distress. She has scattered ulcerations	130
over the entire buccal mucosa.	136
Physical examination and laboratory tests revealed an	147
acutely ill female with acute lymphoblastic leukemia. She is	159
dehydrated. She was seen in hematology clinic.	168
At that time, she was referred to the Mobile Hospital. A	180
white blood count revealed blast cells on peripheral smear.	191
After spending several days in the hospital, patient was	202
started on a protocol of Vincristine and prednisone. The	213
patient was released from the hospital in remission.	223
The patient did well out of the hospital until she	234
contracted a hacking, barky cough that became worse	244
throughout the day and became quite severe. There was no	255
cyanosis. No members of the family have been ill. She has been	267
on penicillin.	270
Physical examination revealed a harsh, croupy cough with	282
inspiratory and expiratory stridor and mild respiratory	293
distress. The epiglottis was normal. The diagnosis at this	304
time is croup. She has had numerous upper respiratory and ear	316
infections the past several months.	321
The child improved rapidly with therapy. The chest had a	333
few rhonchi transmitted from the upper airway but no wheezing	345
or rales and no respiratory distress. Laboratory studies	356
consisting of complete blood count and urinalysis were within	370
normal limits.	373

☐☐☐☐1☐☐☐☐2☐☐☐☐3☐☐☐☐4☐☐☐☐5☐☐☐☐6☐☐☐☐7☐☐☐☐8☐☐☐☐9☐☐☐☐10☐☐☐☐☐11☐☐☐☐12

Paragraphs—Five-Minute Timed Writing

FIVE-MINUTE TIMING—DOUBLE SPACE

Mr. Fellows is an engineer who gives a history of	11
recurrent chest pains while jogging for the past year. He did	23
not pay attention to these pains and did not consult his	34
physician for that period. He had severe symptoms of influenza	46
last week with high fever, cough, and an episode of near	57
syncope. During that time, he had some moments when he would	68
feel his heart skipping beats. He also had an episode of	79
clamminess, coolness, and dizziness. He was brought in to	90
the emergency room of Mobile Hospital and admitted after	101
electrocardiogram revealed an acute inferior wall myocardial	112
infarction. He has been in the intensive care unit since then.	124
His hospital course has been characterized by recurrent	135
ventricular fibrillation beats, which was first treated with	146
lidocaine.	148
The patient had a melanoma removed from his neck, and	159
had carcinoma of the prostate treated by local excision and	170
radiation. He was taking no medications. He had no known drug	182
allergies except to penicillin.	188
When examined in the intensive care unit, the patient	199
appeared to be comfortable. Examination demonstrated no	210
jugular venous distention. There are no carotid bruits. The	221
lungs are clear to percussion and auscultation. On	231
auscultation the first heart sounds are normal. There are no	242
gallops or murmurs heard. The abdomen is soft, flat,	252
nontender. No organs or masses are palpable. There is a	263
fairly recent laparotomy scar. Extremities show no edema,	274
cyanosis, or clubbing. The peripheral pulses are full.	284
Neurological examination is within normal limits.	294
Electrocardiogram on admission shows evidence of acute	305
inferior and possible dorsal infarction with Q waves in II,	316
III, and aVF. In the tracing taken today, this has improved.	327
The cardiac enzymes were normal on admission. The complete	338
blood count cells and hematocrits were normal. Electrolytes	349
were normal. The patient appears to be stable now and present	361
management should be continued.	367

□□□□1□□□□2□□□□3□□□□4□□□□5□□□□6□□□□7□□□□8□□□□9□□□□10□□□□11□□□□12

Paragraphs—Five-Minute Timed Writing

FIVE-MINUTE TIMING—DOUBLE SPACE

Today I received a call from the intermediate facility at   12
Lemon where this patient has been residing, stating that the   23
patient has been lethargic, restless, and incoherent at times.   35
They asked if I would see her, which I did. On examination of   46
the patient, it was quite obvious that the patient was very   57
weak, lethargic, and that she was unable to communicate   68
properly as she had been in the past. During the examination   80
it was quite evident that there were some rales in the lower   92
right chest, and her temperature was elevated at that time. I   104
felt that perhaps this patient had acute pneumonia, and she   115
was brought to the hospital at Mobile.   123

The patient has a long-standing history of rheumatoid   134
arthritis treated by many physicians in the past. She has been   146
and is currently on Relafen for rheumatoid arthritis. Her last   158
admission to this hospital was in January of last year at   170
which time she was admitted for an acute exacerbation of her   182
rheumatoid arthritis. She was also seen by Dr. Kinney for   193
acute gastrointestinal complaint. She was also seen by Dr.   204
Brown for persistent rheumatoid arthritis symptoms.   214

At the time of her gastrointestinal examination by Dr.   225
Brown, it was quite evident that the patient had a large   236
gastric ulcer, which he proceeded to treat.   244

Both her mother and father are deceased. She has a living   256
son in Laveen. Her mother died of cancer, and her father died   268
of congestive heart failure.   274

The patient denies any particular problems with her eyes,   286
ears, nose, and throat. She does wear glasses for reading. The   298
patient denies any history of any neurological problems,   309
hepatitis, or seizures. The patient also denies any history of   321
cardiopulmonary problems such as chest pain or shortness of   333
breath.   335

As stated before, the patient has had some vague upper GI   347
complaints, which through endoscopy revealed a large gastric   358
ulcer. She has been under current treatment with antacids. The   370
patient admits to having rheumatoid arthritis for several   381
years and has been treated off and on by many physicians with   393
many medications.   396

□□□□1□□□□2□□□□3□□□□4□□□□5□□□□6□□□□7□□□□8□□□□9□□□□10□□□□11□□□□12

Paragraphs—Five-Minute Timed Writing

FIVE-MINUTE TIMING—DOUBLE SPACE

This is a black male who presents with the chief complaint	12
of chest pain, cough, and purulent sputum production.	22
The above symptoms have been present for the past several	34
days and have been associated with increased dyspnea. The	45
patient has a long-standing history of chronic obstructive	56
pulmonary disease characterized as chronic bronchitis. He has	68
chronic dyspnea, which has been present for the past several	79
years, essentially at rest. There is also a history of cough	90
productive of about a teaspoon of mucoid sputum generally in	101
the early morning. Over the past days, the sputum production	112
have been more viscous and dark. There has been no hemoptysis.	123
The patient denies any recent history of fever or chills. There	135
has been no significant acute congestive heart failure	146
symptoms, although the patient has had symptoms of nocturnal	157
dyspnea, orthopnea, and peripheral edema.	165
Most recently, there has been a history of pleuritic chest	177
pain, which generally accompanies the cough; but the patient	188
also admits to a chronic history of chest pain, which is	199
localized to the left anterior chest and is relieved by	210
nitroglycerin.	
This patient is being admitted essentially for diagnosis	222
and therapy of his acute respiratory symptoms.	231
The patient has a history of arteriosclerotic heart	242
disease, and there is evidence of an old inferior myocardial	253
infarction. The patient also carries the background diagnosis	265
of chronic alcoholism, alcoholic liver disease, and had	276
delirium tremens in the past. The patient also has had	287
essential hypertension; otherwise there has been no history	298
of rheumatic heart disease, tuberculosis, or neoplastic disease.	310
The patient has had several recurrent pneumonitis episodes	321
in the past, requiring hospital admission.	329
He has had an operation for abdominal adhesions	339
obstructing the small bowel and appendix. Otherwise, the	350
surgical history is unremarkable.	356
His father died of a cerebrovascular accident. His mother	368
died of old age. He has one brother who has had recurrent	379
pyelonephritis; otherwise, the family history is unremarkable	391
for tuberculosis, cancer, or heart disease.	400
The patient currently smokes cigars. He consumes one pint	412
of bourbon per day. He denies allergies, and there has been no	424
significant pulmonary occupational history.	432

□□□□1□□□□2□□□□3□□□□4□□□□5□□□□6□□□□7□□□□8□□□□9□□□□10□□□□11□□□□12

Paragraphs—Five-Minute Timed Writing

FIVE-MINUTE TIMING—DOUBLE SPACE

```
       The patient is a female who was generally well until       11
approximately several hours prior to admission when she            22
eveloped epigastric gnawing hunger-like pains that radiated        34
into her abdomen. This became severe enough that she presented     46
herself to the emergency room at Mobile Hospital this morning,     58
at which time she was evaluated by the emergency room              69
physician. At that time her white count was normal. She had no     81
temperature and no localizing abdominal findings but some         92
tenderness in the epigastrium. She was given an oral              102
preparation to ease her pain and dyspepsia; however, she          113
promptly vomited this. I was called as a surgical backup in       124
regard to this patient, and it was decided to give her Demerol    136
and Vistaril as a sedative, and with the absence of any           147
specific findings that she be allowed to return home and was      159
advised to get in touch with me if her symptoms persist or        171
progressed.                                                       173
       The patient then returned to my office the next morning    185
complaining of abdominal pain, nausea, vomiting, fever, but no    197
diarrhea, and was anorectic. The pain was mostly across both      209
lower quadrants, and she also complained of some dysuria. The     221
patient stated her last normal menstrual period was last week     233
and that she had no abnormal vaginal discharge in the past.       244
       On my examination in the office, the patient was noted     255
to have bilateral guarding, tenderness, and rebound in both       266
lower quadrants of the abdomen. Bowel sounds were hypoactive,     278
and her temperature was elevated.                                 285
       With the findings, I called Dr. Smith to see this patient  297
regarding the possibility of pelvic inflammatory disease and      308
referred her to his office for pelvic examination.                318
Subsequently, following his exam, the patient was admitted to     330
the hospital with a diagnosis of probable pelvic inflammatory     342
disease, and I was asked to see the patient in consultation       354
regarding the possibility of appendicitis.                        363
       She has had the usual childhood diseases. No previous      374
surgery, no previous major medical or surgical illness, no        385
known allergies. She is on no medications at this time.           396
       An acutely ill patient complaining of severe abdominal     407
pain in the lower quadrants. Abdominal exam reveals bilateral     419
guarding, tenderness, and rebound with diminished bowel           430
sounds but no palpable masses or organomegaly. The pain is        441
somewhat worse on the right side. However, I feel that it is      453
very poorly localized. It seems to be mostly confined to the      465
lower quadrants.                                                  468
```

□□□□1□□□□2□□□□3□□□□4□□□□5□□□□6□□□□7□□□□8□□□□9□□□□10□□□□11□□□□12

Numbers and Top Row Keys

Learning Numbers, Three-Minute Timed Writing

Goals

After completing this lesson, you will be able to:

✔ Key numbers and figures.
✔ Use figures for age, weight, height, blood pressure, pulse, respiration, dosage, and temperature.

Skillbuilding Paragraph

Instructions

Key 3 two-minute timings—double space.

```
     The patient saw an eruption on the fingers of both hands.   12
They were pruritic and did not burn. The eruption has            23
persisted despite using Kenalog on her hands. She gives a        34
history of having had a diagnosis of dermatitis on her arms.     46
□□□□1□□□□2□□□□3□□□□4□□□□5□□□□6□□□□7□□□□8□□□□9□□□□10□□□□11□□□□12
```

1 AND 2

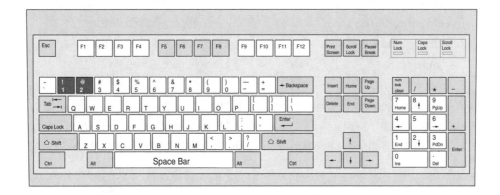

Instructions

Key each line two times. Double-space between each group of two lines. Say the letter first, then key the letter.

Learn the 1 key. Key with the a finger.

```
1  qqq aaa 111 aaa q1q a1a 111 aaa qqq 111 qqq aaa
2  111 aaa q1q a1a 111 q1q 111 111 q1q 111 aid 111
3  ask 111 a1q q1q 111 111 bone 111 pain 111 aorta
4  The patient's pulse is 111 and regular. The
5  11-year-old boy went home to 111 11th Street.
```

Learn the 2 key. Key with the s finger.

```
1  222 sss 222 s2s 222 ss2 22s s2s 222 sss 222
2  222 ss2 22s s2s 222 sss 222 222 scan 222 222
3  asthma 222 gland 222 cell 222 222 anorexia 22
4  The 12-year-old female was admitted. 22222
5  She's in Room 212, section 2 of floor 2.
```

3 AND 4

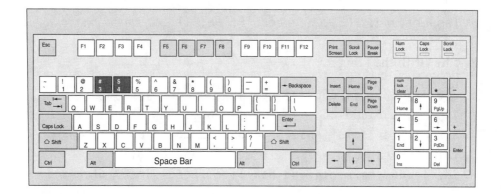

Learn the 3 key. Key with the d finger.

```
1  333 ddd 333 ddd 333 ddd 333 eee 3e3 3e3 333 ddd
2  333 ddd 333 ddd 333 eee 333 333 cornea 333 ear3
3  vital 33 yerba 333 pnea 333 hypoplasia 333 3333
4  This 32-year-old male was in a car accident 33.
5  Weight: 132. The doctor's number is 321-3323.
```

Learn the 4 key. Key with the f finger.

```
1  444 fff 444 ff4 ff4 44f 44f ff4 444 444 fff ff4
2  444 fff 444 fff ff4 4f4 4f4 434 r4r f4f r4r 4r4
3  444 onyx 424 sac 441 rachial 432 nystagmus 441
4  dermatoid 421 gout 444 call 414-444-4343 cecum
5  This is the first admission for this 14-year-old.
```

5, 6, AND 7

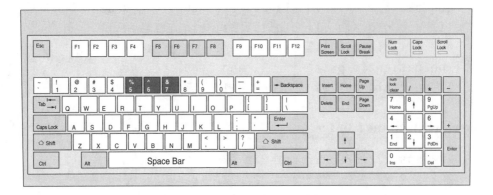

Learn the 5 key. Key with the f finger.

```
1  555 555 f5f 555 ff5 fff 555 f55 55f 5f5 555 555
2  f5f 555 ff5 f55 544 duct 555 tract 515 anemia 525
3  ileus 545 phobia 522 laryngitis 524 pleurisy 542
4  This 55-year-old male has a history of dizziness.
5  Temperature: 105.2 degrees. Pulse: 115.
```

Learn the 6 key. Key with the j finger.

```
1  666 jjj 666 jjj 666 jjj 666 j66 jjj 666 jj6 j6j
2  jjj jjj 666 666 666 6j6 6j6 j66 666; Six 6-bed;
3  Six 6-liter solutions. 6j6 666; 62 mg Tylenol.
4  This 65-year-old was admitted for nocturia.
5  She is 66 years old and has lived here since '66.
```

Learn the 7 key. Key with the j finger.

```
1  777 jjj 777 jjj 777 jjj 777 j77 777 uuu u7u 7u7
2  777 uuu 777 ju7 ju7 7uj 7uj 7j7 7j7 j7j 7j7 j7j
3  This 77-year-old male was admitted for a severe
4  headache and nausea. Blood pressure is 142/72.
5  Pulse: 77. He's been ill for 7 hours.
```

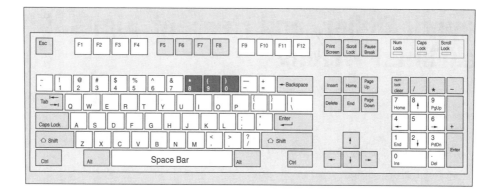

Learn the 8 key. Key with the k finger.

1 888 kkk 888 kkk 8kk 888 k88 kkk 88k 888 888 kkk
2 888 kkk 8kk 888 k88 kkk 8k8 k88 888 888 kkk kk8
3 k88 888 88k 88k 888 k88 888 888 kkk kk8 888 kk8
4 She's in no acute distress. Her physical findings:
5 pulse is 84 per minute. Blood pressure is 122/82.

Learn the 9 key. Key with the / finger.

1 999 111 999 111 999 111 999 119 991 991 991 199
2 999 111 999 111 999 999 191 919 11 99 11 99 191
3 Blood Pressure: 192/68. Pulse: 92.
4 He's lived to be 99 because he won't see doctors.
5 His address is 919 No. 99th Street.

Learn the 0 key. Key with the semicolon finger.

1 000 ;;; 000 ;;; 000 ;;; 000 ;;; 0;; 0;; 000 ;;;
2 000 ;0; 00; 00; 00; 000 ;;; ;0; 0;0 0;0 ;0; ;0;
3 Blood count showed 12,000 white blood cells.
4 This 73-year-old male is alert and cooperative.
5 Blood Pressure: 160/84. Pulse: 120. Height: 71.

The Pound, Dollar, and Percent Signs, Five-Minute Timed Writing

Goals

After completing this lesson, you will be able to:

✔ Key the pound sign.
✔ Key the dollar sign.
✔ Key the percent sign.

AND $

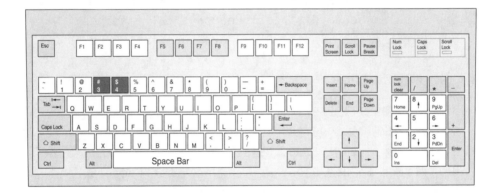

Rule 1

Pound sign: The # (pound sign) means number. Do not space after the #.
Example. #3-0 sutures.

Rule 2

Dollar sign: A dollar sign is used before the amount. Do not space after the dollar sign.
Example. $25.01.
For an even amount do not include cents.
Example. $25

Rule 3

Percent sign: Use of % after the numeral. Do not space between the numeral and symbol.

Example. 2% Xylocaine.

If the numeral is written out, write the (word) percent.

Example. Forty percent of the patients participated in the cancer research.

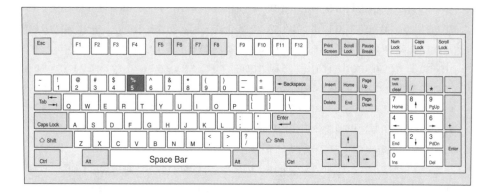

Instructions

Key each line two times. Double-space between each group of two lines.

Learn the pound key. Use the d finger, shift of 3 key.

1 ### ddd ### d#d ##d d#d d#d ##d ### ### D#D #D#
2 ### DDD ### ##D #2-0 Vicryl sutures, #3-0 Tevdek
3 sutures. Note: #3-0 sutures, #3-0 sutures.
4 #3-0 silk sutures #4-0 silk sutures
5 #5-0 multifilament wires #14 Foley

Learn the dollar sign key. Use the shift of the 4 key.

1 $$$ fff $$$ $$$ f$F f F $$$ F F F $F
2 $25 $25.01 The clinic spent $34.02 for bandages.
3 Purchase the Desk Reference at Dallas for $59.09.
4 The patient spent $459.50 for the walker.
5 They were priced at $5.99, $6.78, and $12.89.

Learn the percent key. Use the f finger, shift of the 5 key.

1 fff %%% fff %%% %f% %f% %f% %%f %%f %%% %%% %%%
2 f%% %%% 45% 3.5 mg% 44 vols% 22% lymphocytes
3 The lab report showed: 76% neutrophils, 30%
4 lymphocytes, 1% basophils, and 2% eosinophils.
5 Hemoglobin was 12.6 g, and hematocrit 32%.

This patient was admitted to Mobile Hospital because of   12
chest pain and difficulty breathing. He has been developing   24
progressive shortness of breath over the past several months.   36
He had been bedridden at home for several days prior to   47
coming to the emergency department.   54

Laboratory studies and x-ray findings were consistent   65
with chronic emphysema and bronchitis. The patient has been   77
seen by several specialists.   83

The patient was placed on telemetry, then transferred   94
to ICU by Dr. Charles Foot, who saw him in consultation. The   106
patient improved very slowly. His shakes and chest pain   117
disappeared. The patient continued to have difficulty   128
breathing with exertion.   133

Discharge medications include Inderal 10 mg b.i.d. p.o.   145
and Nitrostat 2.5 mg p.o. I will follow the patient in my   156
office, in one week.   160

□□□□1□□□□2□□□□3□□□□4□□□□5□□□□6□□□□7□□□□8□□□□9□□□□10□□□□11□□□□12

The Ampersand and the Asterisk, Two-Minute Timed Writing

Goals

After completing this lesson, you will be able to:

✔ Key the ampersand.
✔ Key the asterisk.

Skillbuilding Warmup—Two-Minute Timing—Double Space

This man was seen by the doctor with complaints of	11
increasing symptoms of bladder neck obstruction. He complained	23
of the urinary stream requiring longer time to initiate. There	35
is no history of urinary tract infections or hematuria.	46

□□□□1□□□□2□□□□3□□□□4□□□□5□□□□6□□□□7□□□□8□□□□9□□□□10□□□□11□□□□12

& AND *

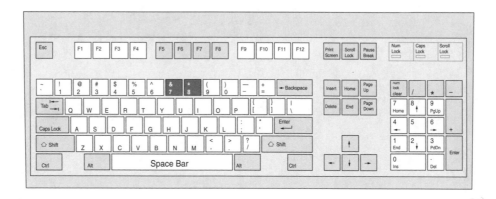

Instructions

Key each line two times, double-spacing between groups of two.

Learn the ampersand key. Use the j finger, shift of the 7 key.

```
1   &&& jjj &&& J&& &&& jjj &&& &jj j&j &&& jjj &&&
2   &&& tumor &&& pain &&& villi &&& memory &&& &&&
3   arthritis &&& insulin &&& dyspnea &&& & &&& &&&
4   The Anderson & Sampson Law firm is located on Elm Street.
5   Brown & Adams will merge with Walker & Kinney.
```

Learn the asterisk key. Use the k finger, left shift of the 8 key.

```
1   *** kkk *** kkk *** KKK *** kkk *** kkk *** kkk
2   *He denies symptoms of weakness or sensory loss.
3   *There has been no confusion or memory loss.
4   *Note: The patient suffered a myocardial infarction.
5   *He left the hospital before being discharged.
```

The Open and Close Parentheses and the Underline, and Five-Minute Timed Writing

Goals

After completing this lesson, you will be able to:

✔ Key the open parenthesis.
✔ Key the close parenthesis.
✔ Key the underline.

(

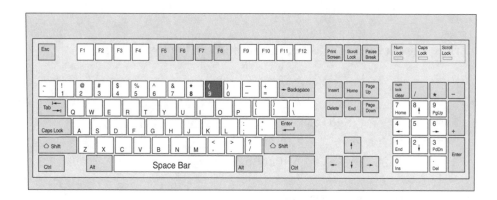

Instructions

Key each line twice, double-spacing between groups of two.

Learn the open parenthesis key. Use the / finger, shift of the 9 key.

```
1  ((( lll ((( (L( lll ((( lll ((( lll ((( lll (
2  lll food ( tremor ( trachea (edema ( fever ((
3  ( bile ( dysuria ( thrills ( gallops ( rhythm
4  ( sinus ( flat ( distress ( headache ( nausea
5  ( typing ( can ( be ( so ( much ( fun ( blood
```

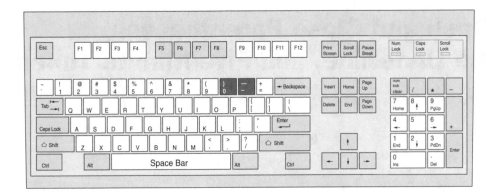

Learn the close parenthesis key. Use the semicolon finger, shift of the zero key.

```
1   ))) ;;; ))) ;;; ))) ;;; ))) ;;; ))) ;;; ))) ;;;
2   ))) ;;; ))) ;;; ))) ;;; );) );) );) ))) ;)) :::
3   ):) ):) ):) ):) ):) ):) :): ):) ):) ))) ):) :):
4   (pulse) (mild) (urethra) (jaundice) (diabetes)
5   (temperature) (amenorrhea) (homeopathic medicine)
```

Learn the underline key. Key with the colon finger, shift of the hyphen key.

```
1   ____ _____ _____ _____    ;;; ____ ;;; ____
2   ___ ___ ___ ___: ___: ___: : ___ : ___
3   Name _____ Medical Record _____
4   Admission Date _____ Surgeon _____
5   Room No. 25 __ Race __ Occupation _____
```

Skillbuilding Warmup—Five-Minute Timing—Single Space

```
        The patient is a Cuban male admitted on January 5 with a    12
diagnosis of hypertrophied tonsils and chronic tonsillitis.         23
Tonsillectomy and adenoidectomy were carried out on January 5       35
with dissection and snare technique.  The patient had an            46
uneventful postoperative course and is to be discharged home        58
with post tonsillectomy and adenoidectomy instructions.  The        70
patient will be seen in the office on February 10.                  80
   □□□□1□□□□2□□□□3□□□□4□□□□5□□□□6□□□□7□□□□8□□□□9□□□□10□□□□11□□□□12
```

The Equal and Plus Signs, Five-Minute Timed Writing

Goals

After completing this lesson, you will be able to:

✔ Key the equal sign.
✔ Key the plus sign.

= AND +

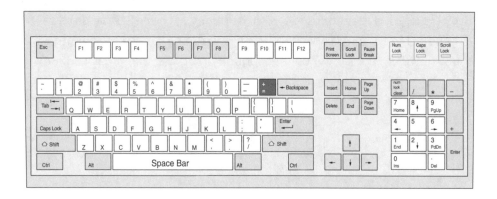

Instructions

Key each line two times, double-spacing between groups of two.

Learn the equal sign key. Key with the semicolon finger.

```
1  === ;== =;= ;;; === ;;= =;= =;= =;= =;= =;= =;=
2  =;= =;= =;= =;= = wheezing = sclerae claudication
3  = hematuria = swelling == lesion == bony ==
4  cardiac == normal == thorax == adenitis == tissue
5  lobelia == midwife == vaccination == acupuncture
```

Learn the plus key. Use the semicolon finger, shift of the equal sign key.

```
1  ;++ +++ ;+; +++ ;;; +++ ::: +++ ;;; +++ ;;; +++
2  ;;; +++ ;+: ++ 3+ protein 1+ prostatic enlargement
3  2+ femorals 2+ pulses. Urinalysis on admission
4  showed 3+ bacteria and epithelial cells. +++ +++
5  2 + 5 = 7 43 + 5 + 22 = 70 1 + 2 + 3 + 4 = 10
```

```
        No previous chest films are available for comparison.      11
The current study shows evidence of congestive heart failure.      23
This is manifested as cardiomegaly, bilateral pleural              33
effusions, and redistribution of the pulmonary vascularity         44
into the upper lobes.  Cardiomegaly with radiographic signs        55
reveal cardiac failure is present.  In addition to the large       66
left pleural effusion, the patient has changes within the          77
left lower lobe.  An enlarged right hilum represents vascular      89
engorgement, rather than a hilar mass.                             97

        Chest film today revealed moderate generalized cardio-    108
megaly.  All the cardiac chambers appear enlarged. There is       119
evidence of mild pulmonary venous hypertension with pulmonary     131
vascular congestion.  The lung fields are otherwise unremark-     143
able.  There are no pleural effusions.  The bony thorax shows     155
only mild osteoporosis.  In summary, there is moderate            166
generalized cardiomegaly with evidence of mild congestion.        177
```

▯▯▯▯1▯▯▯▯2▯▯▯▯3▯▯▯▯4▯▯▯▯5▯▯▯▯6▯▯▯▯7▯▯▯▯8▯▯▯▯9▯▯▯▯10▯▯▯▯11▯▯▯▯12

The Right and Left Brackets, Five-Minute Timed Writing

Goals

After completing this lesson, you will be able to:

✔ Key the right bracket.
✔ Key the left bracket.

}

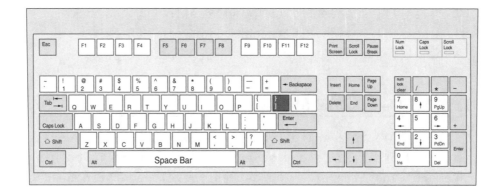

Instructions

Key each line two times, double-spacing between groups of two.

Learn the right bracket key. Reach with the semicolon finger.

```
1  ]]] cord ]]] silk ]]] sutures ]]] wound ]]]]
2  ]]] supine ]]] aorta ]]] kidney ]]] pelvic ]
3  spine ]]] colon ]]] anemia ]]] aphasia ]]] ]
4  throat ]]] logorrhea ]]] verbomania ]]] feet
5  fingers ]]] ears ]]] eyes ]]] nose ]]] baby
```

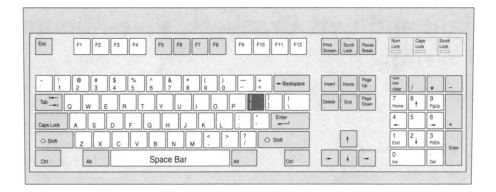

Learn the left bracket key. Shift and reach with the semicolon finger.

```
1  [[[ [[[ [[[ [[[ ;;; [;[ ;[[ [;[ [[[ [[[ [;[ [;[[
2  [[[ [[[ nerves [[[ eyes [[[ ear [[[ clumsy [[[[[
3  CT scan [[[ clonus [[[ optic [[[ cells [[[ nodes
4  [[[ neck [[[ rales [[[ rhonchi [[[ vein [[[ [[[[
5  venal [[[ jaundice [[[ insipid [[[ sleepy [[[[[[
```

FIVE-MINUTE TIMING—DOUBLE SPACE

Debbie is a white female who over the past several days	12
has had progressive and severe headaches unrelieved with	23
Demerol and Tylenol. The patient developed these headaches	34
several days ago, and this is associated with photophobia,	45
neck stiffness, and waking up in the middle of the night.	56
The patient has had nausea associated with the headaches but	68
has not had any vomiting. She has also had a progressive	79
weight loss over the past year despite a vigorous appetite.	90
The patient was seen yesterday in my office and had a severe	102
headache that kept her from work.	108
Neurologic examination was normal. The patient was	119
given intramuscular injection of Demerol to control her pain.	131
However, the pain has persisted despite this heavy medication.	143

☐☐☐☐1☐☐☐☐2☐☐☐☐3☐☐☐☐4☐☐☐☐5☐☐☐☐6☐☐☐☐7☐☐☐☐8☐☐☐☐9☐☐☐☐10☐☐☐☐11☐☐☐☐12

The Exclamation Point and the At Sign, Five-Minute Timed Writing

Goals

After completing this lesson, you will be able to:

✔ Key the exclamation point.
✔ Key the at (or each) sign.

! AND @

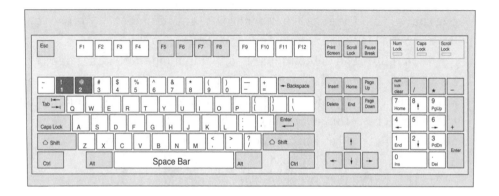

Instructions

Key each line twice, double spacing between groups of two.

Learn the exclamation point. Shift and reach with the a finger.

1 111 !!! aaa 111 !!! !q! !a! !!! !q! 1!1 !1! !! 11
2 !!! 1!1 !a! !q! !!! !a! !a! a!a q!q !!! q!q !! 11
3 No! Yes! Right now! Please help me! Call 911!! 11
4 Immediately! The ambulance is coming! Stop now!
5 This is critical! What a beautiful baby boy!

Learn the at sign. Shift and reach with the s finger.

1 ss ss sw sw s2 s2 s@ @s @s w@w @w2 @@@ s@s @s@ 2@
2 sw@ 75 @@@ 45 @@@ 78 @@@ 11 @@@ 222 @@@ 67 @@@ 90
3 They ordered 12 microscopes @ $45.02 each.
4 We will need 34 of the tourniquets @ $12 each.
5 Bill the patient for 12 aspirins @ $2.30 each.

```
        A physical examination was performed on Jill Scope.        11
Informed consent was obtained from the patient explaining          22
all risks and benefits to the procedure.  The premedication        33
included Demerol and Versed for the colonoscopy and                43
esophagogastroduodenoscopy. The patient was connected to the       55
monitoring devices and was placed in the left lateral              65
position.  Oxygen was provided with a nasal cannula, and           76
intravenous medicine was administered through an intravenous       88
port.  After sedation was achieved, a digital examination          99
was performed, and the colonoscopy was introduced into the         110
rectum and advanced to the cecum.  The cecum was identified        121
by visual landmarks.  The colonoscope was removed while            132
carefully examining the color, texture, anatomy, and the           143
mucosa.  In the rectum, the colonoscope was retroflexed to         154
evaluate for internal hemorrhoids and anorectal pathology.         165
No abnormalities except for one small polyp.                       174

        On EGD, the second part of the duodenum was identified     185
by visual landmarks.  No esophageal mucosal abnormalities          196
were seen.  There were erythema and edema noted throughout         207
the stomach.  The duodenal bulb and second portion were            218
normal.  Retroflexion showed a diminutive fundic gland polyp.      230
Gastritis is the diagnosis.                                        235

        The patient was transferred to the recovery suite in       246
satisfactory condition.                                            250
```

□□□□1□□□□2□□□□3□□□□4□□□□5□□□□6□□□□7□□□□8□□□□9□□□□10□□□□11□□□□12

Punctuation Marks, Five-Minute Timed Writing

Goals

After completing this lesson, you will be able to:

✔ Key punctuation marks accurately.

SPACING AFTER PUNCTUATION MARKS

Comma: Space once after a comma.

Period: Space twice after a period that ends a sentence for readability.

Question mark: Space twice after a question mark.

Exclamation point: space twice after the exclamation point.

Instructions

Key each drill two times. Rekey each error line two times. Double-space after keying each numbered item.

Drill 1: Comma, Period, and Apostrophe

1 Patient's blood pressure is 120/42, temperature 98°, pulse 117, respirations 20 per minute.
2 After the patient had been stabilized, x-ray films were done on the left arm, indicating a fracture of the left humerus.
3 No known history of indigestion, allergies to medication, melena, diarrhea, or hematemesis.

Drill 2: Question Mark, Period, and Exclamation Point

1 It is important to perform emergency surgery now! Why? It is an emergency! The patient was given the wrong medication! Why? Call an ambulance!
2 Call the doctor. She's at the club lifting weights.

Drill 3: Quotation Mark, Period, and Comma

1 The physician said, "Order these tests for the patient: hematocrit, white blood count, and blood urea nitrogen." "OK," I answered.
2 "Will my son be all right?" he asked. "He will be fine."
3 "Are you ill?" I asked. "No," he replied, "but I probably will be soon." "Why?" I asked. "I've been exposed to the HIV virus," he answered.

Drill 4: Dash and Hyphen

1 The patient is a 51-year-old female who was admitted--yesterday--
  to the hospital.
2 The county hospital--a 103-year-old institution--is going broke.
3 The patient--a 14-year-old--complained of a 10-pound weight gain.

Drill 5: Semicolon and Colon

1 Vital signs: Blood Pressure: 120/90; Pulse: 110; Temperature:
  101°; Weight: 62 pounds.
2 Please see to the following: order towels; check lotion supplies;
  and call the day nurse.
3 Things to do: buy shampoo; check with Michael's doctor; clip the
  dog's toenails.

FIVE-MINUTE TIMING—DOUBLE SPACE

The patient was well until yesterday. After lunch and	11
while at work, he developed fluttering of his heart and	22
nausea. A fellow worker recently had the same symptoms and	33
suffered a myocardial infarction. This fear brought the	44
patient to Dr. Sampson's office. In the office, an EKG was	55
performed, which showed paroxysmal atrial tachycardia. He	66
was admitted to the hospital and was digitalized with	76
conversion to a normal sinus rhythm. Past history includes	87
hypertension, depression, and labrynthitis. At present, the	98
EKG shows possible evidence of a previous myocardial	108
infarction.	110
Presently, the patient is having chills with an elevated	122
temperature. Lungs are clear. Heart is in a sinus rhythm,	133
no murmurs or extra sounds are heard. Abdomen, soft, obese,	144
nontender; bowel sounds are good. There is some tenderness	155
over the left hip with ecchymosis. Extremities have no edema.	167
At this time, the EKG showed left atrial enlargement. I plan	179
to keep the patient digitalized and on maintenance digoxin.	190
Serum enzyme tests will be done to rule out a myocardial	201
infarction. At the present time, a complete blood count is	212
being done for his temperature elevation.	220
He is to be in the office 1 week following discharge.	231
He is to be put on a low-fat, low-sodium diet and observed	242
for control of his hypertension.	248

□□□□1□□□□2□□□□3□□□□4□□□□5□□□□6□□□□7□□□□8□□□□9□□□□10□□□□11□□□□12

Figures for Keying Age, Five-Minute Timed Writing

Goals

After completing this lesson, you will be able to:

✔ Use figures for keying age.
✔ Use hyphens correctly.
✔ Use figures for fractions in ages.

Rule:

Use figures for fractions in ages.

4½ years old

4½-year-old child

The preferred style is the symbol for ½ if your computer has the symbol. Also
3-½-year-old is appropriate.

Instructions

Key the following sentences. Use figures for keying age and add the appropriate hyphens. Hyphens are used between numbers and "year-old," for example,
"26-year-old" before a noun. Note: Answers to problems begin in Appendix A.

Example:

This is a 51-year-old female who is well developed and in excellent health.

1   This twenty-two year old male was seen for a problem of bladder difficulty.

2   The seventy-year old male was admitted to Pacific View Hospital for brain surgery and hypertension.

Example:

The patient is a 3½-year-old female who has Down syndrome.

1   This ten and a half year old boy is being admitted for diagnostic testing of a Ewing's tumor of the long bone.

2   Jonnie Hubbard is a four and a half year old who has tonsillitis.

3   The eight and a half year old female patient is suffering from a virus.

Summary Exercise

Key the following sentences, adding hyphens.

1   This patient is a forty-two year old male who presented with fatigue and myxedema.

2　Rosemary Sampson, a ten year old female, was seen at Pacific View
　　Hospital for pneumonia and fever.

3　This nine and a half year old male fell and fractured his left
　　arm.

FIVE-MINUTE TIMING—DOUBLE SPACE

The patient is an 86-year-old woman who was transferred	11
from a hospital in Phoenix. She has known senile dementia	22
and is under conservatorship. While in Phoenix, she	32
experienced painless hematuria. She was evaluated at a	43
hospital in Phoenix, and an intravenous pyelogram revealed	54
transitional cell carcinoma of the bladder. Because this	65
will entail invasive evaluation, she transferred to this area	77
where her family resides. The patient is unable to give an	88
adequate history due to her dementia, and her history is	99
obtained from previous medical records from Phoenix.	109
She has no known tuberculosis or prior cancer. The	120
patient does not smoke or consume alcohol but apparently was	132
a heavy drinker for many years. The patient denies chest	143
pain or dysuria. The patient is an elderly woman appearing	154
her stated age and lying supine in no distress. No	165
organomegaly, masses, or tenderness. There are two scars	176
present, one is on the right side of her abdomen and the	187
other is midline. Rectal examination was performed recently	199
and was unremarkable.	203
The patient, at this time, appears medically stable.	214
Appropriate laboratory studies will be obtained immediately.	225
The patient's evaluation in Phoenix reveled no obvious	236
organic cause for dementia.	241

□□□□1□□□□2□□□□3□□□□4□□□□5□□□□6□□□□7□□□□8□□□□9□□□□10□□□□11□□□□12

Figures for Keying Height, Five-Minute Timed Writing

Goals

After completing this lesson, you will be able to:

✔ Use figures for keying height.

Instructions

Correct the sentence below as you key.

Rule:

Use figures for keying height. Height: 6 feet 7 inches.

Example:

The patient is 6 feet 10 inches and suffers from hypertension.

1   The young male is five feet four inches and is positive for
    pneumonia.
2   The patient is five feet three inches and has a history of urinary
    tract infections.

Figures for Keying Weight, Five-Minute Timed Writing

Goals

After completing this lesson, you will be able to:

✔ Use figures for keying weight.

Instructions

Correct the sentence below as you key.

Rule:

Use figures for keying weight. Spell out pounds and ounces.

Example:

The patient with anorexia weighs only 98 pounds.

1 The patient is on a healthy diet and weighs two hundred twenty pounds.

2 The patient presented to my office; he weighed one hundred thirty pounds.

This is a 60-year-old female with known arteriosclerotic   11
heart disease and coronary artery disease. She has chronic   22
obstructive pulmonary disease and is status post myocardial   33
infarction. She also has known hypothyroidism. She has been   44
maintained on a program of Nitrogard, Synthroid, Lasix,   55
Tagamet, and terbutaline. Recently, there has been a   65
pattern of chest discomfort, epigastric in nature, possibly   76
of gastrointestinal origin. Because of the patient's past   87
history, she is admitted to Mobile Hospital for evaluation.   98

She is a well-developed, well-nourished, obese female.   109
The chest is clear to percussion and auscultation. The first   121
and second heart sounds are of good quality. CBC, FBS, BUN,   132
and electrolytes were within normal limits. EKGs and cardiac   143
enzymes were within normal limits. The patient has   153
gastroenterologic chest pain syndrome.   161

She was seen in consultation by Dr. Good. A gastro-   172
enterology workup was negative; however, the patient   182
continued to complain of right upper quadrant and peri-   193
umbilical pain.   196

The patient denies orthopnea and paroxysmal   205
nocturnal dyspnea. Cardiac risk includes a history of   217
smoking and a positive family history for arteriosclerotic   228
heart disease.   231

The patient was continued on antacids and Tagamet. She   243
will be discharged to be followed by Dr. Good.   252

□□□□1□□□□2□□□□3□□□□4□□□□5□□□□6□□□□7□□□□8□□□□9□□□□10□□□□11□□□□12

Figures for Keying Blood Pressure, Five-Minute Timed Writing

Goals

After completing this lesson, you will be able to:

✔ Use figures for keying blood pressure.

Instructions

Correct the sentence below as you key.

Rule:

Use figures for keying blood pressure. Blood pressure can be spelled out or use B/P if dictated.

Example:

On physical examination, the patient's blood pressure is found to be 198/98.

1   Today her blood pressure is one hundred twenty-eight over ninety-eight.

2   The patient had a CT scan for lumbar spine and his blood pressure is one hundred twenty-four over seventy-four.

Figures for Keying Pulse, Five-Minute Timed Writing

Goals

After completing this lesson, you will be able to:

✔ Use figures for keying pulse.

Instructions

Correct the sentences below as you key.

Rule:

Use figures for keying pulse.

Example:

Pulse: 84.

Use figures for keying pulse.

Example:

The patient's pulse is 82.

1 The patient's pulse upon admission was fifty.
2 Mrs. Mary Sampson is being treated for hypertension; her pulse is sixty-two.

FIVE-MINUTE TIMING—DOUBLE SPACE

The patient is a 59-year-old female who has been admitted	12
to the hospital with chest and abdominal pain. After pre-	23
medication, the endoscope was introduced without difficulty.	34
The esophagus was visualized. The esophagus appeared within	45
normal limits with no evidence of significant esophagitis,	56
esophsgeal ulceration, lesions, or esophageal varices. In	67
the distal esophagus, there was mild esophagitis above a	78
small hiatal hernia. The endoscope was advanced through the	90
stomach to the antrum. The pylorus was easily intubated.	101
A portion of the duodenum was seen and appeared normal.	112
The duodenal bulb was seen and appeared normal with no	123
evidence of duodenitis or duodenal ulceration. There was no	135
evidence of gastritis, gastric ulceration, or lesions. The	146
endoscope was removed. There was no significant inflammation	158
of the hiatal hernia pouch. The patient tolerated the	168
procedure well.	171

☐☐☐☐1☐☐☐☐2☐☐☐☐3☐☐☐☐4☐☐☐☐5☐☐☐☐6☐☐☐☐7☐☐☐☐8☐☐☐☐9☐☐☐☐10☐☐☐☐11☐☐☐☐12

Figures for Keying Respiratory Rate, Five-Minute Timed Writing

Goals

After completing this lesson, you will be able to:

✔ Use figures for keying respiratory rate.

Rule:

Use figures for keying the respiration rate. Respirations can be keyed. Respirations: 40/min.

Instructions

Correct the sentences below as you key.

Example:

Her respiratory rate is 20.

1 He is a well-developed, well-nourished male whose respiratory rate
   is twenty-four.
2 The patient experienced a sudden ringing in the ears, headache,
   dizziness, and a respiratory rate of forty.

FIVE-MINUTE TIMING—DOUBLE SPACE

```
        This 70-year-old female is being evaluated for joint      11
pains.  She has obvious degenerative arthritis of both knees.     22
She fell in the bathtub on January 12 and came to the Mobile      33
Hospital emergency department.  The last several days, she        44
has been unable to walk and has been confined to a wheelchair.    56
        Examination reveals her to have obvious degenerative      67
changes of both knees.  She has pain in the right groin on        78
any attempts at motion.  Neurovascular status is normal.  In      90
reviewing her x-rays, she has a femoral neck fracture on the     101
right.  One of the films showed a fracture of the right hip.     112
The patient will have open reduction, internal fixation with     123
pinning of the hip.  Arrangements will be made, and the          134
problem has been discussed with the patient's husband and        145
sister, as well as with the patient.  Arrangements will be       156
made for open reduction and internal fixation.                   165
```

☐☐☐☐1☐☐☐☐2☐☐☐☐3☐☐☐☐4☐☐☐☐5☐☐☐☐6☐☐☐☐7☐☐☐☐8☐☐☐☐9☐☐☐☐10☐☐☐☐11☐☐☐☐12

Figures for Keying Temperature, Five-Minute Timed Writing

Goals

After completing this lesson, you will be able to:

✔ Use figures for keying temperature.

Rule:

Temperature can be keyed with:

✔ the figures, the degree symbol (°), and F (for Fahrenheit) or C (for Celsius): 98.6°F
✔ the figures and the word "degrees": 98.6 degrees
✔ the figures and the scale's name: 98.6 Fahrenheit

Instructions

Correct the sentences below as you key.

Example:

He developed a temperature of 102.3 degrees.

1 On admission today, the patient's temperature was one hundred
   point six degrees.
2 His temperature is ninety-nine point three Fahrenheit.

This 80-year-old man has been a resident of Brown's | 11
Board and Care since May 10, 2002. He was moved there from | 22
his home because his wife could no longer care for him due | 33
to his severe organic brain syndrome. He was extremely | 44
agitated, combative, and paranoid on admission, but improved | 55
considerably with Thorazine and other medications. Over the | 66
last several days, he has become increasingly lethargic, has | 77
eaten little, and was found to be febrile and congested. He | 88
was admitted to the emergency department yesterday with a | 99
diagnosis of right lower lobe pneumonia seen on x-ray. He | 110
continues to be febrile. He has arcus senilis and is | 121
somewhat dehydrated. | 125

The corner of the right mouth droops. Neck is stiff | 136
but otherwise not remarkable. No thrills or murmurs. The | 147
abdomen shows a left inguinal hernia. In his lower | 157
extremities, the pulses are decreased with edema of the right | 169
foot. The right knee is quite hot and swollen, and there is | 180
pain on movement. I suspect he has possible acute gouty | 191
arthritis of the right knee. I will order a uric acid test | 202
and aspirate the knee. CAT scan has been done, and the | 213
results are not available at the time of this dictation. | 224

☐☐☐☐1☐☐☐☐2☐☐☐☐3☐☐☐☐4☐☐☐☐5☐☐☐☐6☐☐☐☐7☐☐☐☐8☐☐☐☐9☐☐☐☐10☐☐☐☐11☐☐☐12

Metric Measurements and Latin Abbreviations, Five-Minute Timed Writing

METRIC MEASUREMENTS AND LATIN ABBREVIATIONS

Goals

After completing this lesson, you will be able to:

✔ Use figures for keying dosage.
✔ Use Latin abbreviations with periods.
✔ Use metric abbreviations.

Rule:

When keying metric abbreviations:

✔ no period follows unless the abbreviation ends a sentence
✔ use the singular form or if plural is understood, do not add s
✔ change fractions to decimals

Summary of Metric Abbreviations

cc	cubic centimeter	mg	milligram
kg	kilogram	mcg	microgram
g	gram	mL or ml	milliliter

Rule:

Use periods with lowercase Latin abbreviations.

Summary of Latin Abbreviations

a.c.	before meals	ad lib.	as desired
p.c.	after meals	b.i.d.	twice a day
c̄	with	h.s.	at bedtime
n.p.o.	nothing by mouth	p.r.n.	as needed
q.d.	every day	q.h.	every hour
q.h.s.	every bedtime	q.i.d.	four times a day
q.o.d.	every other day	p.o.	by mouth
t.i.d.	three times a day		

Example:

The patient was discharged with a prescription for Evoxac 30 mg t.i.d.

Instructions

Key the following sentences using the rules shown above.

1 This patient is taking thirty-five milliliters of Maalox.
2 She takes twenty milliliters of milk of magnesia daily.
3 The total liquids for the morning are fifty milliliters and seventy milliliters for the evening.

Summary Exercise

Instructions

Correct the sentences below as you key with abbreviations and figures.

Example:

His medications include Naprosyn 30 mg t.i.d., Dyazide 40 mg q.d., Synthroid 40 mg p.c.

1 The patient has been instructed to take Tagamet forty milligrams three times a day before meals.
2 The patient currently takes Carafate twenty milligrams twice a day before meals.

MILLIEQUIVALENT AND CENTIMETERS

Goals

After completing this lesson, you will be able to:

✔ Use figures for milliequivalent.
✔ Use figures for centimeters.

Rule:

Use figures and abbreviation with milliequivalent and centimeters.

Instructions

Correct the sentences below as you key with abbreviations and figures.

The abbreviation "mEq" stands for milliequivalent. Use "liter" if requested.

Example:

The physician prescribed 60 mEq of potassium.

1 K-Lyte is an effervescent tablet that includes potassium and chloride, twenty-five milliequivalents.
2 Serum potassium showed two point eight milliequivalents.

Rule:

Use "x" for the word "by." Space before and after the "x." Use lowercase "x." The abbreviation "cm" stands for centimeter.

Correct the sentences below as you key with abbreviations and figures.

Example:

The lesion is 2.5 x 1 cm on her chest.

1 The scar on the lip is one point three by zero point four centimeters.

2 The mass on her ankle is two by two centimeters.

FIVE-MINUTE TIMING—DOUBLE SPACE

```
     This 2-year-old black male was brought into the emergency    12
department by his parents, who noticed blood in his diaper.       23
The physician removed a blood clot from the child's urethra.      34
However, the child voided grossly bloody urine.  A catheter was   46
passed into the bladder through the urethra without              56
difficulty.  Grossly bloody urine was found within the           67
bladder.  There is no history of trauma.  The child has not      78
felt well for the past week; however, there is no history        89
of recent sore throat or ear infection.  He has had several     100
episodes of tonsillitis in July.                                106

     His mother has been well, although his father has had      117
malaise and a rash.  Past surgical history has been negative.   129
No known allergies.  The child has been on no medication.       140
Diagnosis is gross hematuria.                                   145
```

□□□□1□□□□2□□□□3□□□□4□□□□5□□□□6□□□□7□□□□8□□□□9□□□10□□□□11□□□□12

Prescription Labels, Five-Minute Timed Writing

Goals

After completing this lesson, you will be able to:

✔ Key prescription labels.
✔ Use figures for keying dosage and how many times medicine is to be taken.

Rule:

Labels are preprinted with the name of pharmacy, address, city, state, zip code, area code, and telephone number. You must key in the prescription number and date, the doctor's name, the patient's name, usage instructions, the drug's name, the dosage, the expiration date, and the number of refills.

Instructions

Key the following labels.

Label 1

```
 1   Mobile Drugs
 2   3842 Desert View Drive
 3   Mobile, AZ 92000
 4   (002) 279-0000
 5   Dr. Matthew T. Sampson
 6   RX 20000A October 10, 200__
 7   Sampson, Edna
 8   Take 1 tablet every 4 hours as needed for pain.
 9   Vicodin tablets 500 mg #20
10   Potency Expires 5/05 Refills 0
```

Label 2

```
 1   Mobile Drugs
 2   3842 Desert View Drive
 3   Mobile, AZ 92000
 4   (002) 279-0000
 5   Dr. Matthew T. Sampson
 6   RX 0543XXX September 17, 200__
 7   Sampson, Joe
 8   Take one tablet three times a day with food.
```

```
 9   Naproxen tablets 375 mg #30
10   Discard after 09/03 Refills 1
```

FIVE-MINUTE TIMING—DOUBLE SPACE

It is the first Children's Hospital admission for this	11
6-day-old female infant who was the product of normal term	22
pregnancy. The baby was born after a spontaneous labor and	33
delivery. In the newborn nursery, it was noted that this	44
child has small eyes, bilateral cataracts, peculiarly shaped	56
ears, and a heart murmur. The mother has a febrile illness	67
at six weeks' gestation, characterized by a rash of a two or	78
three days' duration. At that time, the mother had a	88
hemagglutination inhibition test performed, which was	99
positive, but the titer was low. Another hemagglutination	110
inhibition test was done at five months' gestation, which	121
revealed maternal rubella infection.	128
The child had x-rays of the bone, which revealed rubella	140
osteopathy. The child was having tachypnea, tachycardia,	151
and congestive heart failure. The child was digitalized.	162
Since the digitalization, the child's heart rate has slowed	173
down, and she is improving.	178
The child will be discharged today to be followed by	189
Dr. Jean Kind as an outpatient.	195

□□□□1□□□□2□□□□3□□□□4□□□□5□□□□6□□□□7□□□□8□□□□9□□□□10□□□□11□□□□12

Timed Writing Paragraph, Five-Minute Timed Writing

FIVE-MINUTE TIMED WRITING—DOUBLE SPACE

Instructions

Indent each paragraph five spaces.

The patient is an elderly female who was admitted to the	12
hospital with chest pain to rule out myocardial infarction. I	24
was asked to see her for gastrointestinal pain. The patient	35
claims that the discomfort began in the epigastric region	46
with radiation to the back. She took nitroglycerin, which	57
helped but not significantly.	63
She was nauseated and diaphoretic. She had a previous	74
hospitalization for a similar problem with chest pain;	85
myocardial infarction was excluded during that time. Also,	96
she has diverticulum disease and a spastic colon. The patient	108
has had a cardiac catheterization. There is a midline scar	119
from her cholecystectomy. Abdomen is obese.	128

□□□□1□□□□2□□□□3□□□□4□□□□5□□□□6□□□□7□□□□8□□□□9□□□□10□□□□11□□□□12

This patient was hospitalized at Mobile Hospital in	11
January 2003 for prostatic obstruction and a hard, enlarged	22
prostate, as well as many stones in the bladder. At that time,	34
he was found to have a high acid phosphatase. A bone scan	45
was also positive for multiple metastases. The patient was	56
complaining of multiple aches and pains at that time, which	67
were felt to most likely be due to the carcinoma of his	78
prostate gland. The patient's prostate was biopsied and	89
found to be a poorly differentiated adenocarcinoma of the	100
prostate, which is extensive. Many bladder stones were	111
surgically removed, and transurethral resection of the	122
prostate was done. He tolerated the procedure well but	133
refused orchiectomy. He experienced ankle edema for which he	145
was treated with Dyazide. He did have urinary tract	155
infections periodically.	160
The patient was not seen for several months. Later, he	171
returned complaining of arthritic pains, was not eating well,	182
and he said that his urine was passing fine. He had been on	193
Lasix and was having to void frequently but only when he	204
would take the Lasix. He has been having back pain recently.	216
The prostate was found to be 3+, hard, and irregular,	226
especially on the left side. Ann intravenous pyelogram was	237
done, which showed no ureteral obstruction. Bone scan	248
showed improvement.	252

□□□□1□□□□2□□□□3□□□□4□□□□5□□□□6□□□□7□□□□8□□□□9□□□□10□□□□11□□□□12

Percentages and Ratios, Five-Minute Timed Writing

Goals

After completing this lesson, you will be able to:

✔ Use percentages with words and figures.
✔ Key ratios.

Rule:

Do not space between the figure and percent sign.

Instructions

Key the following sentences using figures and percent sign.

Example:

The patient was injected with 2% Xylocaine.

1 The patient received five percent dextrose intravenously.
2 The patient received anesthesia using three percent Xylocaine.
3 Dr. Louis Hubbard, the anesthesiologist, administered zero point five percent Marcaine.

Rule:

Do not space before the colon or after for a ratio.

Instructions

Key the following sentences. Use a colon to separate figures.

Example:

Xylocaine with 1:100,000 was given.

1 The dilution is one:one hundred thousand.
2 Test material in the test tube is one to fourteen.
3 Dilution of serum is one to one hundred twelve.
4 The ear was injected with one to six thousand of solution.

The patient is a well-developed, well-nourished black	11
male child who is in no acute distress. Examination of the	22
head is negative. Tympanic membranes are intact. There are	33
no diseases of the nares, the tongue, or the oropharynx.	44
The uvula is in the midline. The teeth appear to be in good	55
condition. There are no palpable masses. Lungs are clear	66
to percussion and auscultation. There is no cardiomegaly.	77
The heart sounds are normal. The abdomen is soft and non-	88
tender. Liver, spleen, and kidneys are not palpably enlarged.	100
There are no abnormal masses or bruits. There are no	110
structural abnormalities of the back. The testes are bi-	121
laterally descended and are normal. The spermatic cords are	132
normal. There are no inguinal hernias present. The external	144
urethral meatus is slightly stenotic.	151
There is normal range of motion of the extremities.	162
There is no peripheral edema. Rectal examination is negative.	174
There are no abnormal masses. Deep tendon reflexes are	185
present and equal bilaterally. No abnormal reflexes are	196
noted. There is no significant lymphadenopathy.	205

□□□□1□□□□2□□□□3□□□□4□□□□5□□□□6□□□□7□□□□8□□□□9□□□□10□□□□11□□□□12

Roman Numerals, Five-Minute Timed Writing

Goals

After completing this lesson, you will be able to:

✔ Know when to use Roman numerals.

Instructions

Key each line two times.

Rule:

The following specific designations are not capitalized unless they begin a sentence: factor, grade, lead, stage, and type.

Roman numerals are used with the following:

cranial nerves I–XII

Cancer staging:

stage I

stage II

stage III

stage IV

EKG leads:

lead I

lead II

lead III

Blood clotting factor:

factor I–XIII

Use figures with grades for cancer and diastolic murmurs.

Rule:

Do not capitalize grade.

grade 1

grade 2

grade 3

grade 4

cranial nerves 1–12. Note: Roman numerals may be used as well as figures with cranial nerves.

Your patient, Molly, age 2, was seen because of sudden   11
hematuria last night. Examination, except for the mass, is   22
unremarkable. Her history suggests that she has had low   33
grade fever over the past week and has not been as active as   44
usual. When I examined the abdomen, it was easy to outline   55
a firm upper left quadrant mass that felt like a Wilms tumor.   67
Urinalysis was loaded with red blood cells.   75

A half an hour before the intravenous pyelogram, she   86
should be given chloral hydrate. If the intravenous pyelogram   98
verifies that the tumor is attached to the kidney, I recommend   110
surgery as soon as possible.   115

□□□□1□□□□2□□□□3□□□□4□□□□5□□□□6□□□□7□□□□8□□□□9□□□□10□□□□11□□□□12

Spacing with Symbols and Numbers, Five-Minute Timed Writing

Goals

After completing this lesson, you will be able to:

✔ Key symbols and words.

Rule:

Symbols are keyed:

✔ with no space between symbol and referent: 98.6°

Instructions

Key the following sentences. Apply rules previously learned from earlier chapters for keying blood pressure, age, and temperature.

Example:

Purchase the *Physicians' Desk Reference* for $129.05.

1 The patient is a thirty-nine-year-old engineer who awoke with severe chest pain and vomiting.

2 Her blood pressure today is one hundred thirty over eighty.

3 There has been no dizziness, vertigo, or muscle weakness, but the patient's temperature is ninety-eight point six degrees F.

Instructions

If you finish before time is up, start over. Proofread and circle errors. Double-space. Determine gross words a minute for the timing.

```
      This 52-year-old attorney was born in Canada and came to      12
Phoenix several years ago.  He is in good health, quite             23
athletic,and plays football once a week.  He felt well and         34
had been playing football for approximately 30 minutes when,       45
after running, he became dizzy and lost consciousness for one      57
to four minutes.  There was no convulsion, tongue biting, or       68
loss of urine. The patient was brought to the emergency            79
department where electrocardiogram showed premature atrial         90
contractions, and he was admitted for observation.  He denies     102
chest pain and shortness of breath.  He had no excessive          113
diaphoresis nor palpation with activity or at rest.  He has       124
not been on any medication, does not smoke, and uses coffee       135
moderately.                                                       137

      The patient sustained an ankle sprain one year ago,         148
which occasionally swells.  No unhealing lesions, abnormal        159
pigmentations, or eruptions, other than a birthmark on his        170
right thigh.  No previous episodes of syncope, except for         181
fainting as a child because of an emotional upset.                191
```

□□□□1□□□□2□□□□3□□□□4□□□□5□□□□6□□□□7□□□□8□□□□9□□□□10□□□□11□□□□12

Subscript and Superscript, Five-Minute Timed Writing

Goals

After completing this lesson, you will be able to:

✔ Key a subscript.
✔ Key a superscript.

Instructions

Ask your instructor for instructions on setting these. Key the following subscripts and superscripts. Word software uses Alt + P for superscript and Alt + B for subscript. WordPerfect 6.1 uses font, position.

1   T_6 T for thoracic
2   Vitamin B_{12}
3   L_3 L for lumbar
4   Temperature: $98.6°$.
5   Temperature: $37.2°C$.

Suture Materials, Five-Minute Timed Writing

Goals

After completing this lesson, you will be able to:

✔ Use figures for keying suture names.

Rule:

Use figures, the pound sign, and the hyphen for keying suture names.

Instructions

Key the following sentences and apply proper expression of figures, pound sign, and hyphen.

Example:

The wound was closed in layers using #3-0 chromic catgut.

1 The incision was closed with 2-0 Vicryl.
2 The wound was closed using interrupted number two Vicryl in the deep fascia and number three-zero Vicryl.
3 The peritoneum was closed with number two-zero chromic in a running fashion.

The patient is a 60-year-old female who was found by her   11
son-in-law on the floor in a semicomatose condition. The   22
patient was brought to the emergency department for evaluation 34
and was noted to have complete right-sided paralysis. The   45
patient also has deviation of her eyes to the left side with   56
expressive aphasia. Her electrolytes were within normal   67
limits. Her glucose was slightly elevated. The patient's   78
EKG showed a sinus rhythm with no irregularities. The   88
patient is being admitted to the intensive care unit for   99
extensive right-sided cerebrovascular accident.   108

The patient has never been hospitalized and has never   119
had surgery. Her present medications are estrogen and Altace. 131
The patient has no known drug allergies, and she does not   142
smoke cigarettes. She does drink an unknown quantity of wine 154
every day.   156

Her family history is negative for diabetes mellitus,   167
tuberculosis, cancer, or heart disease. There have been   178
several strokes in the family.   184

The patient has had no seizures, blackouts, convulsions,   196
migraine headaches, TIAs, or vertigo. She has not had   207
sinusitis. She does not have upper teeth and has several   218
loose lower teeth. She has no history of thyroid abnormal-   229
ities, asthma, bronchitis, or pneumonia.   237

She is negative for heart disease. She has had a   248
history of hypertension for the last eight years, which has   260
been controlled with medication.   266

She has not had any urinary tract infections, postmeno-   278
pausal bleeding, or arthritis.   284

☐☐☐☐1☐☐☐☐2☐☐☐☐3☐☐☐☐4☐☐☐☐5☐☐☐☐6☐☐☐☐7☐☐☐☐8☐☐☐☐9☐☐☐☐10☐☐☐☐11☐☐☐☐12

Time of Day and Circular Position, Five-Minute Timed Writing

Goals

After completing this lesson, you will be able to:

✔ Key time of day.
✔ Understand circular position.

Rule:

For both a.m. and p.m., use figures with circular position, for example visualizing the operative site as a clock and the figure must be followed by the word "o'clock." For military time, colons are not required. It should be keyed 0845 hours.

Instructions

Key the following sentences using the rule shown above.

Example:

Geraldine Sampson will be admitted to the Mobile Outpatient Clinic at 8:15 a.m.

1 The resident applicants will arrive at one twenty in the afternoon.

2 He is scheduled to speak at ten tomorrow morning.

3 She will speak at eleven in the morning at the auditorium.

4 Sutures were used at the twelve o'clock and six o'clock positions.

The Plus Sign, Five-Minute Timed Writing

Goals

After completing this lesson, you will be able to:

✔ Key figures with the plus symbol.

Rule:

No space before plus symbol.

Instructions

Key the following sentences using the rule shown above.

Example:

The carotid pulse 4+.

1 Prostate two plus enlarged and benign.
2 Carotids two plus.
3 Prostate two plus without nodules.

FIVE-MINUTE TIMING—DOUBLE SPACE

```
        This 60-year-old Caucasian male was recently discharged    11
from Mobile Hospital and readmitted with chest pains.  His         22
previous admission was for severe congestive heart failure,        33
respiratory arrest, and chronic obstructive pulmonary disease.     45
Chest x-ray was abnormal on admission, which showed pneumonia      57
with pleural effusion.  The patient was admitted to telemetry.     69
Enzymes and EKGs were done, which showed no evidence of an         80
acute myocardial infarction.  He was maintained on digoxin,        91
Nitrol, and Haldol.  He was also given bronchodilators.           102
He was seen again in consultation by Dr. Cobb, who had            113
previously evaluated the patient.  An effort was made to          124
ambulate the patient.  However, he became markedly hypoxemic      136
because of pneumonia and had to be transferred to the            146
intensive care unit.  Bronchoscopy was done by Dr. Cobb.         157
Cytology revealed no evidence of carcinoma.  His pulmonary        168
status finally improved.  He was able to eat better and was      179
transferred to the suite.                                        184

        He was seen in consultation by Dr. Deary because of his  195
persistent anemia.  However, this was due to thalassemia,        206
which is long-standing.  The patient was placed in a long-term   218
care facility at the request of his daughter.                    227

        Discharge medications include Lanoxin, Nitrol, and       238
bronchodilators, as prescribed by Dr. Cobb.                      246

        The patient is to be followed in the long-term care      257
facility by the house physician.                                 263
```

☐☐☐☐1☐☐☐☐2☐☐☐☐3☐☐☐☐4☐☐☐☐5☐☐☐☐6☐☐☐☐7☐☐☐☐8☐☐☐☐9☐☐☐☐10☐☐☐☐11☐☐☐☐12

Dates, Five-Minute Timed Writing

Goals

After completing this lesson, you will be able to:

✔ Use figures for keying the date.
✔ Spell out the month.

Rule:

Use a comma after the ordinal number before the year. A comma goes after the year also if it is in the middle of a sentence.

Instructions

Key the following sentences.

Example:

September 9, 2004

1 On 1/5/2001, she had an appendectomy and several months history of chills, fevers, and progressive shortness of breath.

2 This 11-year-old boy with acute lymphocytic leukemia was diagnosed on 07/05/2003.

3 The baby was examined on 08/05/2003.

Rule:

Do not use commas with inverted dates.

Instructions

Key the following sentences with dates inverted.

Example:

21 November 2003

1 This patient was last seen in my office on November 6, 19XX, for a myelogram.

2 The Neurology Conference is scheduled for 11/11/200__ in Washington, D.C.; Dr. Edward Burns will be presenting research data on Alzheimer disease.

3 A CT scan was completed and reviewed on 09/12/200__ and is within normal limits.

The patient is a 50-year-old male with chronic obstruc-   12
tive pulmonary disease, osteoporosis with compression   23
vertebrae, chronic chest pain, cataract of the right eye,   34
arteriosclerotic heart disease, cardiac pacemaker implantation, 46
and aphakia of the left eye, who has been treated for his   57
chronic obstructive pulmonary disease with prednisone.   68

The patient was seen by Dr. Cactus on May 6, 2002. At   79
that examination, the patient was doing well except for   90
experiencing morning nausea to medications. The patient was 102
told to continue the same dose of medicine and continue with 114
increasing activity. This morning the patient experienced   125
tremors and difficulty urinating. He was seen by Dr. Needle 137
in the office. While in the office, he was observed to have   149
a generalized tremor. This tremor has been occurring on   160
infrequent intervals over the past several months. It has   171
been due to chronic anxiety and pain. The tremor was not   182
associated with loss of consciousness, seizures, or postictal 194
state. The patient was evaluated for urinary difficulty,   205
which revealed urinary tract infection.   213

His past history includes transurethral resection of the   225
prostate. The patient is allergic to Demerol. He has a   236
history of endocarditis following cardiac catheterization.   247
The patient has a history of cigarette smoking. He has   258
worked with dry wall construction and has been dyspneic for   269
several years. He is currently being followed by Dr. Louis   280
Hubbard for chronic back pain. The pain is due to his   291
vertebral compression fracture secondary to iatrogenic   302
hyperadrenocorticalism. The physical examination reveals a   313
comfortable, well-developed, well-nourished male in no   324
distress. Head is normocephalic. The right fundus cannot   335
be visualized because of a cataract. Tympanic membranes are 347
not clearly visualized. Extremities reveal diffuse ecchymosis 359
secondary to chronic steroid administration. There is normal 371
male genitalia.   374

□□□□1□□□□2□□□□3□□□□4□□□□5□□□□6□□□□7□□□□8□□□□9□□□□10□□□□11□□□□12

Decimals and Fractions, Five-Minute Timed Writing

Goals

After completing this lesson, you will be able to:

✔ Use figures when keying numbers containing decimals and fractions.

Rule:

Convert fractions to decimals. Place a zero before a decimal that lacks a whole number (for example, 0.5%). Do not space between figure and percent.

Instructions

Key the following sentences applying the rules above.

Example:

The physician injected 0.5% of medication in the ear.

1 The physician injected three-fourths of the solution to the incision.
2 The skin was burned over half of the body.
3 One and three-fourths percent of them are sterile.

She is a 48-year-old woman who comes in today for follow-	12
up of abdominal pain. I saw her a month ago, at which time	23
she was describing reflux symptoms. I started her on Tagamet	35
400 mg b.i.d. She states that the Tagamet has relieved the	46
reflux symptoms. She has had no change in her bowel function.	58
Bowel movements are normal.	63
The patient has been having recurrent gastrointestinal	74
complaints for the last four or five years. She feels that	85
they are progressively getting worse. SHe has undergone at	96
least three colonoscopies because of previous adenomatous	107
polyps in 2000 and a tubular adenoma in 2001. Her last	118
colonoscopy was in December 2003, which was normal. She had	130
an upper GI series done about two years ago, which showed	141
reflux. She has been experiencing some unintentional weight	152
loss with these symptoms.	157
The patient is in no acute distress. Her weight today	168
is 140 pounds, which has decreased 3 pounds from a month ago	180
and 9 pounds from almost a year ago. Abdomen has active	191
bowel sounds, soft, nontender, and nondistended. No masses	202
or hepatosplenomegaly.	206
I am going to refer her to the Smith's Gastroenterology	218
Clinic. She will follow up with me after she has been seen	229
in the clinic.	232

▭▭▭▭1▭▭▭▭2▭▭▭▭3▭▭▭▭4▭▭▭▭5▭▭▭▭6▭▭▭▭7▭▭▭▭8▭▭▭▭9▭▭▭▭10▭▭▭▭11▭▭▭▭12

Drug Names with Numbers, Five-Minute Timed Writing

Goals

After completing this lesson, you will be able to:

✔ Key drug names with figures.

Rule:

Do not begin a sentence with a numeral unless the numeral is part of a medication's brand name.

Instructions

Key the following sentences applying the rules above.

Example:

Dr. Jean prescribed FK-506 for the patient.

1   New drugs presented at the pharmaceutical exhibits were:
    TP-forty, Pentam three hundred, Theo-twenty-four, Oxy five
    and Ovcon-fifty.
2   Current medications for the patient are: Demulen
    one/thirty-five and D.H.E. forty-five.
3   The patient is presently taking Humulin seventy/thirty.
4   The patient received Obetrol-twenty.
5   She was given VP-sixteen.

This 85-year-old female was admitted to Mobile Hospital   11
with a chief complaint of confusion, vomiting, and a fever.   22
The patient had been living on her own and has not been able   33
to care for herself. On the day of admission, her daughter   44
stated that when she telephoned her mother, she did not sound   55
well and was confused. This resulted in her being seen by   66
Dr. Cotton for evaluation and treatment. The patient has a   77
history of melancholia and has been maintained on Sinequan   88
at bedtime. She also had been under the care of Dr. Tension   99
for hypertension and angina pectoris.   106

The patient had been living with six members of her   117
family, bouncing from one home to another during the last   128
few years. She became irritable with her family; she stated   139
that she did not want to be bothered with their problems and   150
moved to a seniors' apartment. Since that time she has been   161
doing fairly well but her physician noted that she is going   172
downhill. The patient is mildly anxious and depressed. She   183
is worried about her discharge. SHe insists on living alone,   195
but she is unable to manage. There is no evidence of   205
psychosis. She is alert, oriented, and memory is intact.   216
The patient is no longer capable of living on her own. If   227
she goes to a rest home, she may like the accommodations. I   238
have taken the liberty of asking her to see Mrs. Cotton at   249
the rest home, which has a top star rating. I think that   260
she will like this facility and would not hesitate to go   271
there on a trial basis for two weeks to a month.   280

▢▢▢▢1▢▢▢▢2▢▢▢▢3▢▢▢▢4▢▢▢▢5▢▢▢▢6▢▢▢▢7▢▢▢▢8▢▢▢▢9▢▢▢▢10▢▢▢▢11▢▢▢▢12

EKG Leads, Five-Minute Timed Writing

Goals

After completing this lesson, you will be able to:

✔ Use figures for keying EKG leads.

Rule:

EKG chest leads can be keyed subscripted. Limb leads are designated by Roman numerals. EKG leads can be keyed on the same line. Example: V1, V2.

Instructions

Key the following sentences.

Example:

Use chest leads V_1 through V_6 or V-1 and V-2.

1 The doctor said to use leads aV_L, aV_R, and aV_F.
2 The nurse attached lead I, lead II, and lead III.
3 The physician presented a seminar on lead I, lead II, and lead III.

Large Numbers, Five-Minute Timed Writing

Goals

After completing this lesson, you will be able to:

✔ Mix figures with words for large numbers.

Rule:

Numbers in millions and billions are used with figures and words.

Instructions

Key the following sentences correctly applying the rule above.

Example:

The Podiatry Clinic cost $3.5 million.

1 It is estimated that two point five million people are without life insurance.

2 Pharmaceutical sales reported a first quarter net income of three point six million dollars.

3 The Eva Sampson Foundation provided one point eight million dollars in grants for medical vocational training and youth organizations.

The patient is a 35-year-old Caucasian male who is three   12
years status post cardiac pacemaker implantation for an   23
apparent heart block. He was referred to my office today for 35
a possible pacemaker malfunction. He also came in today for 46
a workup of chronic abdominal pain and two presyncopal   57
episodes associated with low pulse rate. Apparently, the   68
cardiovascular surgeons had problems obtaining the proper   79
threshold with the pacemaker. Therefore, after the pacemaker 90
was placed, it was removed and a wire was screwed in through 101
a partial thoracotomy. He has had abdominal pain for the   112
past two years. He has also had pain recently under the   123
pacemaker. The patient denies hypertension, diabetes, or   134
pyuria.   135

He had a ruptured disc removed two months ago. He has   146
a mitral valve prolapse. The patient is on disability.   157
Prior to his disability, he was a cabinetmaker. The patient 169
is a well-developed, well-nourished, pleasant male in no acute 181
distress. Carotids are full and equal with no bruits. No   192
thyromegaly. No adenopathy. Breath sounds are diminished   203
bilaterally. No murmurs or thrills. No clubbing, cyanosis, 215
or edema. EKG shows normal sinus rhythm.   223

The patient was admitted to the Telemetry Unit for   233
observation and monitoring. A 24-hour Holter monitor will   244
be worn.   245

□□□□1□□□□2□□□□3□□□□4□□□□5□□□□6□□□□7□□□□8□□□□9□□□□10□□□□11□□□□12

Figures vs. Spelling Out Numbers, Five-Minute Timed Writing

Goals

After completing this lesson, you will be able to:

✔ Know when to spell out a number and when to use figures.

Rule:

Different disciplines have different rules for spelling out numbers vs. using figures. Generally:

✔ spell out the numbers one through ten (unless the number is part of a brand or type name)
✔ if a paragraph contains numbers under *and* over ten, use figures for all
✔ the first number is spelled out when used with two numbers side by side

Instructions

Key the following sentences correctly, using figures or spelling out numbers as appropriate.

Example:

The patient was given fifty 50-mg capsules.

1 The medical school has thirty two-room laboratories.
2 Return twelve one-cup beakers to the warehouse.
3 The art class has sixteen thirty-one-year-olds.
4 Brown's Clinic will print a two-hundred-ten-page manuscript.

Instructions

Key the following sentences correctly, changing figures as appropriate. Spell out a number at the beginning of a sentence.

Example:

The library contains 20 medical dictionaries and 4 radiology word books.

1 The anatomy class has seven physicians and 20 pathologists.
2 We invited fifty Ear, Nose, and Throat residents and seven interns to the Otolaryngology Conference in Arizona.
3 Please order five Penrose drains, seventeen Band-Aids, one package of cotton pads, and twenty alcohol swabs.
4 The five trucks delivered eight gurneys, thirty walkers, and seventy crutches.
5 34 surgeons, ten residents, three interns, and six externs are at the suture class.

The patient is an 84-year-old female who was admitted   11
to Mobile Hospital with acute abdominal pain. Consultation   22
was requested by Dr. M. T. Sampson for her abdominal pain.   33
The patient has significant organic brain syndrome, and very   44
little history is obtained from the patient. The patient was   56
doing well until she developed abdominal pain, nausea, and   67
vomiting. She has had a urinary tract infection that was   78
treated with antibiotics. She has been afebrile. She claims   90
that she has had a hysterectomy and an appendectomy.   100

The physical examination shows an elderly female in   111
moderate distress. Conjunctivae are pink. Oropharynx is   122
edentulous, otherwise benign. Abdomen is soft, quite tender   133
with voluntary guarding. This is in the right upper and   144
right lower quadrants. There is no definite rebound tender-   155
ness. No hepatosplenomegaly. Bowel sounds are present.   166
Rectal examination shows no masses. The patient does have   177
edema in both ankles. SMAC reveals a decrease in potassium   188
and phosphorus. Urinalysis is unremarkable. EKG shows no   199
acute changes. Abdominal echogram did not locate any gall-   210
stones.   211

The patient has right-sided abdominal pain, the etiology   223
of which is not currently clear. She is afebrile, and her   234
white blood count is minimally elevated. I have ordered an   245
abdominal CT scan, lower gastrointestinal series, and an   256
upper gastrointestinal series. Further evaluation will be   267
dependent on the results of those tests.   275

□□□□1□□□□2□□□□3□□□□4□□□□5□□□□6□□□□7□□□□8□□□□9□□□□10□□□□11□□□□12

Plurals of Numbers, Five-Minute Timed Writing

Goals

After completing this lesson, you will be able to:

✔ Key plurals of numbers using figures.

Rule:

Add an "s" to the figure for plural numbers.

Instructions

Key the following sentences, using figures and adding the "s" for plurals.

Example:

The University of Mobile Medical Clinic was built in the 1960s.

1 The laboratories are priced from the low one hundred thirty thousands.

2 Medical costs increased in the nineteen seventies and continued through the mid-nineteen seventies.

3 Robbie had an appendectomy in the early nineteen sixties and, in the mid-nineteen seventies, a coronary artery bypass graft.

This patient was admitted to Mobile Hospital via the 11
emergency department. The patient states that she was 22
walking in her home and slipped from her walker. The patient 34
fell on her coccyx, as well as on her left hip. The patient 45
had substantial pain and was brought into the emergency 56
department. 58

X-rays revealed a questionable fracture of the left hip. 70
The patient's history is very difficult to obtain because she 82
is very hard of hearing. The patient stated that she had 93
surgery on her left hip from an old fracture and a pin insert- 105
tion. The patient also had an appendectomy. She had third- 117
degree burns on her face with obvious facial deformity. 128

Her physical examination revealed an elderly female 139
who had multiple aches and pains. The patient was not able 150
to ambulate and could move around in bed with a lot of 161
difficulty. It is difficult to examine her extremities 172
because of the patient's inability to move around in bed. 183
There was scar over the left hip. The patient had multiple 194
areas of ecchymoses on her left arm and bilateral legs. 205

I do not think that this patient has a fracture of her 216
pelvis or hip; however, I feel that in order to adequately 227
evaluate her, a bone scan should be performed. 236

□□□□1□□□□2□□□□3□□□□4□□□□5□□□□6□□□□7□□□□8□□□□9□□□□10□□□□11□□□□12

Laboratory Values, Five-Minute Timed Writing

Goals

After completing this lesson, you will be able to:

✔ Use laboratory values.
✔ Use figures when keying laboratory values.

Rule:

Laboratory test results are reported with abbreviations, and names of tests are reported using abbreviations.

Instructions

Key the following assignment.

1 Cubic millimeter--cc mm
2 Millimoles per liter--mmol/L
3 Millimeters of mercury--mmHg
4 Milligrams percent--mg%
5 Complete blood count--CBC
6 Lactate dehydrogenase--LDH
7 White blood count or white blood cell--WBC
8 Alanine aminotransferase--ALT
9 Aspartate transaminase--AST
10 Red blood cell or red blood count--RBC
11 Carbon dioxide partial pressure--PCO_2 or pCO_2
12 Oxygen partial pressure--PO_2 or pO_2
13 Chemical symbol for carbon dioxide--CO_2
14 Oxygen--O_2
15 Acid or alkaline--pH
16 Milligrams per deciliter--mg/dl
17 Partial thromboplastin time--PTT
18 Prothrombin time--PT
19 Blood urea nitrogen--BUN
20 milligrams per deciliter--mg/dl

The patient is a 72-year-old married male who was	11
admitted to Mobile Hospital today. He was transferred from	22
Dust Home in Gila Bend where the patient had been staying for	34
the past two months. The patient gives very little history,	45
but does state that he has been nervous and depressed over	56
the past month. He has numerous physical complaints,	66
including a rash on his legs and hemorrhoids. He has been	77
living in Dust Home because his wife is unable to care for	88
him.	89
The patient was admitted because of depression with	100
suicidal ideation. He was in an auto accident, which	110
possibly could have been intentional. At that time, an EEG	121
was done, which was asymptomatic. Upper gastrointestinal	132
series revealed a small hiatal hernia, which was normal.	143
The wife also states that the patient has been voicing	154
suicidal ideation, which the patient denies.	163
The patient has a history of tuberculosis and chronic	174
lower gastrointestinal bleeding with hemorrhoids.	184
Four siblings have suffered from depression, and his	195
son had committed suicide. The patient denies this and	206
states that he died from a heart attack. The patient has	217
six grandchildren.	220
The patient is alert but somewhat uncooperative. He is	232
agitated and tremulous. No evidence of delusional thinking	243
or hallucination, but he tends to deny most problems. There	255
is some mild memory loss. The patient will be started on	266
antidepressants in order to help relieve his depression.	277

□□□□1□□□□2□□□□3□□□□4□□□□5□□□□6□□□□7□□□□8□□□□9□□□□10□□□□11□□□□12

Mechanics I—Language Skills

Abbreviations, Brand-Name Drugs, and Five-Minute Timed Writing

Goals

After completing this lesson, you will be able to:

✔ Key capital letters and shift frequently.
✔ Key brand-name drugs, always capitalizing the first letter.

Rule:

Capitalize brand-name drugs.

Instructions

Key each line two times, double-spacing after each group of two.

Drill 1: Abbreviations

```
1  Accom. ACh ACTA ara-C Astigm. Au A-V BaE BP Ca
2  C-spine CVS DPT Em Fb FBS FTA-ABS Fe F/u Ga Gyn Hb
3  HCG hCG Hct He Hg IgA IgD IgE IgG IgM KUB L&W mCi
4  mg/cc mg/dl mmHg mRNA Na pH Ra RAI Rh TPA Tx WISC
5  INH TPR ACh RIND SGOT SGPT cath CMF Hgb Xrt mEq/L
```

Drill 2: Brand-Name Drugs

```
1  Alphaderm Aristocort Atarax Balnetar Benadryl
2  Indocin Tylenol Zyloprim Achromycin AnalpramHC
3  Keflex Zantac Premarin Seldane Tenormin Vasote
4  Naprosyn Capoten Dyazide Proventil Procardia Lasix
5  Halcion Lopressor Xanax Prozac Cogentin Provera
```

1	The patient is a teacher. She felt the onset	10
2	of abdominal pains below the unbilicus. This pain	20
3	has gotten worse. She has been nauseated and vom-	30
4	ited several times in the past two hours. She de-	40
5	nies fever, chills, or any change in bowel habits.	50
6	She came to the emergency room and was admitted to	10
7	the hospital. She will be seen by Dr. Semicolons.	20
8	The nervous system is composed of billions of	30
9	nerve cells. These nerve cells coordinate activi-	40
10	ties as we speak, move muscles, smell, see, taste,	50
11	hear, and respond to pain and touch. Body temper-	10
12	ature, memory, and association are also controlled	20
13	by the nervous system.	24

□□□□1 □□□□2 □□□□3 □□□□4 □□□□5 □□□□6 □□□□7 □□□□8 □□□□9 □□□□10

Drill 3

1 The patient states that she was started on Ovcon.
2 He was using the drugs Calan and Procardia.
3 She was treated with Cipro, Inderal, Maxzide, and repeated doses of Lasix.
4 The patient was treated with E-Mycin.
5 He will be prescribed Timoptic and Tagamet.

Drill 4

1 Dr. Leukocyte will attend the Society of Gastrointestinal Endoscopy Seminar, in Atlanta, Georgia, at the Gastritis Clinic.
2 Fifty-two patients have been invited to attend the Heart Association dinner.
3 Mary, the dietitian, is presenting a demonstration on the four food groups at the Dietetic Seminar.

ABBREVIATIONS

Goals

After completing this lesson, you will be able to:

✔ Key abbreviations in upper- and lowercase.
✔ Discern which reports do not use abbreviations.

Rule:

Abbreviations are not used for admission, discharge, preoperative diagnosis, postoperative diagnosis, operative title, or consultative conclusion. Periods are not used within or after most abbreviations, abbreviated units of measure, and brief forms, including acronyms.

Instructions

Key the following abbreviations.

	Abbreviation	Meaning
1	Abbreviation	Meaning
2	AB or ab	abortion
3	A, B, AB, O	blood type system
4	AIDS	Acquired Immunodeficiency Syndrome
5	AML	acute myelocytic leukemia
6	bas	basophils
7	BP	blood pressure
8	BX	biopsy
9	Ca	cancer or chemical symbol for calcium
10	CABG	coronary artery bypass graft
11	CCU	coronary care unit
12	D&C	dilation and curretage
13	dl	deciliter
14	DOB	date of birth
15	DTRs	deep tendon reflexes
16	ECG or EKG	electrocardiogram
17	EEG	electroencephalogram
18	EOS	eosinophils
19	F	Fahrenheit
20	FH	family history
21	FU	follow-up
22	GERD	gastroesophageal reflux disease
23	GI	gastrointestinal
24	gtt.	drops
25	Hgb	hemoglobin
26	HCT	hematocrit
27	HX	history
28	ICU	intensive care unit
29	I&D	incision and drainage
30	IUD	intrauterine device
31	K	potassium
32	KUB	kidneys, ureters, and bladder
33	LDL	low-density lipoprotein
34	LMP	last menstrual period
35	met	metastases
36	MI	myocardial infarction
37	monos	monocytes
38	Na	sodium
39	NG	nasogastric
40	NPO	nothing by mouth
41	OR	operating room

42	os	opening; mouth
43	oz.	ounce
44	PDR	Physicians' Desk Reference
45	PE	physical examination
46	pH	hydrogen ion concentration
47	q.n.s.	quantity not sufficient
48	q.p.m.	each evening
49	Rh	rhesus factor or chemical symbol for rhodium
50	R/O	rule out
51	c̄	with
52	sig	label it
53	SOAP	Subjective Objective Assessment Plan
54	tomos	tomograms
55	TURP	transurethral resection prostate
56	Tx	treatment
57	UA	urinalysis
58	UR	upper respiratory
59	VDRL	Venereal Disease Research Laboratory
60	Wt	weight
61	y/o	years old

Word Types, Five-Minute Timed Writing

Goals

After completing this lesson, you will be able to:

✔ Distinguish between words that sound similar.

Instructions

Key and study these definitions and apply them to the exercises following.

	Word	Definition
1	Word	Definition
2	addiction	a habit
3	adduction	movement to the middle
4	aural	pertaining to the ear
5	oral	pertaining to the mouth
6	Camalox	antacid
7	Camelot	a mythic place
8	carpal	pertaining to the wrist
9	corpus	main body part of any organ
10	cerumen	ear wax
11	serum	watery fluid
12	cancerous	pertaining to cancer
13	cancellous	lattice-like structure of bone tissue
14	cholectomy	excision of gallbladder
15	colectomy	excision of the colon
16	corner	angle point
17	coroner	one who investigates unknown causes of death
18	comma	type of punctuation
19	coma	state of deep unconsciousness
20	dysphasia	difficulty in speaking
21	dysphagia	difficulty in swallowing
22	Ball's valve	anal valve
23	bivalve	two valves
24	enervation	lacking nervous energy
25	innervation	supply of nerves to a body part
26	Excedrin	pain medication
27	ephedrine	alkaloid
28	fornix	archlike structure
29	pharynx	passage way within the throat area

30	faint	loss of consciousness
31	feint	something feigned
32	gate	opening to a walk through
33	gait	manner or style of walking
34	gavage	feeding tube
35	garage	where vehicles are stored
36	graft	transplanted tissue
37	graph	presentation of information
38	her suit	wearing apparel
39	hirsute	excessive hair growth
40	scar	healing mark on the skin
41	scarf	covering for the head and neck
42	scirrhous	hard cancer
43	cirrhosis	condition of the liver
44	sycosis	inflamed hair follicles
45	psychosis	condition of the mind
46	sight	to see
47	site	location
48	liter	a unit of volume in the metric system
49	litter	stretcher to transport the sick or wounded
50	liver	large organ in the abdominal region
51	livor	dark spots occurring after death
52	lipoma	tumor consisting of fat cells
53	lymphoma	tumors pertaining to lymph
54	mole	elevated spot growth on the skin
55	mold	fungus growth on plants and objects
56	necrosis	death of tissue
57	nephrosis	condition of the kidney
58	bruit	sound heard on auscultation
59	brute	inability to understand
60	palpitation	abnormal heartbeat
61	palpation	examining the external surface of the body with the hands or fingers
62	plain	simple
63	plane	anatomical positions of the body
64	postpartum	pertaining to after childbirth
65	post partum	after childbirth
66	Perls'	hemosiderin test
67	purls	knitting stitches
68	sitotoxin	poison in food
69	Cytoxan	brand-name drug
70	vein	vessel that carries blood

71	vane	equipment rotated by the wind
72	Valium	drug for anxiety
73	vallum	raised edge of a surface
74	varicella	chickenpox
75	variceal	pertaining to an enlarged artery
76	venous	pertaining to the veins
77	Venus	a goddess
78	vesical	pertaining to the bladder
79	vesicle	bladder containing fluid
80	wound	break in the skin
81	womb	uterus
82	rales	abnormal respiratory sound on auscultation
83	rails	handholds on stairs
84	hypertension	abnormally high blood pressure
85	hypotension	abnormally low blood pressure
86	arteriosclerosis	hardening of the arteries
87	atherosclerosis	hard plaques of fat
88	bare	naked
89	bear	to endure
90	chancre	syphilis lesion
91	canker	ulcer of the lips and mouth
92	corporeal	pertaining to the physical body
93	corporal	a military rank
94	febrile	pertaining to fever
95	feeble	weak

Instructions

Key the following sentences, choosing the correct one of the two similar words.

1 His addiction/adduction to alcohol is unbearable.

2 The 32-year-old woman is suffering from postpartum/post partum depression after the birth of her baby.

3 Dr. Jeffery Sampson, the corner/coroner, investigated a death at the campground.

4 The patient is taking Camalox/Camelot for his stomach problems.

5 The 16-year-old female was in an automobile accident and has been in a comma/coma for three years.

6 Several days ago, Valium/Vallum was prescribed for the patient's anxiety.

7 His uncoordinated gate/gait convinced him to use a cane and walker.

8 Several cancerous/cancellous lesions have metastasized to the liver, brain, bones, and lungs.

9 The lipoma/lymphoma has several fatty cells, which is causing her to consider surgery.

10 The patient's face is excessively hirsute/her suit and has pimples and several scars on the forehead.

11 The physician prescribed Xanax for his sycosis/psychosis.

12 On examination, Mrs. Smith had scirrhous/cirrhosis of the liver, which is causing pain.

13 Cholectomy/Colectomy was performed on the 56-year-old male to remove the gallbladder.

14 Plain/plane sutures were used for the incision.

15 Dr. Robert C. Moss' oral/aural presentation on how to treat Hodgkin's disease was excellent.

16 Cytoxan/Sitotoxin was prescribed for five patients.

17 The patient's skin graft/graph on his chest, legs, arms, and shoulder was successful.

18 A gavage/garage was used to feed the ailing lady.

19 The Perls'/purls test was ordered for the distressed lady in Room 45.

20 A Ball's valve/bivalve was used at St. John's Clinic.

21 The dermatologist removed five moles/mold from her arm.

22 Ephedrine/Excedrin was prescribed for her asthma and hay fever.

23 The physician and the otologist removed cerumen/serum wax from both ears.

24 After examining the pharynx/fornix, the throat was red and very painful.

25 She became faint/feint after hitting her head on the floor.

26 The nurse took blood from the vein/vane for a complete blood count.

27 One liter/litter of saline is enough for her to use.

28 The patient received a liver/livor transplant and is in critical condition.

29 The physician described the bruit/brute sounds as being very clear.

30 Several patients are suffering from nephrosis/necrosis, they see a nephrologist every week for kidney dialysis.

31 Mr. George, a 26-year-old patient, awoke this morning with dysphagia/dysphasia of the throat.

32 The patient is to change the dressing on the wound/womb daily.

33 The patient had her venous/venus organ unclogged by a surgeon.

34 The scar/scarf is infected and antibiotics are being used several times a day.

35 After having surgery, the lovely patient regained her sight/site.

36 The doctor did a palpation/palpitation on his swollen ankles.

37 His variceal/varicella condition is painful, so the physician ordered diagnostic tests for the artery.

38 This young lady was seen today in my office because of enervation/innervation.

39 The doctor described his vesicle/vesical as being filled with excessive fluid.

40 Three corpus/carpal bones will be removed in outpatient surgery.

Instructions

Key the synonym and antonym for each word. Synonyms are words with similar meanings. Antonyms are words of opposite meaning.

	Word	Synonyms and Antonyms
1	pain	throe agony distress comfort
2	agitate	impel calm annoy excite
3	collapse	faint succumb revive fail
4	comatose	unconscious alert torpid stuporous
5	communicate	tell memo conceal sign
6	conflict	disagree concord strife harmony
7	console	blame comfort annoy kindness
8	delusion	reality error illusion fantasy
9	depression	gloom joy poverty sorrow
10	die	live vanish expire depart
11	emotion	feeling apathy reaction reason
12	faint	weak revive pale black out
13	fever	afebrile heat fire mania
14	grief	sadness remorse joy affliction
15	isolate	unite quarantine free exclude
16	insane	sane mad depressed wild
17	lacerate	treat cut mangle suture
18	malady	illness health cold recovery
19	naked	clothed bare palatable manifest
20	obtuse	sensitive stupid apparent happy
21	pseudo	genuine mania false purchased
22	sedate	lively unwell serious calm
23	transparent	turbid clear explicit lucid
24	urgent	grave pressing required unimportant
25	vision	blindness image manifestation hallucination

This is a 66-year-old demented, senile patient who was   11
transferred from Laveen to Mobile to be with her family. The   23
patient was noticed by her daughter, who came to visit the   34
patient after the death of her husband, to have gross hema-   45
turia around the bathroom and in the toilet bowel. The   56
patient did not complain of any pain or bleeding. The patient 68
was brought to the emergency department in Mobile Hospital.   79
She was found to be unable to carry on a conversation. An   90
IVP revealed a large, irregular sessile mass in the urinary   101
bladder. In view of the problem, the patient was transferred 112
to Gila Bend Hospital where cytology was performed for   123
diagnostic purposes and a large tumor was found in the right 134
side of the bladder. The tumor appears to impinge into the   145
right side of the bladder wall. The ureter was unaffected.   156
The pelvic examination showed a tumor in the right side of   167
the patient's bladder, which was confirmed by rectal   177
examination. The patient is a widow and smokes moderately.   188
This patient has a diagnosis of squamous cell carcinoma of   199
the bladder with extensive pelvic invasion. In this kind of 210
situation, I agree with Dr. Hart that the patient is not a   221
candidate for surgery. If anything should be offered to   232
her, the option would be chemotherapy. In the meantime, I   243
will suggest obtaining a liver scan and CT scan of the   254
pelvis. When these procedures are completed, we will decide 266
with the family which therapeutic approach to follow.   276

□□□□1□□□□2□□□□3□□□□4□□□□5□□□□6□□□□7□□□□8□□□□9□□□□10□□□□11□□□□12

Spelling, Word Choice, and Word Division, and Five-Minute Timed Writing

Goals

After completing this lesson, you will be able to:

✔ Correctly spell often-misspelled words.
✔ Choose the correct word from two similarly spelled words.
✔ Divide words correctly.

Instruction

Key each sentence, choosing the correct word. If you need to, use your dictionary for this assignment.

1 The (postoperative, post operative) diagnosis is an inflamed appendix.
2 Ten patients are (all right, alright) after the bus accident.
3 Prepare the surgery (calendar, calender) for Dr. Roger Smith.
4 His (preoperative, pre-operative) diagnosis is carpal tunnel syndrome of the left hand.
5 The (anxious, eager) patient is concerned about her MRI and surgery.
6 After taking the medication, she became very (weak, week).
7 The clinic manager asked (somebody, some body) to get the x-rays.
8 The physician is having a (personal, personnel) consultation with the patient.
9 Sit (hear, here) and listen carefully to her class on stress management.
10 In the Otology Clinic, we have (fewer, less) patients than they have in the Cardiology Clinic.
11 The pharmacy technician (continually, continuously) comes to our clinic.
12 The researcher (accepted, excepted) the grant to study cancer in mice.
13 The doctor (assured, ensured) the family about diabetes mellitus.
14 Treatment will (proceed, precede) after surgery.
15 The (effect, affect) on the arthrocentesis is unknown at this time.
16 A (bone scan, boney scan) was obtained on the patient today.
17 The patient has (herpesvirus, herpes virus).
18 Several children died from E. coli (bacteria, bacterium).

19 Schedule the (venipuncture, venipunction) and (ekg, EKG) for tomorrow.

20 The 26-year-old female patient diagnosed with leukemia is in (remission, re-mission).

21 The chest x-ray revealed (dust cells, dustcells) in his lungs.

22 She had (double vision, doublevision) for several days after the accident.

23 The 26-year-old male patient is suffering from a (concussion, concusion).

24 The (mouth wash, mouthwash) contains chemical compounds and is considered safe for a sore throat.

25 X-rays revealed an (illiofemoral, iliofemoral) fracture.

Instructions

Key the correctly spelled words.

Rule:

Use the dictionary to find the correct words.

1	ability	abilty
2	beleive	believe
3	desert	decert
4	pateint	patient
5	nieghbors	neighbors
6	reveiw	review
7	unfortunatly	unfortunately
8	hospitel	hospital
9	doctor	docter
10	asthma	ashma
11	emphysemia	emphysema
12	heparine	heparin
13	parcell	parcel
14	zifoid	xiphoid
15	callus	calli
16	pioderma	pyoderma
17	polip	polyp
18	sieze	seize
19	releif	relief
20	seperate	separate
21	pancreas	pancreus
22	malignent	malignant
23	relie	rely
24	expinse	expense
25	success	succcess
26	scleiroderma	scleroderma

27	lipocyte	liposite
28	coccygeul	coccygeal
29	gangloin	ganglion
30	thalassemia	thalassima
31	edema	eduma
32	dysurea	dysuria
33	postoperative	post operative
34	abscess	abcess
35	nitrogenous	nitrogeneous
36	preoperative	pre operative
37	nephroscleerosis	nephrosclerosis
38	hysterectomy	hysteractomy
39	adnexa	adneksa
40	areola	areloa
41	nephropeathy	nephropathy
42	keratosis	karotosis
43	pulmonary ademia	pulmonary edema
44	postmature	post mature
45	fallopian tube	fallopien tube
46	ovareian	ovarian
47	purulent	puralent
48	prostrate gland	prostate gland
49	lewkocyte	leukocyte
50	sytotoxic cells	cytotoxic cells

Instructions

The following are common and frequently misspelled words (not entirely in alphabetical order). Key each line twice.

1	accommodate	accidentally	absence
2	accompanying	acknowledgment	achieve
3	acquaintance	acquisition	advantage
4	affidavit	aggressive	aging
5	all right	already	amateur
6	analogous	analysis	apparatus
7	approximate	assistance	auxiliary
8	basically	beginning	believe
9	beneficiary	benefited	biased
10	brochure	calendar	calorie
11	canceled	carriage	catalog
12	chronological	changeable	census
13	coincidence	colossal	commitment
14	committee	connoisseur	condor
15	conscience	conscientious	conscious
16	consensus	consistent	continuous

17 controversy	convenience	deficit
18 definite	descendant	develop
19 development	disappoint	disastrous
20 dissatisfied	dissimilar	discipline
21 either	eliminate	emphasize
22 entrepreneur	environment	enumerate
23 exaggerate	exceed	excellent
24 exercise	exhaustible	exhilarate
25 existence	exonerate	exorbitant
26 extraordinary	eyeing	familiar
27 February	fluorescent	financier
28 forbade	foresee	forfeit
29 gauge	government	gray/grey
30 grievous	gruesome	guarantee
31 heterogeneous	hemorrhage	harass
32 indispensable	incidentally	hygiene
33 innocuous	inoculate	insistence
34 irrelevant	laboratory	liable
35 liaison	library	license
36 lien	likable	liquefy
37 maintenance	mediocre	milieu
38 millennium	misapprehension	mischief
39 misspell	necessary	negotiate
40 obsolescent	occasionally	occurrence
41 offense	omission	oneself
42 ophthalmology	opinion	pamphlet
43 parallel	pastime	patience
44 permissible	perseverance	persistent
45 phenomenal	physician	sincerely
46 sizable	specimen	surgeon
47 susceptible	temperature	technique
48 their	through	unctuous
49 unforgettable	vacillate	Wednesday
50 weird	wholly	yield

Instructions

Divide the following medical words. Check your dictionary or medical dictionary for division of unfamiliar words.

Rule:

Word division is a complex subject. Generally:

✔ try to leave at least three letters at the end of a line, hyphenate, and take three to the next line. Divide words between syllables only.

✔ try not to divide the last word of the paragraph at the bottom of the page
✔ avoid keying more than two hyphens in a row at the right edge of a paragraph
✔ do not divide proper names, abbreviations, or the number from a street name in an address
✔ do not divide words of five or fewer letters

1	aphasia	16	ultraviolet
2	atheroma	17	sympathectomy
3	cephalalgia	18	mesentery
4	encephaloma	19	euphoria
5	hyperemesis	20	ova
6	deaf	21	necrosis
7	circumscribed	22	claustrophobia
8	ossify	23	paranephritis
9	psychiatrist	24	pharyngitis
10	gingivitis	25	iridalgia
11	uremia	26	plasmapheresis
12	postpartum	27	bronchiectasis
13	febrile	28	leukapheresis
14	sclerectomy	29	retroperitoneal
15	precancerous	30	urethritis

Instructions

Key each phrase below, using a slash (/) to show how it should be divided.

1 2409 Fleetwood Street.
2 2056 Bush Avenue
3 can't, won't
4 page 32, page 40
5 12:15 p.m.
6 ova
7 ovum
8 deaf
9 CMS
10 FICA
11 UNICEF
12 USA
13 3 o'clock
14 B.A.

Charlie is a healthy individual who is employed at Dale's	12
Shop. Prior to the injury of his right ring finger, he had no	23
problems with his right hand. On the date of injury, his	34
right ring finger got caught between a saw and a brick, which	45
caused amputation of the right ring finger. He was taken to	56
Mobile Hospital where he was evaluated, and an attempt was	67
made to replant the finger but this was not possible. He	78
was, subsequently, followed at Laveen and continued to work	89
in a modified status. In June 2001, he began to have numb-	100
ness and tingling in the thumb, index, and middle fingers of	111
the right hand. There was concern about whether or not he	122
might have carpal tunnel syndrome. He did undergo a	132
Celestone injection at Laveen but with no significant benefit.	144
His pain began to slowly worsen, and he desired a second	155
evaluation and treatment. He complained of a sensation of	166
tightness at the site of the amputation. He had pain in the	177
amputated finger site that radiated up into his shoulder.	188
He noticed color change and swelling. He was initially	199
treated nonoperatively and there was some improvement in his	210
symptoms. He continued to have hypersensitivity at the	221
amputation site suggestive of possible neuroma formation, as	232
well as the development of a hypertrophic scar. He underwent	244
a bone scan on September 9, 2001, which revealed no evidence	256
of dystrophy. However, there was evidence of a right fourth	267
digit neuroma.	270

▭▭▭▭1▭▭▭▭2▭▭▭▭3▭▭▭▭4▭▭▭▭5▭▭▭▭6▭▭▭▭7▭▭▭▭8▭▭▭▭9▭▭▭▭10▭▭▭▭11▭▭▭▭12

Eponyms and Acronyms, Five-Minute Timed Writing

Goals

After completing this lesson, you will be able to:

✔ Capitalize eponyms.
✔ Capitalize acronyms.

Note: The trend is to omit the possessive form of eponyms. Examples of eponyms: Alzheimer disease, Tourette syndrome, Down syndrome, Bell palsy.

Acronyms are keyed in all capital letters. Examples of acronyms: GERD, TURP, ESRD, AIDS.

Instructions

Key the following sentences, capitalizing the eponyms and key in acronyms in all capital letters.

1 A foley catheter was inserted in the urinary tract.
2 The 76-year-old man is suffering from alzheimer disease and bell palsy.
3 Dr. Robert Frome used the chamberlen forceps to assist with the delivery of the baby girl.
4 The mri scan revealed a lesion on her left lung.
5 Several drugs are used to treat aids: one is zdv.

CAPITALIZATION

Do not capitalize words derived from personal and geographic names when they have a special meaning or when they are used as an adjective, as in the gram-negative bacteria and pasteurization.

Personal example: My aunt has an appointment at the clinic. Aunt is not capitalized.

Geographic names: french fries.

Use lowercase for disease names except when there are eponyms in the name. Example of lowercase diseases: chickenpox, mumps, and measles.

Capitalize eponyms. Do not capitalize common nouns, adjectives, and prefixes that follow the eponym.

Example of eponyms: Alzheimer disease, Down syndrome and Tinel sign.

The trend is to omit the possessive form of all eponyms.

Virus names are not capitalized unless an eponym is with the virus name. Example: Epstein-Barr virus, Marburg virus, Norwalk virus, and Ebola virus.

EPONYMS

An eponym is a name derived from a person's name. To find an eponymous term in the dictionary, look up the second term first. (For "Foley catheter," look up "catheter," then "Foley.") Key the following eponyms.

1 Addison anemia
2 Babinski reflex
3 Bravais-Jacksonian epilepsy
4 Pfannenstiel incision
5 Glisson capsule
6 Wilms tumor
7 Down syndrome
8 Alzheimer disease
9 Bowman glands
10 Bell palsy
11 McMurray test
12 Cushing syndrome
13 Colles fracture
14 Dupuytren contracture

ACRONYMS

An acronym is a word formed from the first letter or letters of several words of a compound term. Acronyms are keyed in uppercase letters. Key each acronym and the words from which it is derived.

1 FDA (Food and Drug Administration)
2 MRI (magnetic resonance imaging)
3 CPR (cardiopulmonary resuscitation)
4 NSAID (nonsteroidal anti-inflammatory drug)
5 WBC (white blood cell or white blood count)
6 CBC (complete blood count)
7 SOAP (Subjective Objective Assessment Plan)
8 RICE (Rest Ice Compression Elevation)
9 CABG (coronary artery bypass graft)
10 CNS (central nervous system)
11 CT (computerized tomography)
   CAT (computerized axial tomography)
12 PET (positron emission tomography)
13 DSA (digital subtraction angiography)
14 SPECT (single photon emission tomography)
15 DVI (digital vascular imaging)
16 PDR (Physicians' Desk Reference)
17 LEEP (loop electrocautery excision)

18 TUMT (transurethral microwave thermotherapy)
19 RFA (radio frequency catheter ablation)
20 ARMD (age-related macular degeneration)

FIVE-MINUTE TIMING—DOUBLE SPACE

```
        The father is a 30-year-old male who has heart disease      11
for which he takes nitroglycerin.  He had a positive tuber-         22
culin skin test with a negative chest x-ray over a year ago,        33
for which he was treated with INH.  The children in the             44
family were not skin tested.  The mother is 25 years old, and       56
had a cholecystectomy at age 22 for a stone impacted in the         67
common bile duct.                                                   70

        There are two siblings, brothers, ages 9 and 2.  The        81
9-year-old is mentally retarded of unknown etiology.  The           92
2-year-old had neonatal jaundice that was said to be secondary     104
to an incompatibility between the mother and child's blood         115
types.  He has had no further problems with jaundice.  There       127
is no other heart disease, kidney disease, epilepsy, anemia,       138
or clotting disturbances.  There have been no children who         149
died in infancy or childhood.                                      155

        There is no known gastrointestinal or liver disease.       166
There is a history of diabetes mellitus in the maternal            177
grandmother and during the mother's gestation.  The father         188
is an engineer who is on disability because of heart disease.      200
The mother is an attorney.                                         205
```

□□□□1□□□□2□□□□3□□□□4□□□□5□□□□6□□□□7□□□□8□□□□9□□□□10□□□□11□□□□12

Instructions

If you finish before time is up, start over. Proofread and circle errors. Double space. Determine gross words per minute for the timing.

Genus Names

Goals

After completing this lesson, you will be able to:

✔ Capitalize and use the initial for the name of a genus.

Rule:

Capitalize the initial for the genus name. Do not capitalize species name.

Example:

M. bovis

Instructions

Key the following sentences, correctly applying the above rule.

1 The patient is suffering from n. meningitidis.
2 Several people contracted s. enteritidis from the food served at the picnic.
3 The infant has pneumonia and h. influenzae.
4 X-rays showed m. tuberculosis in both lungs.

Names with Single Letters

Goals

After completing this lesson, you will be able to:

✔ Capitalize names with single letters.

Instructions

Key the following sentences, capitalizing both the name and the single letter following it.

1 The diagnosis is australian x disease.
2 Dr. Paulette Sampson performed a roux-en-y jejunal loop incision.
3 She was given cytosar-u for leukemia.
4 Discharge medications are: micro-k and pen-vee k.
5 Be sure to pick up slow-k, vira a, and wyamine e at the pharmacy.

Names of Instruments, Five-Minute Timed Writing

Goals

After completing this lesson, you will be able to:

✔ Capitalize eponymous names of instruments.

Instructions

Key the following sentences, capitalizing eponymous names of instruments.

1 Order one bailey-morse knife.
2 The laboratory assistant autoclaved the bard-parker dermatome.
3 A demonstration will be given on the wolf-schindler gastroscope.
4 Dr. Charles Protein is using a calhoun-merz needle.
5 A glisson sling will be used for the left arm.

FIVE-MINUTE TIMING—DOUBLE SPACE

This girl has had recurrent acute throat infections with	12
joint and limb pain. She has been taking penicillin daily.	23
There has been no joint pain since August, but she still has	35
sore throats.	37
This patient is a well-developed, well-nourished 10-	48
year-old girl who does not appear acutely ill. Head:	58
negative. Ears: negative. Nose: open and clear. Pharynx:	69
chronically inflamed. Throat: Chronically inflamed tonsils	80
and adenoids. Cervical adenopathy. Chest: clear to ausculta-	92
tion and percussion. Heart: not enlarged; no murmurs.	102
Abdomen: negative.	105

□□□□1□□□□2□□□□3□□□□4□□□□5□□□□6□□□□7□□□□8□□□□9□□□□10□□□□11□□□□12

Proofreading and Capitalization, Five-Minute Timed Writing

Goals

After completing this lesson, you will be able to:

✔ Proofread accurately.
✔ Use proofreader's marks.

The proofreading stage is the final chance to catch errors before releasing a document, so it is important to proofread slowly and carefully. You must check for many types of errors: spelling, grammatical, typographical, formatting, and words incorrectly divided. Read right to left for typographical errors. The following are proofreader's marks.

Capitalize	(Cap) or ≡	alzheimer
Close up	⌢	oss ify
Delete	✗	feebrile
Insert	∧	ultrviolet
Move left	⊏	⊏ This patient
Move right	⊐	⊐ This patient
Lowercase	(lc) or /	The Psychiatrist
Subscript	∧	H2O
Superscript	∨	Footnote 3
New Paragraph	¶	¶ This patient
Spell out	○ or (sp)	The (2) patients
Let it stand	(stet) or . . .	The two patients
Add a space	(#)	Thetwo patients
Transpose	∼	hte two patients
Add quotation marks	⌄" ⌄"	The doctor said, "She is well."
Add comma	⌄	The doctor who is . . .
Add period	⊙	. . . to the room She then
Add semicolon	⌄;	. . . yesterday therefore . . .
Add colon	⌄:	. . . two things first
Add hyphen	⁼∧	word dividing hyphen
Set italic	_____	this patient
Set bold	∼∼∼	this patient

Instructions

Insert the correct proofreader's marks in the following exercise:

1	Insert	She is ick.
2	Close up	to gether
3	Transpose	recieve
4	Add a space	put on thefloor
5	Delete	medications is/are
6	Lower case	Hemoglobin
7	Move to the left	Her appointment is at 2:15 p.m.
8	Move to the right	He is an excellent physician for dermatology.
9	Superscript	101o temperature
10	Let it stand	Goiter is enlarged.
11	Paragraph	Suture class is at 6 p.m.
12	Capitalize	hiv positive
13	Add comma	The patient who had surgery is named George.
14	Add colon	Please buy towels; lotion; and bandages.
15	Add hyphen	The hyphen is a word dividing mark.
16	Add period	He's gone
17	Set italic	You should have given this patient the medication!
18	Add quotation marks	Did he say, All is well?
19	Set bold	Refer to Section 426 of the manual.
20	Add semicolon	She's graduated therefore, she's working now.
21	Spell out	B/P

Instructions

Key the following sentences *with* the errors, then proofread and use proofreader's marks. Correct the errors from the copy you have marked.

1 Thept is afour month old baby boy.
2 The temperature was one ten degrees
3 The bold count was elevated
4 There has been a sor throat and cough.
5 I heard no riles upon examination.
6 The baby had just been discharged from the hopital to home.
7 He recieved antebiotics for 1 week.
8 Upon sischarge she had been taking laseen.
9 I consulted with her pedatrician Dr. heart.
10 The cry was somewhat coarse.
11 I would obtain an cardiogram on Nonday.
12 His height is 68".

13 Please put the check in the en velope.

14 Doctor john sampson will shcedule appointments on mon and fri.

15 contact the pt immediately.

16 she is in seriou condition with neumonia.

17 mrs. murrays' ven is hand to find.

18 She is a specialist in sichiatry.

19 dr athea sampson who is a cardiothoracic surgeon performed sugery yesterday on a thiry two year old lady.

20 Patient remainied stable on medications tht had been institued in ccu following a holter monitor survey,.

21 Patient was discharted on may 14,

22 The patient is su ferring from arterial hypertension and is being advised from the physician to lose witht and red uce fat in his diet.

23 Schedule the patient on monday for a cardiac mri and called the physician immediately with the results.

24 sgot and sgpt are enzyme tests that can be used for the liver.

25 Dr. mark was consulted and the patient was transferred to the ccu.

Instructions

Key the paragraph below *with* the errors. Then proofread and prepare a final, corrected copy.

1   This sixty-year-old lady was admetted with

2 fever, vomitting, tachypnea, tachcardia, diarrhea

3 and leukocytosis follwing approximately a weak of

4 flu-like syndrome, Whe had been under treatment

5 for colitis for 3 yeras.

6   There is also hostory of streak 4 years prior

7 to this admission with complete recoverey from a

8 left-sided paralysyst. On admission her lungs

9 were clear. Patient reamined stable on

10 medications. Diagnositc testing: Admitting cbc

11 fourteen thoused, wbc fifteen thousand two

12 hundred hematocrit fort bun eight.

13   Electrocardiogram on admission showed

14 tachycardia. Chest X-ray on admission showed

15 cardiomegaly.

16   Pt discharged from the hoptial to home on

17 june 12

Instructions

Key the paragraph below with errors. Then proofread and prepare a final, corrected copy.

```
      The patient is a 25-year-old- hispanic male with left-      11
sided weekness.  Two evenings ago, the patient developed          22
sudden onset of dizzimess, and vertigo which lasted several       33
minutes.  He also developed timgling and weekness in the          44
left arm and leg.  This left-sided weakness gradually clared       56
overnight; although, he still says his left arm fatigues          67
with exertion.  At that time, the patient had a headache          78
which was not severe.                                             82

      The patiemt had no head trauna; although, he had a          93
bruise on his head.  The patient was not sleep deprived, and     105
he was not abusing medications.  The patient has had head-       116
aches and sore neck muscles while driving his truck.  The        127
patient is a chromic stutterer.  There is no other serious       138
illness.  His mother suffers from migraime headaches.            148

      Gate is normal.  ct scan with contrast is normal.          159
Cervical spime and skull x-rays are negative.  eeg is normal.    171
Electrolits and liver function tests are normal.  The patient    183
had a tia in the cerebral artery.  The patient should be         194
placed on medications.                                           198
```

□□□□1□□□□2□□□□3□□□□4□□□□5□□□□6□□□□7□□□□8□□□□9□□□□10□□□□11□□□□12

CAPITALIZATION

Goals

After completing this lesson, you will be able to:

✔ Use capitalization

Capital Letters

Instructions

Capitalize the first word of every sentence.

Example: 1. There are no heaves, thrills, or murmurs.

Capitalize proper nouns.

A proper noun names a person, place, or thing.

Examples:

Names of persons: Robert, Anita, Parry, Lisa, Mr. Moss, Mrs. Young, Dr. Mary Sampson, Evie Sampson, MD, Matthew Thomas Sampson, MD

Names of places: San Diego, China, Mobile, Arizona, France, Mobile Hospital

Names of things: Zocor capsule, Aquaplast splint, Ann Arbor clamp, Vistec sponge, Tuke saw, Pugh nail

Capitalize geographic names.

Examples:

the Bay Area, Pacific Ocean, Gulf of Mexico, Lake Erie, the West Coast, San Diego County, Stone Mountain, Third World, Hoover Dam, Mississippi River

---

Capitalize holidays, days of the week, the months, and calendar events.

Examples:

Easter, Hanukkah, Fourth of July, September, New Year's Eve, Friday, Yom Kippur, Kwanza, Passover, Thanksgiving Day, Holy Week, Cinco de Mayo, October

Capitalize trade names of drugs. Do not capitalize generic names.

The drug company and the United States Adopted Names Council give the generic name. Generic drug names are keyed in lowercase letters.

The Food and Drug Administration selects the trade name for the drug. The first letter of trade-name drugs is capitalized.

Examples: Trade names of drugs. Generic names are in parentheses.

Valium (diazepam)

Prilosec (omeprazole)

Premarin (estrogen)

Trimox (amoxicillin)

Zocor (simvastatin)

Instructions

Key the following sentences and underline words that should be capitalized.

1 i think that an emg conduction study will work on that ulnar nerve.

2 This 58-year-old caucasian male is admitted to the hospital because of pain in the left shoulder.

3 In october of 2005, he was started on digoxin and nitroglycerin tablets.

4 He was treated with radiation therapy during the past year at the va hospital in phoenix, arizona.

5 the patient was rehydrated with iv fluids and was started on iron therapy with ferrous sulfate.

6 A follow-up ct scan performed prior to mary's discharge from the hospital indicated rather marked destruction of temporal lobes bilaterally.

7 mrs. smith does remark that she does not feel that nanci hears well.

8 behavioral audiometry is planned in the future by dr moss.

9 Initial evaluation at mobile emergency department revealed chloride 100, potassium 2, and bun 16.

10 An aterial blood gas revealed PH 7.43, with a base excess of -2.2.

The patient is a 50-year-old male who presented at the	11
hospital in a semicoma state. He had overdosed on Tylenol	22
with Codeine and had ingested large quantities of alcohol.	33
He was seen and treated by the emergency department physician.	45
He was treated with ipecac syrup and had an episode of emesis.	57
He was admitted to the ICU for observation. The patient had	68
a blood alcohol level of 250. The patient is very drowsy but	80
is readily aroused and does not respond rationally and co-	91
herently but immediately drops off to sleep again.	101

He had a severe injury in a car accident two months ago,	113
at which time, he had amputation of his right forearm and an	125
above-knee amputation of the right leg. The patient states	136
he has been well and has had no serious illnesses or other	147
surgery.	149

The patient has been depressed, resulting in his present	161
admission. At the present time, the patient also complains	172
of severe discomfort and pain in his right lower stump and	183
pains in his right upper extremity.	191

I have discussed with the patient healing of the above-	203
knee amputation before prosthesis can be fitted. He has	214
agreed to call me next week and come into the Brown's	224
Rehabilitation Center and begin therapy. I have asked him	235
if he would be willing to participate in an inpatient program	247
for prosthetic.	250

☐☐☐☐1☐☐☐☐2☐☐☐☐3☐☐☐☐4☐☐☐☐5☐☐☐☐6☐☐☐☐7☐☐☐☐8☐☐☐☐9☐☐☐☐10☐☐☐☐11☐☐☐☐12

Mechanics II—Grammar and Punctuation

Nouns, Five-Minute Timed Writing

Goals

After completing this lesson, you will be able to:

✔ Identify nouns.

Rule:

Nouns:

✔ A sentence must have a subject and a verb that expresses a complete thought. The subject of a sentence names a person, place, or thing. The subject is a noun or pronoun.
 A person: nurse, doctor, child, woman, Dr. Sampson
 A place: hospital, office, city, Phoenix, Alaska
 A thing: forceps, otoscope, stethoscope, computer, cardiogram

Punctuation Review

Rule:

End punctuation and abbreviations:

✔ space twice after a period at the end of a sentence
✔ do not space after a period that ends a line
✔ use a period after most abbreviations; this varies
✔ use a period after an initial
✔ do not space after a period within abbreviations

Example:

A lipoma is a fatty tumor. Subject is lipoma. This is a complete sentence.

Incomplete thought: A fatty tumor. More information is needed for a complete sentence.

Instructions

Key and underline the following sentences. If the words do not form a sentence, do not underline.

1 The father has heart disease
2 The thyroid was enlarged.
3 Child with diabetes.
4 Bertie takes nitroglycerin daily.
5 This female developed acute bronchitis associated with dry cough and back pain.

Instructions

Key the following sentences, underlining only those words that function as nouns.

1 During the winter, Ruth worked on her research study.
2 The physician lectured on AIDS at Columbia University.
3 The doctors flew to California for the symposium.
4 Kim was promoted to radiology secretary.
5 After a trip to Atlanta University, Roosevelt accepted the otolaryngology residency position.
6 Parry showed his medical card to the receptionist.
7 Karen was admitted to Mobile Medical Clinic for a diagnostic test.
8 The temporal bone class will be in Brown Hall on Saturday morning.
9 This young female with Tourette syndrome was admitted today after an episode of hemoptysis.

Proper Nouns

A proper noun names a person, place, or thing, and begins with a capital letter.

Example:

Names of persons: Anita Young, Grayelin Young Jr.

Names of places: Mobile Hospital, San Diego, CA

Names of things: Western blot, Tagamet pill

Instructions

Key the following sentences, underlining the proper nouns twice and other nouns once.

1 Dr. Jean Sampson teaches at Mobile University, but she is a research assistant in the afternoon.
2 Mrs. Mary Leukocyte purchased a new CT scan for the clinic.
3 Dr. Beach recommended Mary because of her honesty and excellent attendance.
4 The patient, Bob, lives in Yuma, Arizona.
5 Mrs. James Rubin has a history of hypertension and diabetes.
6 Mary and Sheree went to the medical library on Bush Street in San Francisco.
7 The secretary wrote a letter of congratulations to the president of the medical society in Chicago, Illinois.
8 The Dodson Radiology Medical Group is moving to Arizona in the spring.
9 The dietitian spoke at a meeting of the Red Cross in New York.
10 Dr. Frank and Dr. Berger will join the medical staff for a luncheon.

This 45-year-old black man has severe chronic obstructive   12
pulmonary disease and has been followed by Dr. Deary. He is   23
in the outpatient clinic for a gastrointestinal workup and   34
abdominal pain. His pulmonary status has been stable and   45
cardiac arrhythmias have not been a major problem since the   56
patient was switched from Lopressor to verapamil. Currently,   67
he is coughing up small amounts of nonpurulent mucus and   78
states that his breathing is stable. He does become short of   89
breath while walking a short distance and is unable to climb   100
stairs. Recent medications have included prednisone and an   111
Alupent nebulizer inhaler, which the patient states makes   122
him sick to his stomach. Digoxin has been discontinued, and   133
he is taking Theo-Dur. The patient is allergic to penicillin   145
and Demerol.   147

He is currently denying any cephalgia or changes in   158
hearing. His vision is fair to poor. He is not aware of any   170
chest pain. The abdominal pain is in the midline, is severe   181
at times, and does not seem to be related to eating. He   192
denies any difficulty passing urine. His mild ankle edema is   204
relieved by intermittent use of Oretic.   212

The patient is a well-developed, adequately nourished   223
gentleman who appears somewhat older than his stated age.   234
He is alert and oriented. He is afebrile. Expiratory   245
wheezes are heard bilaterally. The right nipple is somewhat   257
irritated and crusted. The abdomen is benign to palpation   268
with healed surgical incisions. The patient's medications   279
will be continued, and, hopefully, he will not experience an   291
exacerbation of his wheezing.   297

☐☐☐☐1☐☐☐☐2☐☐☐☐3☐☐☐☐4☐☐☐☐5☐☐☐☐6☐☐☐☐7☐☐☐☐8☐☐☐☐9☐☐☐☐10☐☐☐☐11☐☐☐☐12

Pronouns, Five-Minute Timed Writing

Goals

After completing this lesson, you will be able to:

✔ Identify pronouns.

Rule:

✔ A pronoun is a substitute for nouns

Pronouns

us	him	yours	me	my	mine	myself
them	I	you	he	she	it(s)s	yourself
theirs	we	they	some	every	who	itself
their	which	that	what	this	that	yourselves
himself	such	whoever	his	her	their	themselves

Possessive pronouns show ownership. Possessive pronouns are: my, your, his, her, their, our, its.

Combinations with *-self* and *-selves* are also pronouns (such as *himself* and *themselves*).

Example: <u>He</u> attended the diabetic conference.

Instructions

Key the following sentences, underlining each pronoun.

1. The patient had her throat sprayed with Cetacaine.
2. Her rugal folds were normal.
3. The physician prepared his manuscript on AIDS in the United States.
4. We prepared the patient for the endoscopy.
5. Her esophagus was examined, and its entire length was normal.
6. They drove the patient and his mother to the emergency room.
7. We received their x-rays yesterday.
8. The physician showed them how to administer her anesthetic.
9. You may have hemorrhoids, and he may recommend surgery.
10. The doctor may prescribe pain medication; she will instruct you how to care for yourself.

Key the following sentences. Underline the nouns twice and the pronouns once.

1   The nurse took your temperature to check for fever.
2   The endoscope was withdrawn and no abnormalities were seen.
3   Her throat is sore, and she feels groggy from the anesthesia.
4   He will assume his official duties next week.
5   Antibiotics are given to control a bacterial infection.
6   She canceled her mammogram appointment until next week.
7   She said, "You are at risk for pneumonia."
8   They released the medical records without authorization.
9   Gila Clinic provided many services for his bypass operation.
10   We reviewed their diagnostic tests and medical history.

Objective Pronouns

Objective pronouns are: them, it, him, her, you, us, me. Objective pronouns are used as direct objects and indirect objects of verbs.

Example:

She will buy them tomorrow.

Instructions

Key the following sentences. Underline the pronoun, choosing the correct pronoun.

1   Did you give (I, us) the x-rays from Dr. George?
2   The surgeon will ask (her, me) to cough.
3   The physician will give (your, you) the injection.
4   These CT scans were done by (me, I).
5   Please call (her, hers) before you leave the office.
6   Her sister wants to sit between Bob and (me, I).
7   Is this lab report for (him, he)?
8   The doctor wanted (them, they) to continue to exercise.
9   Check with (they, them) now.
10   The physician interviewed my friend and (me, they).

Robbie was diagnosed as having stage II Wilms tumor on   11
September 10, 2000. He underwent resection of the tumor and   22
a combination of chemotherapy with vincristine and radiation   33
therapy to the tumor bed. He was placed on the Wilms tumor   44
protocol. A routine follow-up x-ray revealed lung metastases   55
on January 16, 2001. A follow-up chest x-ray revealed that   66
the metastases had grown in spite of recent courses of   76
vincristine. Because of the aggressive nature of the tumor,   87
a new plan of therapy was instituted. Robbie was to start   98
on the drug after an evaluation of other sites of metastases.   110
Vital signs were normal. Robbie was in no distress.   120

On the day of admission, the CT scan of the liver was   131
obtained because of a prior liver scan which was suspicious   142
for a tumor. The CT scan revealed multiple hepatic   152
metastases. Robbie's blood counts were too low to start the   164
therapy. For this reason, he was treated with IV antibiotics   176
for two days prior to the start of chemotherapy. Chest x-rays   188
revealed growth of the metastatic lesions, but follow-up chest   200
films revealed decrease in size of the metastases. Other than   212
difficulty with IV therapy, Robbie tolerated the chemotherapy   224
very well. Because of Robbie's metastases, surgical therapy   236
is not feasible. The plan is to try to shrink the metastatic   248
lesion of the liver and lungs with chemotherapy and radiation.   260
The parents appear to understand the situation. The patient   272
was discharged to the care of his family. They received   283
strict instructions to call if he runs a fever or appears ill.   295
He will be followed in hematology services.   303

□□□□1□□□□2□□□□3□□□□4□□□□5□□□□6□□□□7□□□□8□□□□9□□□□10□□□□11□□□□12

Verbs, Five-Minute Timed Writing

Goals

After completing this lesson, you will be able to:

✔ Recognize verbs in sentences.

Rule:

Verbs:

✔ A verb is a word that expresses action or state of being. Almost every sentence has a subject and a verb.

Example: They <u>attended</u> the radiology conference in San Francisco.

Instructions

Key the following sentences, underlining the verbs.

1 A myelogram is an x-ray of the spinal cord.
2 She took large doses of penicillin for infection.
3 The patient was distressed and febrile for several days.
4 Initial evaluation revealed cardiomegaly.
5 The patient's blood pressure was elevated, and she was treated with antihypertensive medication.
6 She has had dyspnea and migraine headaches.
7 The patient underwent a biopsy for a lesion that was removed from the left breast.
8 He is currently on chemotherapy.
9 Examination of her bladder was within normal limits.
10 Sally will receive methotrexate treatment today.

Instructions

Key the following sentences. Underline the word functioning as a noun once and the verb twice.

1 This boy is very quiet, but he is not depressed.
2 She is in a special education class and enjoys jogging and working on her computer.
3 The boy is experiencing more weakness and has increasing difficulty with self-feeding.
4 She has a rash on her arms and is being treated with Keri lotion.
5 The patient is taking no medication and reports occasional constipation.
6 Ultrasound showed multiple gallstones.

7   Cholangiograms were taken and no cholelithiasis was found.

8   The patient is not very cooperative in giving a history.

9   The patient is lethargic, subdued, and not delusional.

10   She denied vomiting, fever, and constipation.

Subject and Verb Agreement

Instructions

Verbs must agree with subjects in person and number. If the subject is singular, the verb should be singular.

Example:

I prefer to pay my hospital bills by VISA.

"I" is the subject and "prefer" is the verb.

If the subject is plural, use a plural verb.

Example:

Mary and Grayelin are working for Dr. Smith.

"Mary," "Grayelin" are subjects and "are" is the plural verb.

Key the following sentences. Select the correct verb in parentheses.

1   She (was, were) at the hospital.

2   Judy and John (is, are) returning for a MRI.

3   Where (is, are) the pathology reports?

4   Motrin and Valium (was, were) prescribed.

5   The patient (were, was) taken to surgery for an arthroplasty.

6   The physical examination (show, shows) erythroderma.

7   She (was, were) treated with chemotherapy.

8   A patient (was seen, were seen) with the complaint of asthma.

9   You and I (have, has) been selected to participate in a pain study.

10   There (were, was) two residents in the clinic.

Rule:

Helping verbs express such things as ability or possibility and are joined to the main verb in a sentence. Some common helping verbs are have, can, could, may, might, shall, and will.

Example: He has <u>decreased</u> hearing bilaterally.

Instructions

Key and underline the main verbs in the sentences below.

1   His hemoglobin had fallen to 9.5 g.

2   He was discharged last week on Theo-Dur 300 mg b.i.d.

3   The patient was placed on bed rest and I.V. fluid.

4   Bob has a negative family history for heart disease.

5   Rhonci were heard throughout the chest.

John, a 62-year-old male who was seen at the request of   11
Dr. Corn, complained of a sore right foot. The patient stated   23
that his right foot had always been painful, and he had   34
previously been treated palliatively by a podiatrist. His   45
left foot also gave him discomfort but to a lesser degree.   56

The patient's chief complaint consisted of thickened   67
and enlarged toenails, especially the right hallux nail. The   79
patient's toenails are hypertrophied, extending in dorsal and   91
lateral planes. The patient's left hallux toenail is also   102
dystrophic and hypertrophied and extending in a dorsal plane.   114
The diagnosis is onychomyosis. All toenails were markedly   125
hypertrophied and complicated with mycotic infections.   136
Treatment is conservative debridement bilaterally with   147
Betadine solution and dressing. The patient is a pleasant   158
man in no distress.   162

□□□□1□□□□2□□□□3□□□□4□□□□5□□□□6□□□□7□□□□8□□□□9□□□□10□□□□11□□□□12

Adjectives and Plurals, Adjective Suffixes, and Five-Minute Timed Writing

Goals

After completing this lesson, you will be able to:

✔ Recognize adjectives.
✔ Form plurals of medical terms.
✔ Recognize adjective suffixes.

Adjective Suffixes

See the medical dictionary for adjective suffixes. Adjective suffixes describe a word root.

The suffixes below are adjective endings.

Suffix	Example	Definition
-ac	cardiac	pertaining to the heart
-al	cecal	of or like the cecum
-ar	ulnar	relating to the ulna
-ary	urinary	relating to, occurring in urine
-form	villiform	having the form of a villi
-ic	bulimic	of, relating to bulimia
-ical	anatomical	of or relating to the anatomy
-ile	febrile	pertaining to fever
-ive	addictive	causing or characterized by addiction
-ous	venous	characterized by veins
-oid	fibroid	resembling, forming a tumor
-ory	stimulatory	relating to a stimulant

Key the adjective suffixes and nouns in the following assignment.

1 bucca
2 biogenic
3 angina
4 malar
5 sterile
6 oat-cell
7 uremia
8 retina
9 retinal

10 thorax

Example:

The patient has advanced chronic obstructive pulmonary disease.

Underline tha adjective suffixes in the sentences below.

1 This 87-year-old black female patient has arteriosclerotic heart disease.

2 This Caucasian male had a perforated duodenal ulcer.

3 The patient was treated with intravenous fluids.

4 The patient underwent an endoscopic carpal tunnel release of the right hand.

5 Mary enters the hospital for a vaginal hysterectomy.

6 She is on hypertensive medication.

7 The patient is a cachectic woman in acute distress.

8 The prognosis is poor for this woman with advanced metastatic carcinoma.

9 The patient has been treated for congestive heart failure.

10 He gives a history of having a myocardial infarction.

Adjectives

Rule:

An adjective describes a noun or pronoun. The adjective qualifies *what kind of* noun or pronoun, *which* noun or pronoun, or *how many* nouns or pronouns. See the following examples (the adjectives are in **bold**): **cardiology** office, **busy** place, **medical** record; **this** CT scanner, **that** echogram, **these** hematology reports; **one** x-ray, **several** patients, **30** Valiums.

The articles *a, an,* and *the* are also used as adjectives even though they are different from typical adjectives.

Example: The physician prescribed 30 mg of Prevacid.

Instructions

Key the following sentences. Underline the words that function as adjectives in the following sentences.

1 The arthroscopic procedure is used to diagnose knee problems.

2 The patient had one chest x-ray taken last Tuesday.

3 Those radiology books are located in the library.

4 An interested doctor will provide treatment for her serious problem.

5 Several residents assisted the surgeon with a radial keratotomy.

6 The information you requested on musculofascial disease can be found in the bookcase.

7 Dr. David Rad will be the graduation speaker for Mobile University School of Medicine.

8 All the medical transcriptionists met to learn about the new computer.

9   The patient is an obese female who was admitted to the hospital with severe abdominal pain.

10 The evaluation failed to show any evidence of a malignant lesion.

Singular and Plural Endings

Instructions

Use the following table for singular and plural endings. Use your medical dictionary if you need help.

Forming Plurals

Singular Ending		*Plural Ending*	
a	vertebra	ae	vertebrae
u	cornu	ua	cornua
us	bronchus	i	bronchi
inx	meninx	inges	meninges
um	atrium	a	atria
anx	phalanx	anges	phalanges
oma	lipoma	omata	lipomata
on	spermatozoon	a	spermatozoa
is	crisis	es	crises
ix	varix	ices	varices
ma	stigma	mata	stigmata
en	lumen	ina	lumina
ax	thorax	aces	thoraces

Singular ending:

Example: The diagno*sis* is bronchopneumonia.

Plural ending:

Example: His skin showed no rash or petechi*ae*.

Key the following sentences, choosing the singular or plural form as appropriate.

1   The patient was admitted with (carcinoma, carcinomas) of the brain, liver, spine, and left shoulder.

2   The (ganglion, ganglia) is in the carotid artery.

3   The patient is suffering from (encephalitis, encephalitides) of the cerebrum.

4   After surgery, the patient's (crises, crisis) were depression and insomnia.

5   The physician examined his left (naris, nares) and saw a tumor.

6   The (delirium, deliria) was caused by exhaustion.

7   The x-ray of the knee joints showed (bursa, bursae).

8   The swollen left (epididymis, epididymides) caused pain.

9   The (septum, septa) of the heart cavities are blocked.

10 The left and right (bronchi, bronchus) were found to be infected.

Instructions

Key the following sentences, choosing the correct form. Underline plural words, and circle singular words.

1   He has many (ganglia, ganglion) in the brainstem.

2   Two (ilia, ilium) bones were x-rayed yesterday.

3   The (iris, irides) of the left eye is green.

4   The (lunula, lunulae) of her fingernail is sore.

5   Her (maxilla, maxillae) bone of the upper jaw was fractured in an automobile accident.

6   The (meninges, meninx) of the spinal cord has become inflamed.

7   His (nares, naris) are filled with a discharge.

8   The patient has (nephritis, nephritides) of the left kidney as well as hypertension.

9   Several patients have (neuritides, neuritis) that affect the eyeball.

10 Dr. Russell Sampson, the dermatologist, plans to remove three (nevi, nevus) from her neck.

FIVE-MINUTE TIMING—DOUBLE SPACE

```
        This is a 55-year-old male followed by my office with a        11
cardiac pacemaker.  He has pericarditis and coronary artery            22
disease.  The patient has been evaluated for right upper               33
quadrant pain in the past.  He has been evaluated extensively          45
for multiple cardiac problems and has had cardiac catheter-            56
ization, which showed a prolapsing mitral valve.  He has had           67
multiple abdominal evaluations for abdominal pain, including           78
upper GI series, lower GI series, and abdominal CT scan, with          90
no definitive diagnosis.                                               95

        The patient's past history shows a transurethral re-          106
section of the prostate.  In 2002 he had an episode of endo-          117
carditis.  He has had advanced chronic obstructive pulmonary          128
disease since 2002, managed with steroids.  The patient has           139
abdominal discomfort, back pain, and has had a questionable           150
syncopal episodes; She is admitted for further management.            161
There is no abnormal jugular venous distention.  The carotids         173
show good quality upstroke.                                            178

        The extremities show no evidence of phlebitis or edema.       189
The admitting electrocardiogram shows a pattern of atrial             200
fibrillation.  Because of a questionable cardiac arrest               211
situation, I would repeat an electrocardiogram, serum enzymes,        223
and cardiac monitoring.                                               227
```

□□□□1□□□□2□□□□3□□□□4□□□□5□□□□6□□□□7□□□□8□□□□9□□□□10□□□□11□□□□12

Adverbs, Five-Minute Timed Writing

Goals

After completing this lesson, you will be able to:

✔ Recognize adverbs.

Rule:

✔ An adverb describes a verb, an adjective, or another adverb. Adverbs will tell you when, where, and how.

Examples:

1 The patient was taken to the OR this morning.
   WHERE: OR this morning
2 The patient wsa discharged on September 20, 2005.
   WHEN: discharged on September 20, 2005.
3 The spleen was palpated 2 cm below the left costal margin.
   HOW: palpated below the left costal margin

Instructions

Key the following sentences, underlining the adverbs.

1 The dietitian carefully prepared the menu for the diabetic.
2 Mrs. Weddington humbly accepted the award for working with disabled children.
3 The Radiology Clinic quickly moved to the third floor.
4 Ship the vaccine immediately to the clinic.
5 The audit of the medical office clearly revealed it to be financially independent.
6 We rarely have time to volunteer in the pharmacy.
7 Our medical staff is working efficiently on the cholesterol project.
8 Please return the patients' charts immediately.
9 She was in satisfactory condition after the chondrectomy.
10 As you key the medical reports you must carefully analyze your data.

Conjunctive Adverbs

Conjunctive adverbs describe the relation of the ideas in two clauses. The clauses are separated by a semicolon, and the conjunctive adverb is often followed by a comma.

Rule:

Conjunctive adverbs:

✔ relate main clauses

Some Conjunctive Adverbs

accordingly	furthermore	moreover	similarly
also	hence	namely	still
anyway	however	nevertheless	then
besides	incidentally	next	thereafter
certainly	indeed	nonetheless	therefore
consequently	instead	now	thus
finally	likewise	otherwise	undoubtedly
further	meanwhile		

Instructions

Key the following sentences, underlining the conjunctive adverbs.

1   Her operation was successful; however, she will not be discharged.
2   The medical assistants' meeting was not over until 3:30 p.m.; consequently, we missed the demonstration.
3   You may take the book on pregnancy; however, please return it next week.
4   The doctor presented a lecture on anemia; further, she agreed to discuss it with our staff.
5   The presentation on hearing will be at 10 a.m.; undoubtedly, we will attend.
6   Many nurses were angry that the rules on use of radioactive materials were not being followed; accordingly, we will have another meeting with the technician.
7   Inoculation is ultimately far cheaper than caring for a sick child; nevertheless, many people cannot afford vaccinations.
8   She broke her right arm; furthermore, she fractured her left leg.
9   We will have to run the tests; otherwise, we may be sued.
10 He did not go to the physician; he went to the acupuncturist instead.

This patient was in her usual state of excellent health	11
until a few years ago when she presented for evaluation of	22
hemorrhoids at Mobile Clinic. She underwent a colonoscopy,	33
which revealed several small polyps, and she was told to have	44
a follow-up examination in one year. In 2002, she underwent a	56
colonoscopy examination, and a small adenoma was found in the	68
rectum. Pathology revealed a tubular adenoma, and she was	79
told to have a colonoscopy in one year. Since that time, she	91
has been feeling quite well with normal bowel movements. She	102
takes Perdiem daily, and has no complaints of alteration of	113
her bowel habits. She denies any continued hematochezia.	124
There is no family history of colon cancer. Her past medical	136
history is noncontributory. She is quite healthy with no	147
history of heart disease, lung disease, kidney disease, or	158
liver disease. She has no known drug allergies. She is	169
single, and has a son and daughter. She is a legal secretary.	181
In general, she is a well-appearing woman in no acute	191
distress. Her sclerae are anicteric, and her oropharynx is	202
clear. Her neck is supple with full range of motion, with	213
no thyromegaly or adenopathy. The lungs are clear to	223
ausculation and percussion. Cardiac examination reveals a	234
regular rate and rhythm, without any murmurs, rubs, or	245
gallops. The abdomen is soft and nontender, with no organo-	257
megaly and no masses. The extremities are without edema.	268
I have explained the risks, benefits, and alternatives of a	279
follow-up colonoscopy. If on the other hand, she has one	290
small polyp, one could consider follow-up in three to five	301
years.	302

□□□□1□□□□2□□□□3□□□□4□□□□5□□□□6□□□□7□□□□8□□□□9□□□□10□□□□11□□□□12

Prepositions, Five-Minute Timed Writing

Goals

After completing this lesson, you will be able to:

✔ Recognize prepositions.

Rule:

✔ A preposition is a word that shows relationship to other words in a sentence. A preposition connects a noun, a pronoun, or a word group functioning as a noun to another word in the sentence.

Example: <u>During</u> the morning session, we listened <u>to</u> the diabetic educator.

Prepositions

about	beneath	in spite of	round
above	beside	instead of	since
according to	between	into	through
across	beyond	like	throughout
after	by	near	till
against	concerning	next to	to
along	despite	of	toward
along with	down	off	under
among	during	on	underneath
around	except	onto	unlike
as	except for	out	until
aside from	excepting	out of	up
at	for	outside	upon
because of	from	over	with
before	in	past	within
behind	in addition to	regarding	without
below	inside		

Instructions

Key the following sentences, underlining the prepositions.

1 Tuberculosis is not likely because of the negative skin test results.

2 The bleeding seems to be from an artery.

3 The patient needs to be examined for these lesions.

4 The patient had pneumonia while in the hospital for an appendectomy.

5 This patient has a history of locking of her left knee.

6 She had surgery on her left knee and is in pain.

7 He will return to the clinic in two weeks for evaluation of his hand.

8 I suspect that she will be able to work within six weeks after surgery.

9 On examination he was weak, and he could stand only with support.

10 The patient has no tenderness about the right wrist.

FIVE-MINUTE TIMING—DOUBLE SPACE

Betty M. Tibia is a 16-year-old female who has had re- 11
current episodes of otitis media and tonsillitis for the past 22
several years. She is admitted for a tonsillectomy and 33
adenoidectomy. No past history except for recurring otitis 44
media, upper respiratory infection, and tonsillitis. She has 55
had all her immunizations. No family history of diabetes, 66
tuberculosis, or hypertension. 72

The adenoids were removed with the adenotome and forceps. 84
The soft palate was elevated by placing catheters through 95
each nostril and bringing them out the mouth and holding them 107
tight. Using the forceps, the adenoid tissue could very 118
easily be removed at this time. Inspection with a mirror 129
showed the adenoid tissue to be adequately removed. Bleeding 141
was controlled with sponge pressure. The right ear was first 153
examined; drum was dull. Myringotomy was made anterior to the 165
long arm of the malleus, and a large amount of very thick, 176
gluey material was aspirated from the middle ear. A tube 187
with an attached wire was placed through the myringotomy 198
opening and left in position. A similar procedure was done 209
on the left ear, and a large amount of gluey material was 220
aspirated from the middle ear. A tube was placed in the left 232
myringotomy opening. Sterile cotton was placed in each canal. 244
The patient was in good postoperative condition at the end of 256
the procedure. 259

□□□□1□□□□2□□□□3□□□□4□□□□5□□□□6□□□□7□□□□8□□□□9□□□□10□□□□11□□□□12

Conjunctions, Five-Minute Timed Writing

Goals

After completing this lesson, you will be able to:

✔ Understand and use conjunctions.

Rule

✔ A conjunction is a word that joins together words, sentences, phrases, or clauses.

Conjunctions

and	nor	for	yet	but
or	so	after	because	in order that
than	when	although	before	now that
that	whenever	as	even if	once
though	where	as if	if	rather than
till	whereas	as long as	if only	since
unless	even though	as though	wherever	so that
until	while	both ... and	neither ... nor	either ... or
as ... as	whether ... or	not ... but	not only ... but also	

Example: (word joined is *and*)

Bill and Mary completed the manuscript. A period is at the end of the sentence.

Example: (phrase joined)

During the morning and throughout the night, the surgeon performed an appendectomy. Use a comma after a phrase. During the morning and throughout the night, is a phrase.

Example: (independent clauses)

There has been no joint pain, but she has a sore throat.

Two independent clauses joined by a conjunction make a compound sentence.

Make sure what follows *but* is an independent clause. but: she has a sore throat.

Ask yourself if this is an independent clause. Yes, add the comma before *but*.

Instructions

Key the following sentences, underlining the conjunctions.

1   The patient was seen for a hip problem, and the surgeon recommended a hip replacement.

2   Dr. Jeffey placed ventilation tubes in the ear, so Jerry is feeling better.

3   The diagnosis is severe otitis media, yet the clerk scheduled no appointment.

4   Because of the patient's dizziness, she has been seen by a neurologist.

5   Mary is using a nasal saline solution and will return to the clinic tomorrow.

6   Her left ear revealed inflammation of the tympanic membrane, but the ear canal is also swollen.

7   Rhinoplasty will be performed, but the insurance company has to give authorization before surgery.

8   After the patient had a chest x-ray, his blood tests came back negative.

9   When Charles came to the emergency room with epistaxis, thrombi were removed from his nose.

10 Now that he is on antibiotics, pain medications, and oxygen, the physician will see him tomorrow.

Interjections, Five-Minute Timed Writing

Goals

After completing this lesson, you will be able to:

✔ Understand and use interjections.

An interjection expresses strong feelings. If a sentence ends with strong feelings, end it with an exclamation point.

Example: Call the poison center. Quickly!

Instructions

Key the following sentences, underlining the interjections.

1 Oh! I broke my arm!
2 Well, take the specimen to pathology immediately.
3 Now, your surgery is scheduled for Tuesday.
4 Oh, please hurry!
5 Ah! I understand now!
6 Oh, call a doctor now!
7 Well, you've had a remarkable recovery!
8 Dear me! The emergency room is on fire!
9 Oh, it can be done.
10 Yea, we won!

FIVE-MINUTE TIMING—DOUBLE SPACE

```
        Maria is a 45-year-old white female who fell at home.      11
The patient was taken to the emergency department for evalua-       23
tion and was found to have a fractured left hip and left            34
wrist.  The patient is being admitted to Orthopedic Service         45
where she underwent casting and internal fixation of her hip.       57
The patient developed complications in the postoperative            68
period, including chest pain, diaphoresis, and possible             79
pulmonary embolus.  The patient did have a lung scan that           90
showed no evidence of embolization.  Cardiac enzymes showed         101
no evidence of myocardial infarction.  The EKG revealed a           112
normal sinus rhythm and ventricular tachycardia.  She has           123
maintained normal BUN and creatinine.  Her urinalysis revealed      135
bacteria secondary to a Foley catheter.  The patient was            146
placed on antibiotics for urinary tract infection.  She will        157
have physical therapy to rehabilitate her gait.                     166

        The patient's past medical history includes a cholecyst-    178
ectomy.  The patient also has a history of congestive heart         189
failure and takes Lanoxin.  She does have osteoarthritis of         200
the spine and has been taking Tylenol and Nalfon.                   210

        Family history is negative for diabetes mellitus,           221
tuberculosis, cancer, or heart disease.  She has never had          232
blackouts, seizures, or convulsions.  The patient does have         243
occasional spells of wheezing and is well controlled on Slo-        255
phyllin.  She has no recent weight gain or loss.  The patient       267
is menopausal.                                                      270
```

□□□□1□□□□2□□□□3□□□□4□□□□5□□□□6□□□□7□□□□8□□□□9□□□□10□□□□11□□□□12

FIVE-MINUTE TIMING—DOUBLE SPACE

```
        The patient is a well-developed Caucasian male who          11
appears somewhat older tha his stated age.  He is in no acute       22
distress. He does have difficulty turning his neck and com-         33
plains of pain in the left shoulder.  He is fully alert and         44
oriented.  Vital signs are stable.  Temperature 98.9 degrees,       56
pulse 85, blood pressure 140/70, and respirations 22.  The          67
sclerae are clear.  Conjunctivae are perfused.  Fundoscopic         78
examination is unremarkable.  The ear canals are clear.  The        90
nasal mucosa is erythematous.  An upper denture is present.         101
No pharyngeal masses are encountered.  The neck is erythema-        113
tous on the right side due to his radiation therapy.  He has        125
limited motion of his neck and complains of pain toward the         136
left shooulder.  A few wheezes are heard in the chest.  The         147
abdomen is soft and benign to palpation with no organomegaly.       159
The extremities are without edema, cyanosis, or clubbing.           170
```

□□□□1□□□□2□□□□3□□□□4□□□□5□□□□6□□□□7□□□□8□□□□9□□□□10□□□□11□□□□12

Clauses, Five-Minute Timed Writing

Goals

After completing this lesson, you will be able to:

✔ Recognize dependent clauses.
✔ Recognize independent clauses.

Dependent Clauses with Commas

Rule:

Use a comma after the dependent clause. A clause is a group of words that cannot stand alone. The clause does not express a complete thought. An independent clause is a sentence. A dependent clause may be at the end of a sentence, or it may begin a sentence. Commas are used to separate clauses, phrases, and groups of words. Subordinating conjunctions are used with dependent clauses. Subordinating conjunctions are used with independent clauses to connect the dependent clause. Subordinating conjunctions introduce a dependent clause. A dependent clause can begin a sentence.

Subordinating Conjunctions

when	whenever	that	once
if	as	while	until
because	whereas	where	since
though	before	so	till
after	than	although	so that
for	as if	whether	unless

Dependent Clause

<u>After induction of anesthesia</u> is a dependent clause. The dependent clause is not a sentence. Use a comma after the dependent clause.

After induction of anesthesia, the abdomen was prepared and draped. The dependent clause and independent clause form a complete sentence. The abdomen was prepared and draped. A compete sentence. Independent clause. A dependent clause does not always begin a sentence.

Example:

She attached the report for the intravenous pyelogram results.

Insert commas in the following sentences if needed.

1 If our feelings are confirmed I would suggest initiating chemotherapy on Monday morning.
2 If radiation therapy is indicated it should be started on Saturday.
3 As you know you detected Bob's enlarged liver during a routine examination.
4 I was exhausted after the colonoscopy.
5 When seen last week he had been having enuresis.

Instructions

Key the following dependent clauses, adding an independent clause to complete the sentence.

1 After examining the patient,
2 While you were waiting at the clinic,
3 Although she reports emesis,
4 If her tests are negative,
5 Until her condition improves,
6 So that we can begin treatment,
7 Until I see the physician,
8 Since several months ago,
9 Because of the serious illness,
10 When the surgeon arrived,

Instructions

Key and underline the subordinate clause two times, and underline the main clause one time.

1 Because he suffers from claudication, he will have an examination.
2 Before the patient's aneurysmectomy, he had an infection.
3 Return to the Trauma Service when he is stable.
4 Whose decision was it that he should undergo surgery?
5 After an injection of radiopaque substance, an x-ray is used to locate the tumor.
6 So that you are aware, we plan to use Haldol.
7 Even though Jean is under observation for a rare disorder, she's chipper.
8 After the experimental drug is approved, we'll prescribe it.
9 When this is done, let's go to lunch.
10 Though he had been a heavy smoker, he quit.

Key the following sentences, underlining only independent clauses.

1   After they cleared him for surgery, he was taken to be shaved.
2   Until the motorcycle accident, he'd never sustained a fracture.
3   Now that the patient has had prostate surgery, he is doing well.
4   If the doctor's diagnosis is atherosclerosis, why won't he help her?
5   Because of swollen and twisted veins in the legs, she cannot walk.
6   Although the patient is suffering from emotional stress, she handles it well.
7   Since developing pericarditis, she is not feeling well.
8   When the physician ordered an MRI for her heart, she passed out.
9   The patient is having coronary bypass surgery so that he can feel better.
10 Sammie enjoyed jogging on the treadmill, though it made her tired.

Instructions

Key the following dependent clauses, adding an independent clause to complete the sentence and any punctuation.

1   After examining the patient in the clinic,
2   After evaluation,
3   Before she was hospitalized,
4   When the surgeon arrived,
5   Because of the serious illness,
6   After she had adenopathy,
7   While you were consulting with the patient,
8   Unless she was given medication,
9   If her tests are negative,
10 Though she reports emesis,

INDEPENDENT CLAUSES WITH COMMAS

Rule:

Independent clauses, which are two sentences, are joined by coordinating conjunctions.

Coordinating conjunctions are: yet, so , nor, or, but, and for

The comma is used before the conjunction in independent clauses.

Example:

There is some fungus, but we see no evidence of pruritus. *There is some fungus* is an independent clause. *We see no evidence of pruritus* is an independent clause. Use a comma before the conjunction because the two sentences are independent clauses.

Instructions

Key each of the sentences and add commas.

1 The left tympanic membrane was infected and the buccal mucosa was covered with ulcerations.

2 Mary has rheumatoid arthritis and her joints are inflamed and painful.

3 We can schedule surgery appointments or we can transcribe operative reports.

4 He does not take antibiotics for he is unaware of any allergies.

5 Her head is without trauma but her forehead showed a reddish bruise.

FIVE-MINUTE TIMING—DOUBLE SPACE

The patient is a cachetic 85-year-old female with mild	11
respiratory distress, and she developed progressive	21
difficulty with swallowing and increased lethargy. The	32
patient was admitted to the emergency department, and Dr.	43
Cactus performed the history and physical. The patient was	54
given IV normal saline. She had mild hyperventilation and	65
metabolic alkalemia. The patient did well on therapy, and	76
her dehydration improved.	81
Head is normocephalic. Pupils equal, round, and reactive	93
to light. She does have a nasal cannula in place. Throat	104
shows a large amount of food material with mucus. There is	115
no evidence of inflammation. Neck is supple. There is no	126
thyroid enlargement, and no carotid bruits are heard. Chest	137
is clear to auscultation and percussion. No rales or rhonchi	149
are heard. There is a regular sinus rhythm. Heart sounds are	161
somewhat distant. Her peripheral pulses are full. Abdomen	172
is soft. No hepatosplenomegaly or palpable abdominal masses.	184
No masses are present in her breasts. Rectal examination is	196
negative. The patient does have right-sided hemiparesis with	208
contractures of her upper and lower extremities. Skin is	219
without decubitus ulcers. She is nonverbal. The patient	230
does appear to have diminished gag reflex and is probably	241
having recurrent bouts of pneumonia.	248
She made marked improvement within three days and was	259
discharged to her daughter's home where she will be followed	271
on an outpatient basis.	275

□□□□1□□□□2□□□□3□□□□4□□□□5□□□□6□□□□7□□□□8□□□□9□□□□10□□□□11□□□□12

Phrases, Five-Minute Timed Writing

Goals

After completing this lesson, you will be able to:

✔ Use prepositional phrases.

A phrase is a group of related words that lack a subject, verb, or both. A prepositional phrase shows relationship to other words in a sentence. Use a comma after a prepositional phrase.

Prepositions

inside	of	in	over	below	onto	with	except
behind	through	above	along	since	before	between	under
on	for	off	across	during	toward	until	around
beneath	at	by	like	off	within	up	near
without	upon	after	beside	among	about	into	from
to	inside						

Example:

<u>On the day of admission</u>, he did consent <u>to being taken to the doctor's office for an examination</u>.

Instructions

Key the following sentences, and underline the phrases.

1 That patient had a thorough evaluation for senile dementia.
2 He has not been eating during this time and refused to obtain medical help.
3 There is acrocyanosis in the nailbeds.
4 The patient had been confined to his home for the last two years.
5 On review of medical records, the patient had a BUN of 95.

Instructions

Key the following sentences, underlining the prepositional phrases.

1 There were no gallstones in the gallbladder.
2 There are several masses within the lung fields.
3 She no longer had carpal tunnel syndrome after the operation.
4 The heart and pulmonary vessels are within normal limits.
5 The patient underwent removal of a polyp several months ago.
6 After satisfactory reduction, the limb was put in a cast.
7 He has been started on Demerol for pain.
8 The patient lives at home with his daughter.
9 He went into congestive heart failure at the office.

10   The patient had carcinoma of the lungs attributable to fifteen
     years of smoking.

Instructions

Key the sentences below, and underline the phrases.

1   George Dwon, our first patient, was born in Mobile Hospital.
2   The four patients who were given blood transfusions are doing
    fine.
3   Seven of the medical students who graduated from West Bridge
    Academy are female.
4   William Bilirubin died, twenty days after his heart transplant,
    surrounded by his family.
5   The intern in the Radiology Room read x-rays of the spine.
6   Which physician of those on call will be in the emergency room
    this weekend?
7   Dr. John Leuk, acting as secretary, answered the phone.
8   Those patients flew from San Diego to New York for a study on
    AIDS.
9   The patient sat, looking very irritated, by the nurse.
10 Bruce wanted the poster about autotransfusion displayed across the
    street.

FIVE-MINUTE TIMING—DOUBLE SPACE

```
        Liz is a 25-year-old white female who has had progressive    12
and severe headaches, unrelieved with Demerol.  The patient          23
developed these headaches five days ago, and this is                 33
associated with photophobia, neck stiffness, and waking up           44
in the middle of the night with a headache.  The patient has         55
had nausea associated with the headache but has not had any          66
vomiting.  She has also has a progressive weight loss over           77
the past year of 10 to 15 pounds, despite a vigorous appetite.       89
The patient was seen in my office and had a severe headache          100
keeping her from work.  Neurologic exam was normal.  The             111
patient was given intramuscular injection of Demerol to              122
control her pain.  However, her pain has persisted despite           133
this heavy medication.  Because of her weight loss, acute            144
onset of severe headache, and especially a headache that             155
wakes her at night, the patient is being admitted to the             166
hospital for evaluation of these multiple problems.  She has         178
had nevi removed from her right leg that required surgery.           189
There was no evidence of carcinoma in these nevi.  The patient       201
had an appendectomy, tonsillectomy, and adenoidectomy.  She          212
has been labeled as borderline diabetic.  She also was noted         224
to be jaundiced and underwent a proctosigmoidoscopy and              235
barium enema for gastrointestinal distress.  The patient has         247
been taking Fiorpap for her headache without relief.  She            258
takes no other medications and has no known allergies.  The          269
patient works as a teacher and works long hours.  She is             280
single and lives with her 4-year-old daughter.                       289
```

      □□□□1□□□□2□□□□3□□□□4□□□□5□□□□6□□□□7□□□□8□□□□9□□□□10□□□□11□□□□12

Comma Review, Five-Minute Timed Writing

Goals

After completing this lesson, you will be able to:

✔ Use commas correctly.

Three or more commas:

Rule:

Use commas to separate three or more items in a series.

Example:

The uterus, ovaries, and mammogram appeared normal. Three items—uterus, ovaries, and mammogram—are separated by two commas. Note that no comma comes after mammogram, the last item in this series.

We learned from Dr. Smith that he had written four books, six articles, eight workbooks, and seven suture manuals. Four items—four books, six articles, eight workbooks, seven suture manuals. Commas are used between three items in this series.

Instructions

Insert commas in the following sentences.

1 The side effects of Benadryl are drowsiness tremors and digestive upset.
2 There was evidence of dehydration loss of skin turgor sunken eyes and dry mucous membranes.
3 The patient presented to my office with a three-day history of abdominal pain nausea and inability to retain fluids.
4 Headaches diarrhea stomach pain vomiting and erythema are adverse reactions to omeprazole.
5 The patient denies hematuria change in bowel habits or rectal bleeding.

Instructions

Key each of the following sentences, adding commas where appropriate.

1 The patient has been treated for a malignant tumor and he is asymptomatic.
2 She has mononucleosis and her baby has a sore throat.
3 Because she has a malignant tumor she will go to the hospital.
4 This doctor who examined him yesterday diagnosed a Wilms tumor and hyperemesis.
5 Her moles reappeared but she had them removed.
6 The baby whose mother is blind was born with hyaline membrane disease.

7 There is some fungus but we see no evidence of pruritus.
8 Mary has rheumatoid arthritis and her joints are inflamed and painful.
9 He had no chest pain but his blood results are elevated.
10 The doctor ordered myelograms and the procedure revealed pressure on the nerve and spinal cord.

Commas with appositives:

Rule:

An appositive is a word or phrase that identifies a noun or pronoun in a sentence. The appositive follows the noun or pronoun in a sentence. Use a comma before and after the appositive.

Example:

The gynecologist, Hermann Johann Pfannestiel, invented the Pfannestiel incision. *Hermann Johann Pfannestiel* is an appositive that follows the noun *gynecologist.*

Instructions

Key the following sentences, and use commas for the appositives.

1 Dr. Moss who graduated from Stanford University has a two-year appointment to teach oncology at Mobile Cancer Center.
2 The patient Mary Burns had her first course of chemotherapy two weeks ago.
3 Mary Moss the coder is an associate professor at Mobile Technical College.
4 This 14-year-old boy James Buccal was diagnosed with Wilms tumor.
5 Eliza Burns a research associate at Mobile National Laboratory worked on a sample of DNA cells.

Commas with dates:

Rule:

The month is spelled out in a sentence. Do not use a comma when the month and year do not have a date. Use a comma after the year.

Example:

He was admitted on October 4, 2005, and discharged on October 8.

Rule:

The comma is used before the conjunction in independent clauses.

Conjunctions are: yet, so, nor, or, but, and for

Example:

The patient was discharged on May 21, 2004, but he was readmitted on May 22.

Commas with addresses:

Rule:

Use commas to separate the address from the city and the city from the state in a sentence. A comma is not used before the zip code.

Example:

The American Medical Assistant Conference will be held in Wright Hall, 2540 Desert Lane, Mobile, AZ 82000-0000.

An Overview of Commas

Instructions

Key the following sentences, insert commas, and spell out the month.

1 He was discharged on 10/17/2003 on ampicillin and a high caloric supplement.

2 At 10:30 am on 06/01/2001, the patient had cardiorespiratory arrest and was pronounced dead.

3 He was readmitted in May 2001 for morphine and Thorazine.

4 The radiation therapy was completed, and the patient did well until 01/16/2001, when a routine chest film showed several lung metastases.

5 The Children's Hospital and Health Center is located at 2205 Winter Drive Mobile AZ 82000-0000.

Commas with degrees, titles, Jr and Sr:

Rule:

Use a comma when the academic degrees, titles, Jr., or Sr. follow the person's name.

Example:

David Rad, MD, PhD, professor of oncology, attended the radiology conference in San Diego.

Note: The title of the person is not capitalized when it follows the name. The title *professor* is not capitalized.

FIVE-MINUTE TIMING—DOUBLE SPACE

```
        This 40-year-old Hispanic female came to the office with    12
severe depression, irritability, vertigo, and difficulty with      24
her speech.  The patient has a chronic history of osteoarthri-      36
tis with gouty arthritis in the left knee.  She has had a           47
gradual increase in weight.  She has been treated for mild          58
hypertension with very poor results.  Currently, she is on          69
Diuril, Ativan, Fioricet, and Antivert for vertigo.  The            80
patient was seen by Dr. Sampson for her vertigo, which has          91
been a chronic condition.  She was hospitalized in May of          102
2002 for exhaustion, headaches, and change in personality          113
to rule out cerebral problems.  No family history of cancer,       125
diabetes, hypertension, or tuberculosis.  The patient has          136
noted shortness of breath, but this is associated with her         147
weight gain.  She has had no chronic cough, hemoptysis,            158
nausea, diarrhea, hematuria, dysuria, or pyuria.  Blood            169
pressure is 140/90.  Pulse is 80 and regular.  Respirations        180
are 19.  Temperature is 98 degrees.  Weight is 240 pounds.         191
```

□□□□1□□□□2□□□□3□□□□4□□□□5□□□□6□□□□7□□□□8□□□□9□□□□10□□□□11□□□□12

Semicolon, Five-Minute Timed Writing

Goals

After completing this lesson, you will be able to:

✔ Use semicolons correctly.

Rule:

Use a semicolon to join two related independent clauses when no conjunction joins the clauses.

Example:

He was referred to the emergency department; he was found to be hypotensive.

Instructions

Key the following sentences; insert semicolons.

1 The fasciotomy incision is healing well the leg is larger than normal.

2 The patient was medicated with Demerol the dressings were removed.

3 A thick coat of Betadine ointment was applied over the wound the bandages covered the wound.

4 There is no evidence of clubbing the peripheral cyanosis is present.

5 The stool is brownish on the fingertip external hemorrhoids are present.

Use commas with a semicolon.

Rule:

Use a semicolon after the first independent clause, and a comma after the parenthetical element. A parenthetical element interrupts the sentence. Parenthetical elements are: however, therefore, nevertheless, after all, for example, moreover, of course, consequently.

Example:

The patient denies any substance abuse; however, she has a history of obtaining over-the-counter pills.

Instructions

Key the following sentences; insert commas and semicolons.

1 He is on maintenance chemotherapy therefore he comes in today with no particular problems.

2 The patient is in poor condition therefore he will not survive.

3 That exam included a bronchoscopy consequently no diagnosis was made.

---

4   Cardiac examination was unremarkable of course the rhythm was regular.

5   She has had a myocardial infarction however she denies shortness of breath.

Instructions

Key the following sentences, supplying needed semicolons.

1   The child previously had leukemia unfortunately, he had a relapse.

2   The medical center has offices in Phoenix, Arizona San Diego, California Mobile, Arizona and Miami, Florida.

3   Dr. Holsy Sampson is an otologist he retired in 1992.

4   Temporal bone labs were held in Chula Vista California Gila Bend, Arizona Dallas, Texas and San Diego, California

5   Jean is transferring to the Surgery Department in San Diego she will be a medical receptionist.

6   The Pulmonary Department has six openings for technician positions therefore, they will be hiring six technicians.

7   The department head recommended in-service training however, we read the CPT manual.

8   The Radiology Clinic invited Dr. Charles Leuko, director of radiology Dr. Mary Bun, president of surgery and Dr. Jake Endo, a chemist to attend the conference.

9   The patient was admitted to surgery it will take two hours.

10 The physical medicine conference is at Brown Clinic will you come?

This is a 42-year-old female who was admitted to Mobile	11
Hospital because of severe shortness of breath and acute	22
pulmonary edema. The patient has underlying coronary artery	33
disease with previous myocardial infarction and congestive	44
heart failure. The patient underwent coronary artery bypass	55
surgery. She did well, with resolution of her shortness of	66
breath. She has hypertension, type 2 diabetes mellitus, and	77
chronic obstructive pulmonary disease. The patient was noted	89
to have mild hyperkalemia and azotemia while on Lasix and	100
potassium. Lasix and potassium were stopped, and the BUN	111
normalized. She was maintained on digoxin, aspirin, and	122
Adalat. In May of 2002, she had problems with dizziness and	133
unsteadiness of gait. Evaluation was nonrevealing, and it	144
was thought that she might have TIAs. Two months prior to	155
admission, she had began to have diaphoresis, dyspnea,	165
dysuria, and pyuria. On the day of admission, she woke up	176
at 5:30 a.m. with dyspnea. She was severely distressed. The	188
paramedics were called, and she was brought to Mobile Hospi-	199
tal. She was given oxygen and Lasix. Her blood pressure was	211
200/100. Chest x-ray revealed acute pulmonary edema. After	223
treatment with nitrates, IV Lasix, and oxygen, her blood	234
pressure dropped to 160/90. The skin was diaphoretic.	245
Fundoscopic examination showed AV nicking. Lung examination	256
revealed rales. Cardiac examination showed a gallop with a	267
grade 3 systolic ejection murmur. Extremities showed ankle	278
edema 3+. Hemoglobin A1c test was normal except for an ele-	290
vated cholesterol and triglycerides.	297

□□□□1□□□□2□□□□3□□□□4□□□□5□□□□6□□□□7□□□□8□□□□9□□□□10□□□□11□□□□12

Colon, Five-Minute Timed Writing

Goals

After completing this lesson, you will be able to:

✔ Use colons correctly.

Rule:

A colon is used after a sentence to show what follows. A colon is mainly used to direct attention to something, such as a list, explanation, or quotation. Double space after the colon. Capitalize the word following a colon if it is a proper name or begins a complete sentence.

Example:

Please bring the following items with you: a medical dictionary, a laptop computer, and a cell phone.

Rule:

A colon is used after the salutation in a business letter.

Examples:

Dear Dr. Hubbard:

Ladies and Gentlemen:

To Whom It May Concern:

Rule:

Colons are used in expression of time.

Examples:

5:10 p.m.

7:30 a.m.

Rule:

Colons are used with ratios and dilutions.

Example:

1:100,000

Rule:

Colons follow the headers and subtopics in medical reports. Headers and subtopics are keyed in all capital letters.

Examples:

CHIEF COMPLAINT:, DISCHARGE DIAGNOSIS:, PRESENT ILLNESS:, PAST HISTORY:, REVIEW OF SYSTEMS:, HEENT:, ALLERGIES:, SOCIAL HISTORY:, FAMILY HISTORY:, PHYSICAL EXAMINATION:, MEDICATIONS:, EXTREMITIES:, LABORATORY VALUES:, SKIN:

Key the following sentences, and insert colons.

1   Dr. Hubbard prescribed the following medications Tagamet 800 mg, Fioricet 275 mg, Prilosec 20 mg, and Prevacid 30 mg.

2   The pharmaceutical display will be held from 1015 a.m. to 430 p.m.

3   He is survived by his wife Beulah, his mother Alice, brothers Tom and David, sisters Jan and Nanci and numerous cousins.

4   The lidocaine solution was diluted 1100,000.

5   DISCHARGE DIAGNOSES
    1. Hypertension.
    2. Myocardial infarction.
    3. Diabetes mellitus.
    4. Pneumonia.

Instructions

Key the following sentences, inserting colons where required.

1   The medical staff meeting will be at 745 a.m.

2   Two patients are scheduled for lab work at 1145 and 1050 a.m.

3   Vital signs blood pressure 120/70. Weight 140. Respirations 70. Pulse 78.

4   Preoperative diagnosis Hysterectomy and appendectomy.

5   Several residents were recommended Mary Smith, David Rad, Donald Sampson, and Anita Young.

6   Grayelin Young will speak at the 630 p.m. meeting.

7   Two nurses attended the Oncology Meeting Billi Jo and Janie Wing.

8   The doctor gave her diagnosis Keloids.

9   She feels strongly about alternative medicine it gives patients choices.

10 The patient requested only one doctor you.

Instructions

Key the following sentences, inserting correct punctuation.

1   The progress notes are not signed therefore leave a note for the doctor

2   The otorhinolaryngology residents plan to arrive at 815 am we intend to finish at 615 pm

3   The surgery grand rounds begin at 715 we should be prompt

4   The surgeon will be completing the operation and the anesthesiologist will administer the local anesthesia

5   Dr John Sully a pediatrics professor at the University of Mobile Medical School will speak on immunizations

6   He answered the questions he received many responses.

7   The physician ordered the following tests sodium potassium AST glucose and hemoglobin.

8   Postoperative diagnosis Appendectomy

9   He said the following she is having respiratory difficulty she
    will be admitted to the clinic.

10 Allergies None Smoking None Alcohol None

FIVE-MINUTE TIMING—DOUBLE SPACE

Samuel is an 85-year-old male seen by Dr. Jean Cactus.	11
The patient is a resident at Cupcake's Care Facility and is	22
being treated for pneumonia. He has been lethargic and has	33
a history of acute agitation, controlled by Navane. Current-	45
ly, he is off all sedatives due to his pulmonary condition.	56
On review of the nursing record, the patient was noted	67
to be confused, and when approached by the nurses, he became	79
very combative. The patient will not talk, and rotating him	91
has been quite difficult because of his combativeness. His	102
electrocardiogram revealed atrial fibrillation with rapid	113
ventricular response.	117
On observation, the patient was extremely withdrawn. He	129
was not responsive to commands and would not grab the	139
physician's fingers when asked to; he had difficulty making	150
his needs known. His judgment was impaired. He could not	161
understand the nature of his illness or cooperate with his	172
physician or treatment plan.	178
Apparently, the patient has irreversible senile dementia,	190
and he is incapacitated. He is agitated when approached, and	202
he will need one-to-one nursing care until he is able to	213
adjust to the nurses and unfamiliar surroundings in the	224
facility. He has been controlled on Navane, and it is	235
recommended that he receive Navane Concentrate. He does not	247
appear acutely agitated and combative at the present time.	258

□□□□1□□□□2□□□□3□□□□4□□□□5□□□□6□□□□7□□□□8□□□□9□□□□10□□□□11□□□□12

Parentheses and Italics, Five-Minute Timed Writing

Goals

After completing this lesson, you will be able to:

✔ Use parentheses correctly.
✔ Use italics correctly.

Rule:

Parentheses are used to enclose:

✔ information not essential to the meaning of the sentence
✔ letters and figures labeling items in lists

Example: The medical journals (which arrived yesterday) are in her office.

Rule:

Italics are used to:

✔ mark the titles of books, journals, newspapers, and other published material

Instructions

Key the following sentences, adding parentheses and italics as needed.

1 The patient lives on 25 Home Avenue the one who is depressed.
2 The following books were sent: 1 a medical dictionary, 2 a medical typing book, and 3 a surgery book.
3 A group of physicians will be traveling to Washington they have their tickets.
4 The patient in Room B the one who asked for ice cream will have surgery tomorrow.
5 The doctor subscribed to the Radiology Journal.
6 Read the Work Magazine.
7 Please return both magazines: The Surgery Word and Tumor Journal.

This 45-year-old male entered my office with a complaint	12
of severe left-sided, sharp stabbing pain that radiates	23
through the testicle and left groin. He has had frequency of	35
urination. He has never had a kidney stone or discoloration	46
of urine. The patient noted the onset of constant pain,	57
which became severe. The patient was seen in the office with	69
hematuria, dysuria, and pyuria. The diagnosis is probable	80
left ureteral stone, and he was prepared for an IVP. The pain	91
became more severe, and he was unable to retain codeine. The	103
pain could not be controlled with oral medications so he was	114
hospitalized. A recent electrocardiogram was normal. No	125
shortness of breath, chronic cough, or hemoptysis. The	136
physical examination reveals a male who is in distress with	147
left-sided pain. The skin is warm, moist, and with good	158
turgor. Thyroid is not enlarged. No rales or rhonchi are	169
heard. No murmurs. Testicles are not tender. Deep tendon	180
reflexes are symmetrical as is muscle strength and motion.	191
Vital signs are: weight 250 pounds, height 69.5 inches,	202
temperature 97, pulse 80, respirations 20, and blood pressure	214
140/80.	215

□□□□1□□□□2□□□□3□□□□4□□□□5□□□□6□□□□7□□□□8□□□□9□□□□10□□□□11□□□□12

Apostrophe, Five-Minute Timed Writing

Goals

After completing this lesson, you will be able to:

✔ Use apostrophes correctly.

Rule:

The apostrophe is used to show the possessive of nouns or to show that a letter has been omitted. Apostrophes are used before the gerund.

Example: Mary's reading bothered me.

Examples:

patient's doctor
the baby's head
donor's blood
Example: Because of the patient's senility, she was unable to keep weight off her elbow.

Instructions

Key the following sentences, adding appropriate apostrophes.

1 The patients doctor did not prescribe Valium.
2 The patients daughter could not be reached by telephone.
3 This 15-year-old female patient has Tourettes syndrome and was admitted to the Childrens Medical Center.
4 Due to the patients symptoms, a cholesterol test was ordered.
5 Because the patients cholesterol had increased, he was placed on a special diet.
6 This is not the first visit at the Childrens Medical Center for the baby.
7 The babys mother has been studied and has negative test results based upon her evaluation.
8 Mrs. Browns father did not die of pneumonia.
9 The family history was updated with information obtained on sickle cell anemia studies in Mrs. Champions relatives.
10 The mutation of the genes came from Mrs. Cytes mothers side of the family.

Mr. Gross is a 68-year-old male widower admitted to	11
Mobile Hospital on February 23, 2002, for carcinoma of the	22
right upper lung with metastasis to his spine. The patient	33
has been followed and seen in consultation by Dr. Cotton,	44
who evaluated the patient in January. Since this hospitali-	56
zation, the patient underwent an operation for anterior	67
vertebral body replacement with diskectomy. The patient	78
reports frustration and depression related to his lung cancer	90
and pain. he is on disability from his employment due to	101
chronic pain; although, he denies that this was a significant	113
problem in the past.	117

The patient has been having crying spells, and this is	128
noted in Dr. Cotton's initial history and physical notes.	139
The nursing notes indicate depression in the evenings. The	150
patient is on Sinequan, Atican, and Tylenol. He denies any	161
history of hallucinations or difficulties with his memory.	172
He denies any significant family conflicts and feels that he	184
has a emotional support from his family. The patient	194
describes that he has been sleeping better and has a good	205
appetite.	207

No evidence of past psychiatric illness or treatment.	218
He is allergic to penicillin.	224

□□□□1□□□□2□□□□3□□□□4□□□□5□□□□6□□□□7□□□□8□□□□9□□□□10□□□□11□□□□12

Mechanics III—Capitalization

First Letter of a Sentence, Five-Minute Timed Writing

Goals

After completing this lesson, you will be able to:

✔ Capitalize the first letter of a sentence.

Example: This 32-year-old female had a long history of left knee pain.

Instructions

Key the following sentences, capitalizing the first word of each.

1 the doctor performed a blepharectomy to correct the left blepharoptosis.

2 the patient was alert, friendly, and complained of an earache.

3 she was admitted to the Mobile Hospital for dizziness, weakness, and severe depression.

4 zocor was prescribed to lower his cholesterol, and he is seeing a cardiologist.

5 this 60-year-old female was admitted with hypertension, diabetes, tachycardia, and dyspnea.

FIVE-MINUTE TIMING—DOUBLE SPACE

```
        The patient was treated in the emergency department with    12
IV Lasix, Nitro-Bid, and sublingual Nitroquick for angina           23
pectoris.  A Foley catheter was placed, and the patient             34
diuresed rapidly.  The patient was admitted to the intensive        45
care unit where she was seen in consultation by Dr. Samuel L.       57
Sampson.  Serum enzyme tests showed no evidence of myocardial       69
infarction.  The patient was started on Nitro-Bid IV and IV         80
heparin.  The patient was maintained on oral NitroQuick and         91
oral digoxin.  Chest x-ray showed clearing of the pulmonary        102
edema, and the patient was breathing comfortably.  The patient     114
was moved to telemetry.  The patient remained weak but was         125
not having chest pains or shortness of breath.  Her blood          136
gasses showed a PO₂ of 73, PCO₂ of 45, and a pH 7.42 on room       147
air.  Those blood gases were reviewed by Dr. John Sampson.         158
The patient was discharged on May 10 with prescriptions for        169
digoxin 0.75 mg p.o. q.d., Lasix 40 mg p.o. q.d., albuterol        180
2 inhalations q.6h., and NitroQuick 0.6 mg p.o. (per Dr.Edward     192
Burns).  She was placed on a low-fat diet.  A follow-up            203
appointment for a thallium 201 scintigraphy test was scheduled     215
with Dr. John Sampson on May 15.  Follow-up appointment in         226
Cardiology Clinic in four weeks with Dr. Edward Burns.             236
```
The blood gasses line reads: gasses showed a PO_2 of 73, PCO_2 of 45, and a pH 7.42 on room air.

□□□□1□□□□2□□□□3□□□□4□□□□5□□□□6□□□□7□□□□8□□□□9□□□□10□□□□11□□□□12

Business Applications, Five-Minute Timed Writing

Goals

After completing this lesson, you will be able to:

✔ Capitalize the first letter of a salutation.
✔ Capitalize the first letter of a complimentary closing.
✔ Capitalize reference initials.
✔ Capitalize the first letter of each word of a company name.

Instructions

Key the following sentences, capitalizing as appropriate. Capitalize the first letter of the salutation, names, and titles in the salutation. *Example:* Dear Dr. Sykes:

1 dear dr. jones:
2 dear dr. smith:
3 dear dr. moss:
4 dear dr. sampson:
5 dear nurse ardell:

Capitalize the first letter of complimentary closing. *Example:* Truly yours,

1 sincerely,
2 sincerely yours,
3 cordially,
4 very truly yours,
5 respectfully yours,

Key reference initials in all capital letters. (Reference initials are sometimes typed in all lowercase letters.) If there are two sets of reference initials, type them in the same style for speed. *Example:* EMS:SS

1 eem:es
2 rcm:pdm
3 aly:gy
4 eep:zb

Capitalize company names. *Example:* Aljo Medical Clinic

1 mobile medical clinic
2 laveen cardiology clinic
3 gila memorial hospital
4 maricopa county mental health clinic
5 county health department

This 13-year-old girl entered the Urgent Care Clinic,	11
having fallen off a horse and having inability to weight bear	23
on the right leg. The patient had injured her right hip	34
previously, approximately two weeks ago. She was up and	45
around walking with complaints of pain but able to ride her	56
horse. She has had a history of injuring her back in the	67
past. No history of paralysis. The patient was examined at	78
the Urgent Care Clinic and found to be unable to weight bear,	90
in severe pain on lifting either the right or left leg, with	101
all the pain being referred to the right sacroiliac joint.	112
There is no evidence of fracture on any of the x-rays, and no	124
evidence of bruising. The patient is confused about her fall,	136
but there was no loss of consciousness at any time. The	147
patient has had no previous hysterical reactions, no previous	159
history of loss of consciousness, or severe injury.	169

There is no family history of tuberculosis, cancer,	180
diabetes, hypertension, or allergies.	187

Deep tendon reflexes are symmetrical as is muscle	198
strength and motion. The patient does have severe pain to	209
the right hip on straight leg raising of both right and left	220
legs, severe pain over the sacroiliac joint on pressure, and	231
no bruises. The ankle jerks are symmetrical. The patient	242
has good strength in both legs but pain on movement against	253
pressure of the great toe and forefoot in flexion and	263
extension.	265

CBC and urinalysis were all within the range of normal.	276
She will be treated with Tylenol with Codeine, regular diet,	287
and activity as tolerated at home. She was discharged to	298
home in good condition. She will be followed by Dr. Cactus	309
in the office.	312

□□□□1□□□□2□□□□3□□□□4□□□□5□□□□6□□□□7□□□□8□□□□9□□□□10□□□□11□□□□12

Proper Names and Street, City, State Names; Five-Minute Timed Writing

Goals

After completing this lesson, you will be able to:

✔ Capitalize names and addresses.

Example:	Evie Sampson MD
	39 Dust Drive
	Mobile, AZ 00000-0000

Instructions

Key the following addresses, capitalizing as appropriate.

1 mr parry d moss
   2401 desert drive
   mobile az 00000-0000

2 mrs anita l young
   2201 cactus lane
   mobile az 00000-0000

3 matthew t sampson md
   mobile medical clinic
   2201 cactus lane
   mobile az 00000-0000

4 jehanne q switzer md
   director biology lab
   4545 success place
   taos nm 04040-0000

5 professor mary labonne
   accurate medical transcription college
   1111 academia drive ste 1
   honolulu hi 66466-0000

The patient is a 70-year-old Caucasian female with	11
organic brain syndrome who was admitted to the hospital for	22
right-sided abdominal pain. She was referred to Dr. Blow for	34
persistent congestive heart failure. An abdominal CT scan	45
was done three days ago; the patient went into acute pulmonary	57
edema. The procedure was discontinued, and the patient was	68
returned to her room, at which time she suffered a cardiac	79
arrest. Cardiopulmonary resuscitation was instituted and was	91
successful. The patient was intubated and placed on a	101
respirator and diuresed. The patient has been weaned from	112
the respirator over the past three days. The most recent	123
blood gases were excellent. Sputum, blood, and urine	133
cultures have been obtained. Present medications include	144
digoxin and Ancef.	147
The patient is a thin, frail, elderly female with an	158
endotracheal tube in place. Head, eyes, ears, nose, and throat	170
are unremarkable. Neck is supple. There is no thyromegaly.	181
There is no adenopathy. Carotids are full and equal with no	193
bruits. The chest exam revealed bronchial breathing heard	204
at the base. There are no rales or rhonchi noted. Heart	215
shows normal sinus rhythm. Abdomen is soft. There is vague	227
right-sided tenderness. The bowel signs are active. Chest	238
x-ray on admission showed cardiomegaly. Three days after the	250
cardiac arrest, the patient had congestive heart failure with	262
pulmonary edema. Today, a repeat chest x-ray shows cardio-	273
megaly with no evidence of pulmonary congestion or pulmonary	284
edema.	285

□□□□1□□□□2□□□□3□□□□4□□□□5□□□□6□□□□7□□□□8□□□□9□□□□10□□□□11□□□□12

Titles and Business Correspondence, Five-Minute Timed Writing

Goals

After completing this lesson, you will be able to:

✔ Capitalize titles in business correspondence.

Examples:

1 Dr. David Rad, Professor of Laughter
   3904 Laugh Drive
   Mobile, AZ 00000-0000

2 David Rad, PhD
   Director of Radiology
   3904 Success Drive
   Mobile, AZ 00000-0000

Instructions

Key the following sentences. The title is typed on the same line as the name, separated from the name by a comma. The title may be typed on the second line of the address if the title is too long. In complimentary closing signature lines, the title is typed after the name or below the name.

1 dr. mary rose, professor of surgery
   mobile medical clinic
   2201 cactus lane
   mobile, az 00000-0000

2 samuel sampson, md
   chief of pediatrics
   mobile university hospital
   2202 cactus lane
   mobile, az 00000-0000

3 dr. mary pansey
   professor of otolaryngology
   mobile medical clinic
   2201 cactus lane
   mobile az 00000-0000

4 geraldine sampson, md
   chief of cardiology
   mobile university medical center
   2202 cactus lane
   mobile, az 00000-0000

5 brian capp, phd
   professor of advanced musical therapy
   esaleen center
   2400 esaleen drive
   big sur, ca 91111

Leave four blank lines between the closing and the signature lines.

1 sincerely,

   hosey hubbard, md, professor of rheumatology

2 sincerely yours,

   edward d. burns, md
   chairman of department of neurology

3 respectfully yours,

   eliza burns, md, associate dean of hematology

4 sincerely,

   dr. josephine d. williams, dean of continuing medical education

5 yours truly,

   charels bili, md, surgeon of orthopedics

The patient is a 45-year-old married gentleman with	11
known hypertension. His cerebrovascular accident history	22
dates back to June of 2001, at which time he had episodes of	33
dizziness. He underwent angiography and left carotid endar-	44
terectomy. The patient's wife was told that the patient	55
should stop smoking, take medications, and be treated	65
medically. He was placed on a low cholesterol diet and had	76
his blood pressure controlled with various medications. In	87
January 2002, the patient suffered a cerebrovascular accident	99
with aphasia and a right hemiparesis. There was limitation	110
of function; however, his right lower extremity had enough	121
strength so that he could be rehabilitated at Mobile Hospital	133
and was able to walk with a walker. His aphasia improved	144
with obvious word omissions and occasional difficulty to find	156
appropriate words during conversations. His right upper	167
extremity and right lower extremity had been rehabilitated.	178
Initial evaluation performed by Dr. Magic in April of	189
2002 revealed mild congestive heart failure with an elevated	200
blood pressure and right hemiparesis as well as aphasia. He	211
was placed on a regimen of digoxin, Inderal, and diazepam.	222
Aspirin was ordered for antiplatelet activity. He remained	233
stable until August 20, 2002, when his wife noted an episode	244
of unresponsiveness that lasted several minutes and was	255
associated with paralysis of his right side. He was seen in	266
the office on August 21, 2002, with hypertension.	276
Subsequently, the patient had a similar episode that did not	287
resolve, and he was brought to Mobile Hospital with a stroke	298
of the left parietal area. The patient had a CT scan, which	309
revealed an infarct with the patient's paralysis of the	320
right side. The patient developed difficulty with his food	331
intake and mild aspiration during his hospitalization. The	342
patient was discharged to home where his wife will care for	353
him.	354

□□□□1□□□□2□□□□3□□□□4□□□□5□□□□6□□□□7□□□□8□□□□9□□□□10□□□□11□□□□12

Envelope Address, Five-Minute Timed Writing

Goals

After completing this lesson, you will be able to:

✔ Key an envelope address in all capital letters.

Instructions

Capitalize all letters of the address on an envelope. No punctuation for an envelope.

Key the titles MR, MRS, or MISS before the name.

Examples:

MR HOLCIE SAMPSOON

MRS MARY SAMPSON

MISS EDNA SAMPSON

The return address begins on the second line down from the upper left corner. Begin typing three spaces from the left edge. To type the address of the addressee, indent halfway across the envelope and begin typing eight lines down from the bottom of the return address. Type the following addresses in envelope form. Use zip and 4 code. Example: 00000-0000. See the figure below.

```
1   Dr Mary Glucose
    3940 Virus Lane
    Mobile AZ 00000-0000
2   Dr Matthew Sampson
    Mobile University
    3890 Rubella Street
    Mobile AZ 00000-0000
```

```
MARY GLUCOSE MD
3940 VIRUS LANE
MOBILE AZ 00000-0000




                    MATTHEW T SAMPSON MD
                    SCHOOL OF MEDICINE
                    MOBILE UNIVERSITY
                    3890 RUBELLA STREET
                    MOBILE AZ 00000-0000
```

Recommended Postal Service Style for Envelopes

Address all envelopes in capital letters without punctuation. Zip+4 codes are used on all mail.

Example: International Mail

MR GEORGE TIBA
4250 MAPLE AVENUE
5000 ACAPULCO

MEXICO

Example: U.S.

MRS MABLE ROOF
6975 LAKE AVE
LAVEEN AZ 63011-2000

MR JOE SAMPSON
ATTN SAMPSON PHARMACY
3940 DESERT AVE
LAVEEN AZ 63011-2000

Instructions

Key the address in uppercase for an envelope. Leave one space between the city name and the two state abbreviations and the Zip+4 code. An incorrect zip code can delay delivery of your mail. Foreign postal codes are placed in front of the city on the same line. Double space between the city and foreign country.

Use a No. 10 envelope. Key your name for the return address. Key the following assignment.

1 Mr. Grayelin Young Jr.
   5402 Frostbite
   Mobile, AZ 60100-0000

2 Mr. Bobbie Sole
   5001 Heart St
   5001 Toluca
   Mexico

3 Minnie Hart, MD
   Medical Insurance Dept
   Mobile Hospital
   3952 Desert St
   Mobile, AZ 60100-0000

4 Mobile Hospital
   Att Sally Curve
   3952 Desert St
   Mobile, AZ 60100-0000

How to fold a letter.

1. Fold a third of the letter up the page and then crease.
2. Fold up to the top to about ½ inch, the last folded edge goes in first.
3. Insert in the envelope.

This 49-year-old, black, right-handed male is admitted to   12
the hospital because of pain in the left shoulder and arm.   23
The past history indicates that he has had a large cell   34
carcinoma of the right lung, which was treated with radiation   46
therapy. He describes this pain in the neck, shoulder, and in   58
the elbow. He has noted pain in the wrist; however, he has   69
noted numbness in the little finger with tingling. He states   81
that coughing and any jarring, or sudden motion accentuates   92
the pain.   94

His past history has included a heart attack in October,   106
and he was started on digoxin and nitroglycerin. He has been   118
dyspneic for years. He denies surgery. He has a severe   129
allergy to penicillin with almost an anaphylactic reaction.   140

The patient is sitting in bed, alert, oriented, and   151
cooperative. He appears to be in some distress with pain,   162
and the patient impresses me as not being a complainer.   173
Examination of the head is unremarkable. The neck is tender   184
in the left paraspinal region. I do not feel any nodes. The   196
thyroid is not enlarged. No carotid bruits are heard. The   207
pupils are round, equal, reacting to light and accommodation.   219
No nystagmus. Chest examination shows rhonchi in the right   230
upper portion of the chest. Cardiac examination shows a   241
normal sinus rhythm.   245

Deep tendon reflexes appear to be present throughout and   257
reasonably brisk. No Babinski responses are noted. Motor   268
testing shows weakness of the left hand and weakness of wrist   280
flexion that causes pain. There is no atrophy. There is   291
tenderness to the ulnar nerve at the elbow. An electro-   302
myography or nerve conduction studies will be necessary to   313
investigate ulnar nerve.   318

□□□□1□□□□2□□□□3□□□□4□□□□5□□□□6□□□□7□□□□8□□□□9□□□□10□□□□11□□□□12

Holidays, Days of the Week, and Months

Goals

After completing this lesson, you will be able to:

✔ Capitalize holidays.
✔ Capitalize days of the week.
✔ Capitalize months.

Example: The Brown Clinic will be closed on Thursday because it is Thanksgiving Day.

Instructions

Key the following sentences, capitalizing words as appropriate.

```
1   the books will arrive monday.
2   the center is open monday, wednesday, and friday.
3   make an appointment for wednesday.
4   this office will be closed to celebrate martin luther king day.
5   the doctor will be on vacation for the month of april.
```

Timed Writing—Double Space, Five-Minute Timed Writing

FIVE-MINUTE TIMING

This black female was referred to me by the Mobile Clinic	12
because of a long history of hypertrophic adenoids and	23
tonsils. The child was adopted by her present parents as an	34
infant.	35
She has had almost no medical problems. Mother denies	46
that the child has frequent colds to suggest that she has	57
nasal sinusitis and yet she developed enlarged adenoids and	68
tonsils. She has difficulty with speech development. In	80
addition to the speech problem, she has also had difficulty	91
with chronic mouth breathing and snoring at night.	101
Mother denies frequent upper respiratory infections and	113
does not recall the child ever being treated for tonsillitis.	125
No detailed family history is obtainable. No previous surgery,	137
and no serious illnesses.	142

☐☐☐☐1☐☐☐☐2☐☐☐☐3☐☐☐☐4☐☐☐☐5☐☐☐☐6☐☐☐☐7☐☐☐☐8☐☐☐☐9☐☐☐☐10☐☐☐☐11☐☐☐☐12

Races and Nationalities, Five-Minute Timed Writing

Goals

After completing this lesson, you will be able to:

✔ Capitalize names of races.
✔ Capitalize names of nationalities.

Example: This 22-year-old Cuban has leukemia.

Instructions

Key the following sentences, capitalizing names of races.

1 This 60-year-old asian entered the hospital with dyspnea and edema.

2 The 32-year-old native american female has thyroid disease and a history of cardiac arrhythmia.

3 She is a 43-year-old german female with lupus erythematosus.

4 This 56-year-old spanish male was admitted for coronary artery bypass surgery.

5 This 47-year-old african-american male has tachycardia and difficulty swallowing.

This 47-year-old Asian male is being evaluated for tachy- 12
cardia. He has not had previous episodes of tachycardia but 24
has had a long-standing history of hypertension and angina 35
pectoris. He has been overweight for a number years and has 47
been on Diamox and Tenormin to control his hypertension. In 58
addition, he has had osteoarthritis of the knees and gouty 69
arthritis, which has bothered him and is aggravated by his 80
excessive weight. 83

The patient was hospitalized three years ago for hyper- 95
tension and nervousness with depression. He recovered and 106
has been doing well except for poor control of his hyper- 117
tension due to his weight. 122

There is no family history of cancer, diabetes, tubercu- 134
losis, or hypertension. The patient is apprehensive due to 145
his tachycardia. He is not having any hyperpnea. The skin 156
is warm, moist, and with good turgor. His lungs are clear to 168
auscultation and percussion. The pharynx is benign. No 179
cervical adenopathy is present. Thyroid is not enlarged. No 191
liver, kidneys, or spleen masses are palpable. No hernias are 203
present. No dysuria, hematuria, or pyuria. No history of 214
fainting, convulsions, or paresthesia. No nausea, vomiting, 226
diarrhea, or constipation. 231

☐☐☐☐1☐☐☐☐2☐☐☐☐3☐☐☐☐4☐☐☐☐5☐☐☐☐6☐☐☐☐7☐☐☐☐8☐☐☐☐9☐☐☐☐10☐☐☐☐11☐☐☐☐12

State Postal Abbreviations

Goals

After completing this lesson, you will be able to:

✔ Capitalize state postal abbreviations.

Instructions

Set appropriate tab stops. Key the following state postal abbreviations and common abbreviations.

1	AL	Alabama	AK	Alaska	
2	AZ	Arizona	AS	American Samoa	
3	CA	California	AR	Arkansas	
4	CT	Connecticut	CO	Colorado	
5	DC	District of Columbia	DE	Delaware	
6	FM	Federated States	FL	Florida	
7	GA	Georgia	HI	Hawaii	
8	GU	Guam	IL	Illinois	
9	ID	Idaho	IA	Iowa	
10	IN	Indiana	KY	Kentucky	
11	KS	Kansas	ME	Maine	
12	LA	Louisiana	MH	Marshall Islands	
13	MD	Maryland	MA	Massachusetts	
14	MP	Northern Mariana	MN	Minnesota	
15	MI	Michigan	MO	Missouri	
16	MS	Mississippi	NE	Nebraska	
17	MT	Montana	NH	New Hampshire	
18	NV	Nevada	NM	New Mexico	
19	NJ	New Jersey	NC	North Carolina	
20	NY	New York	OH	Ohio	
21	ND	North Dakota	OR	Oregon	
22	OK	Oklahoma	PR	Puerto Rico	
23	PW	Palau	SC	South Carolina	
24	PA	Pennsylvania	TN	Tennessee	
25	RI	Rhode Island	UT	Utah	
26	SD	South Dakota	VA	Virginia	
27	TX	Texas	WA	Washington	
28	VT	Vermont	WI	Wisconsin	
29	VI	Virgin Islands			
30	WV	West Virginia			
31	WY	Wyoming			

Common Abbreviations

Key these abbreviations in all capitals.

1	AVE	Avenue		14	TPKE	Turnpike
2	BLVD	Boulevard		15	APT	Apartment
3	CTR	Center		16	RM	Room
4	CIR	Circle		17	STE	Suite
5	CT	Court		18	N	North
6	DR	Drive		19	S	South
7	EXPY	Expressway		20	E	East
8	HWY	Highway		21	W	West
9	IS	Island		22	NE	Northeast
10	LN	Lane		23	NW	Northwest
11	RD	Road		24	SE	Southeast
12	SQ	Square		25	SW	Southwest
13	ST	Street				

Religions, Five-Minute Timed Writing

Goals

After completing this lesson, you will be able to:

✔ Capitalize religions.

Example: The Methodist preacher performed the wedding.

Instructions

Key the following sentences, capitalizing the names of religions and their followers.

1 The catholic priest visited the AIDS patient at Cactus Hospital.
2 The 26-year-old female who is jewish collapsed.
3 The cancer patient attended the buddhist gathering.
4 They attended an islamic service at the hospital chapel.
5 The 32-year-old lutheran minister is undergoing radiation for a tumor on his left lung.

FIVE-MINUTE TIMING—DOUBLE SPACE

```
        Rose is a 35-year-old woman who had been coughing for      12
several weeks.  She had become dyspneic and developed wheezing.  24
She has not been responding to treatment with bronchodilators     36
and tetracyclines.  She was dyspneic at rest and afebrile.        47
There was a gurgling sound with respirations.  She has sinus      58
tachycardia.  Breath sounds were absent over the right base and   70
decreased bilaterally, otherwise, with no audible rales.          81
        Pulmonary function studies show decreased vital capacity.  93
Electrocardiogram showed left atrial enlargement and left        104
ventricular hypertrophy. Serum digoxin level was normal.         115
Erythrocyte sedimentation rate was normal.  Urine showed         126
albumin.  Blood sugar and BUN were normal.  Chest x-ray          137
showed only chronic changes in both lungs.                       145
        The patient was treated with bedrest, inhalation therapy, 157
bronchodilators, oral tetracycline, diuretics, and digoxin.      168
Her blood pressure was adequately controlled, and she was        179
maintained on her usual psychotropic medications consisting      190
of Sinequan at bedtime.                                          195
        She has also been treated for epistaxis associated with   207
poorly controlled hypertension.  No known familial illnesses.    219
The patient is single and lives with her parents.  She does      230
not use tobacco or alcohol.                                      235
```

□□□□1□□□□2□□□□3□□□□4□□□□5□□□□6□□□□7□□□□8□□□□9□□□□10□□□□11□□□□12

Languages

Goals

After completing this lesson, you will be able to:

✔ Capitalize languages.

Example: Mary's degree is in Italian.

Instructions

Key the following sentences, capitalizing the names of languages.

1   Mary is pursuing a career in english and german.
2   Two years of spanish is required in order to attend the University.
3   She will go to Paris to study french and the PRC to study chinese.
4   The Language Institute of Mobile is offering italian, greek, japanese, and portuguese.
5   She received her BA in swahili.

Names of Organizations and Departments, Five-Minute Timed Writing

Goals

After completing this lesson, you will be able to:

✔ Capitalize the words *association*, *organization*, or *institution* if they are part of the official name.
✔ Capitalize the names of organizations.
✔ Capitalize names of departments of a hospital.

Example: Sarah is attending the *American Association of Medical Assistants Convention* in Mobile, AZ.

Instructions

Key the following sentences, capitalizing the names of organizations and departments.

1 Mr. John Coastal was admitted to the cardiology department for chest pains, dyspnea, tachycardia, and hypertension.

2 The secretary read the minutes at the temporal bone society.

3 The radiologist administered a CAT scan in the radiology division.

4 Mary got the job heading the society of medical transcriptionists.

5 Mary returned to the infectious disease clinic because of encephalitis.

```
          This 39-year-old female has been having irregular      11
bleeding, and at times, it has been very heavy with clots of     22
blood.  She has had very severe menorrhagia leading back to      33
January.  Her period was fifteen days late.  Another time, it    45
was 20 days late.  Pap smear has been done, which was reported   57
as class II.                                                     59
          Review of systems include no previous headaches, no    70
earache, and no sore throat.  No chest pain, hemoptysis,         81
dyspnea, or edema.  No dysuria, pyuria, or hematuria.  Her       92
uterus appears to be slightly enlarged and has a small           103
posterior cervical cyst.  The are no masses in the adnexa.       114
Thyroid is not enlarged.  No lymphadenopathy.  Chest is clear    126
to auscultation and percussion.  No evidence of cardiac          137
enlargement.  No murmurs are detected.  There are no masses,     148
tenderness, or tumors noted in both breasts.  There are          159
hemorrhoids present internally and externally.                   168
          Her mother and brother died of diabetes.  She has had no  180
previous surgery.  She has four children, living and well.       191
She is healthy appearing female in no acute distress.            201
          The patient had an abdominal hysterectomy, bilateral   212
salpingo-oopherectomy, and appendectomy with abdominal           223
exploration.  She has progressed very well following surgery.    235
          She has been instructed in her postoperative care and  246
activities at home.  She is to see Dr. Sampson in three weeks    258
in the office.                                                   261
```

□□□□1□□□□2□□□□3□□□□4□□□□5□□□□6□□□□7□□□□8□□□□9□□□□10□□□□11□□□□12

Double Space, Five-Minute Timed Writing

The patient is an attorney who was admitted to Mobile	11
Hospital with cerebral hemorrhage secondary to abuse of crack.	23
She was initially brought to Pacific Hospital after she had	34
developed an acute headache and had become unresponsive. A CT	46
scan revealed a right cerebral hematoma with blood in both	57
ventricles. Several days later, the patient underwent a	68
craniotomy for a large cerebral hematoma. Subsequent to this	80
surgery, the patient was comatose. She has a perforated	91
gastric ulcer which required surgery. The patient was found	102
to have an abdominal abscess which was surgically drained.	113
There was recurrent bronchitis and atelectasis of the left	124
lobe of the lung requiring bronchoscopy.	132
She eventually regained consciousness ten days later.	143
Her neurologic exam revealed a diminished gag reflex; but	154
she appeared to be alert and oriented to person and place. She	166
complained of blurry vision and difficulty elevating her arms	178
or legs. The plantar reflexes were downgoing. Her sensory exam	190
appeared normal. Her prognosis for recovery is considered to	202
be quite good. The patient was discharged to home in good	213
condition.	215

□□□□1□□□□2□□□□3□□□□4□□□□5□□□□6□□□□7□□□□8□□□□9□□□□10□□□□11□□□□12

Formats I

Centering and Memoranda, Five-Minute Timed Writing

Goals

After completing this lesson, you will be able to:

✔ Center type.
✔ Use memoranda formats.

Instructions

To center, key words at the left margin then click the center icon using Word for Windows. Key the following exercises, horizontally centering each line on the page. Instructor will show you how to center.

```
1   Dr. Evie W. Sampson
    Announces the opening of her new office
    at
    3801 Cactus Lane Street
    Mobile, AZ 62033-0000
2   Principles of Medical Keyboarding
    Seminar
    by Jean Moss
    Instructor
```

MEMORANDA

Begin keying the memorandum seven lines from the top of the paper. The headings of the memo (TO, FROM, DATE, and SUBJECT) are keyed in all capital letters followed by a colon. These headings are keyed double-spaced. The body of the memo begins two lines below the SUBJECT: line. Memoranda are *not* keyed with paragraph indents; single-space within a paragraph, and double-space between paragraphs. Double-space after the final paragraph to add reference initials, the words "Attachment" or "Enclosure," "c:," or Distribution. These final four items should be keyed single-spaced.

A distribution list is found at the end of a memorandum when there are several individuals listed. Names are listed alphabetically, but they may be listed by rank in the organization. Use a template for formatting a document, such as a memorandum. Instructor will show you how to use a template. E-mails are also similar to memoranda.

Key the following memoranda in the correct format. Set a tab sufficient to clear the subject line or use the template. Study the sample memoranda below and then key. Proofread your copy and correct errors.

Example Memorandum

```
Line 7
MEMO TO:     Mary Success, MD—Distribution below              5
DS
FROM:        Robert Smith, MD                                10
DS
DATE:        May 18, XXXX                                    14
DS
SUBJECT:     ACHIEVING SUCCESS                               19
TS

You are one of the most important persons in the world. Day   30
by day, concentrate your thoughts on achieving the highest    41
goal that is possible to attain. In this endeavor to succeed, 52
many people make mistakes that hold them back and if persis-  63
ted in, will be their downfall. There are certain fundamentals 74
to follow if you are to enjoy success and happiness. You must  85
be willing to sacrifice something to achieve your goals.      95
DS

Confidence in your ability to succeed is the additional factor 107
for success. Individuals are born with a need to succeed in   118
their endeavors. To become successful, one must plan, and one 129
must discipline oneself to achieve goals. Celebrate small or  140
large goals and be proud of your achievements. Success comes  151
with positive thinking, applying knowledge, and attaining     162
skills.
DS

EM                                                           163
DS

Distribution List:                                           166
     Joyce Boil                                              169
     Ruby Fever                                              172
     Sara Foot                                               175
□□□□1□□□□2□□□□3□□□□4□□□□5□□□□6□□□□7□□□□8□□□□9□□□□10□□□□11□□□□12
```

Key the memorandum below. Study the sample before keying. Proofread your copy and correct errors.

Memorandum 1

DATE:	Use current date	5
TO:	Mrs. Ruby Palsy, Education Department	15
FROM:	Mrs. Mary Mass, Director of Health Information	26
SUBJECT:	Proofreading Seminar	33

A Proofreading Seminar will be presented by Jan Bruit,   44
director of Medical Transcription. Your staff is welcome to   55
attend.   56

New techniques for proofreading and proofreaders' marks will   67
be discussed. Attached is the agenda for the seminar. Please   78
call Mrs. Ruthie Brown for reservations at 400-2999, ext. 20.   90

ks   91

Attachment   93

Instructions

Key the following memorandum. Study the sample before keying. Proofread your copy and correct errors.

Memorandum 2

<u>Mobile University Medical School</u>   6

Memorandum   8

DATE:	Use current date	13
TO:	ALL Employees--Distribution below	22
FROM:	Morris Femur, MD, Director of Health Institute	33

SUBJECT: CONFIDENTIAL AWARENESS BROCHURES   41

Enclosed are copies of the Confidential Awareness Brochures   53
that are to be distributed to all employees immediately.   63

Please remember that we are distributing these brochures to   74
comply with the rules of the Medical Board.   82

es   83

Distribution: 85
    Cindy Brown, MD   89
    Charles Tibia, MD   93
    Randy Patella, MD   97

□□□□1□□□□2□□□□3□□□□4□□□□5□□□□6□□□□7□□□□8□□□□9□□□□10□□□□11□□□□12

Key the following memorandum. Proofread your copy and correct errors.

Memorandum 3

DATE:	February 4, 200X	6
TO:	Dr. Louis Hubbard, Rheumatology Division	16
FROM:	Mary Smith, Research Director	24
SUBJECT:	STRESS REDUCTION	30

The Rheumatology Division is invited to attend a seminar on	41
Stress Reduction.	44
This seminar will be presented by Dr. Mary Cocci, director of	56
the Health Institute.	60
Call Mrs. Jean Scan at 000-111-1111, ext. 11, for a	70
reservation.	72
pk	73

Instructions

Key the following memorandum. Proofread your copy and correct errors.

Memorandum 4

DATE:	July 1, 200__	5
DS		
TO:	Employees	9
DS		
FROM:	Dr. Doris Algia, Chief of Radiology	19
DS		
SUBJECT:	RADIOLOGY CLINIC	25
DS		

The Radiology Clinic's new address is 2552 Cactus Road,	36
Mobile, AZ, 00000-6207. Our new telephone number is	46
000-444-5555.	49
Effective July 10, 200__, the Radiology Clinic will be open	60
from 8:00 a.m. to 5:30 p.m.	66
DS	
pk	67

□□□□1□□□□2□□□□3□□□□4□□□□5□□□□6□□□□7□□□□8□□□□9□□□□10□□□□11□□□□12

Simplified Memorandum

The simplified memorandum's format is essentially similar to the standard memorandum format, with the following exception: the words *DATE, FROM,* and *SUBJECT* are omitted. Key the following memoranda in the correct format.

Example Simplified Memorandum

Instructions

Study the example first and then key. Proofread your copy and correct errors.

```
Line 7
Use current date

DS
TO: Jessica King, MD, Director of Medical Education
    Alice Hubbard, MD, Director of Continuing Education

DS
CARPAL TUNNEL SYNDROME STUDY

DS

Helen Carpal is a right-handed female patient who reports feeling a
sharp and burning pain involving the bilateral wrists with numbness
and a tingling extending into the elbow. She is presently employed
as an assembler. She was evaluated by an orthopedic surgeon. The
patient was advised that she was suffering from bilateral carpal
tunnel syndrome. Wrist splints were recommended. The patient wore
splints while sleeping and noted her condition did not worsen. The
patient was referred to another physician for an EMG and nerve con-
duction velocity testing. Physical therapy was provided for her at
the orthopedic clinic. There is some improvement in her condition.
She will be monitored in this research study.

DS
ah
```

Simplified Memorandum 1

Instructions

Key the following memoranda. Proofread your copy and correct errors

Use current date	3
Mary C. Medulla, M.D.	7
Marvin J. Kwell, M.D.	11
THE ART OF LISTENING	15
Mrs. Willie Bone presents a class on The Art of Listening.	26
Ways to improve your listening skills are to listen carefully	37
while the other person is speaking and remain quiet. Look at	48
the person who is talking to you; your eyes can tell you as	59
much as do your ears. Concentrate on what is being said in	60
verbal and nonverbal communication.	77
Learn not to prejudge what the speaker is saying because	88
unconsciously you tune out what is being said.	97
kf	98
Attachment	100
Distribution:	102
Mr. Perry Artery	106
Mrs. Jimmie Incision	111

□□□□1□□□□2□□□□3□□□□4□□□□5□□□□6□□□□7□□□□8□□□□9□□□□10□□□□11□□□□12

Simplified Memorandum 2

Use current date	3
Sarah Cell, RN	6
Brian Megaly, RN	9
TIME MANAGEMENT	12
A Time Management video will be shown every Friday at noon in	24
the library. It is 20 minutes long. Several videos are	34
available to be checked out from the office. Call Mrs. Molly	45
Litho at 277-CARE for information.	51
The video is to be returned in five days.	59
tbm	60

□□□□1□□□□2□□□□3□□□□4□□□□5□□□□6□□□□7□□□□8□□□□9□□□□10□□□□11□□□□12

This 55-year-old Caucasian male was seen in the emergency   12
department complaining of breathing difficulty. He did   22
improve after receiving an aerosol treatment. He does have a   33
complicated past history that includes an inoperable pulmonary   45
sulcus tumor of the right upper lung. Subsequently, he received 57
radiation treatments while in the hospital. He had presented   68
at Mobile Hospital in June with arthritic symptoms and was   79
treated for arthritis. He now feels that he can no longer   100
travel to Mobile Hospital for further treatment and desires   111
to obtain medical care here in Gila Bend. He lives in Gila   122
Bend. He has had great difficulty breathing, although he had   133
not been expectorating purulent sputum. He has been aware of   144
chilly sensations and is quite dyspneic at night. he is   155
allergic to penicillin manifested by tightness in his throat   166
and wheezing.   168

Current medications include Esidrix, Micro-K, and amino-   179
phylline. He is also using codeine for chronic pain in his   190
right shoulder.   193

Physical examination at this time is remarkable. His   204
mouth and throat are free of lesions. The neck is supple.   215
Breath sounds are remarkable for an accentuation of high-   226
pitched breath sounds in the upper chest. The breath sounds   237
are otherwise diminished. No wheezes or rales are currently   248
noted. The heart tones are distant. The abdomen is soft and   259
benign to palpation, and there is no peripheral edema. A   270
chest x-ray demonstrates a density at the right lung apex,   281
and this is in the region of the tumor where he received   292
radiation therapy.   295

He has been given a course of Vibramycin. He will   306
return to see me in follow-up in one week. Attempts will be   317
made to obtain his medical records from Mobile Hospital.   328
SMAC profile is being drawn in the emergency department and   339
faxed to my office.   343

☐☐☐☐1☐☐☐☐2☐☐☐☐3☐☐☐☐4☐☐☐☐5☐☐☐☐6☐☐☐☐7☐☐☐☐8☐☐☐☐9☐☐☐☐10☐☐☐☐11☐☐☐☐12

Minutes and Agendas, Five-Minute Timed Writing

Goals

After completing this lesson, you will be able to:

✔ Prepare and key minutes.
✔ Prepare and key agendas.

MINUTES

Minutes are taken by an attendee of a meeting and later formatted into a record. The record contains the following: the title, the date the meeting was held, the members present, the members absent, a note on the reading of the previous meeting's minutes, sections on subjects discussed at the meeting, a note on the adjournment of the meeting, and closing lines.

The title and the word "MINUTES" are keyed in all capital letters and centered on the page; the word "MINUTES" is underlined. Each section heading is keyed in all capital letters and underlined, followed by a colon.

Double-space after the word "MINUTES." Single-space between sections and paragraphs. Single-space the text within a section. For the closing material, double-space before the line "Respectfully submitted," then triple-space to the writer's name. Double-space again to add the typist's initials.

Key the sample minutes in correct format. Proofread your copy and correct errors.

MEDICAL EDUCATION ADVISORY COMMITTEE   10

DS

<u>MINUTES</u>   17

DS

<u>DATE</u>:   18

The Medical Education Advisory Committee meeting was called to   30
order at 2:45 p.m., Wednesday, February 10, 200__, at Mobile   41
Medical Clinic, Room 201.   46

DS

<u>MEMBERS PRESENT</u>:   49

Joan Oma, Jimmy Cocci, Henry Oste, Bobby Plasma, Betty Brain,   60
Birdie Nerve, Geraldine Petrie, Ann Marie Ventral, Beverly Pain   72
and Jean Dorsal   75

DS

<u>MEMBERS ABSENT</u>:   78

Pamel Tome, Vickie Lateral, Trent Superior, and Anita Cele.   89

DS

<u>MINUTES</u>:   91

Minutes for the January 10, 200__, meeting were reviewed and   102
accepted.   104

DS

<u>MEDICAL KEYBOARDING COMMITTEE</u>:   110

The focus of the Medical Keyboarding Committee is the Medical   121
Keyboard Club. Posters will be made and distributed to the   132
classrooms. The club is to promote excellence, leadership, and   144
educational opportunities. Field trips will be taken to   155
medical facilities.   159

DS

<u>CAREER DAY</u>:   161

Career day was discussed. The focus of the next meeting will   172
be a Career Fair. Twenty companies have agreed to participate.   184
Tony Gait, MD, is the speaker for Career Day.   193

DS

<u>ADJOURNMENT</u>:   195

The meeting was adjourned by the president at 4 p.m.   205

DS

Respectfully submitted,   209

TS

_____

Patty Bony, Recording Secretary   215

DS

ec   216

□□□□1□□□□2□□□□3□□□□4□□□□5□□□□6□□□□7□□□□8□□□□9□□□□10□□□□11□□□□12

AGENDAS

The agenda is keyed before the meeting. It tells information that will be discussed at the meeting. The agenda includes name, date, time of meeting, location of meeting, roll call, committee reports, reports of officers, new and old business, announcements, and adjournment.

Instructions

Key the following agenda. Center the headings, and double-space after the headings. Key Roman numerals to number the list. Leave five spaces after the Roman numeral. Proofread your dopy and correct errors.

Agenda

```
                    AGENDA                                6
DS
                MOBILE MEDICAL CLINIC                     14
DS
        MEDICAL EDUCATION ADVISORY COMMITTEE             23
DS
    February 10, 200__                                    27
DS
I. Call to Order                                         30
DS
II. Roll Call---Introduction of Guests                  38
DS
III. Approval of Minutes---January 10, 200__            47
DS
IV. Officers' Reports---Treasurer's Report              55
DS
V. Committee Reports---Membership and Workplace Needs   65
DS
VI. Old Business---Association of Medical Keyboarding   75
DS
VII. New Business---Medical Keyboarding Club            84
DS
VIII. Announcements---Career Day---Tony Gait, MD,Speaker 95
DS
IX. Adjournment                                         98
□□□□1□□□□2□□□□3□□□□4□□□□5□□□□6□□□□7□□□□8□□□□9□□□□10□□□□11□□□□12
```

Tom is a 65-year-old male with severe chronic obstructive 12
pulmonary disease who was brought by an ambulance to the 23
emergency department. Yesterday, this patient had expecto- 34
rated brownish mucus. He talked with me on the telephone, 45
and I initiated a course of tetracycline. However, he 55
developed difficulty breathing with increased cough, although 66
there was no additional mucus. He had a sharp, stabbing chest 78
pain and contacted me at about 8 p.m. He had Darvocet-N 50 89
at home and was advised to try this for pain relief. He did, 100
and the pain was not alleviated. The emergency department 111
physician found the patient to be in no acute distress. He 122
was complaining of anterior chest pain and seemed to have 133
chest wall tenderness on the right. Chest x-ray revealed a 144
questionable infiltrate in the right lung, but review of this 155
film with Dr. Pima, the radiologist, does not reveal any 166
significant change compared to films obtained on the patient's 178
recent admission. Rib films on the right side were also 189
nonrevealing, and there was no evidence of a recent rib 200
fracture. 202

Vital signs were stable, and physical examination was 213
not significantly changed from the past. Tom's discharge 224
medication included Prelone, Lopressor, Lasix, potassium 235
chloride supplement, and Theo-Dur. 242

The patient is disabled from construction work where he 253
was exposed to asbestos. He denies cephalgia or changes in 264
vision or hearing. He has not had any episodes of difficult 275
swallowing. His appetite is poor. He is aware of a sharp 286
anterior chest pain that radiates to the right lateral chest 297
wall. This is aggravated by deep breathing and coughing. He 309
denies nausea and vomiting. Bowel habits are regular every 320
day. He denies dysuria, although this had been a recurrent 331
problem in the past. 335

□□□□1□□□□2□□□□3□□□□4□□□□5□□□□6□□□□7□□□□8□□□□9□□□□10□□□□11□□□□12

Formats II

Block Letter, Five-Minute Timed Writing

Goals

After completing this lesson, you will be able to:

✔ Key and format a standard block letter.

Instructions

Set 1-inch margins or 1.25 as in Word. Key the following letters in the block format. When you have finished, proofread and mark all errors. Rekey and make the corrections.

Business letters and personal-business letters are written in a formal style. If the writer's style is too informal or is inappropriate for the forum, the information in the letter may be disregarded. When writing business letters, be sure to address recipients by their full names. Be clear, concise, and polite.

Two formats for business and personal-business letters are block and modified block format. This lesson discusses the block format. In the block format, begin keying all information at the left margin.

Letters are always keyed on 8½-by-11-inch paper. Leave 1-inch margins on all sides. If company letterhead stationery is used, the return address need not be added, because that information will appear preprinted on the stationery. If you are using blank paper, this is the personal-business letter, and you will need to add your return address.

BUSINESS LETTER

Business letters have certain standards in content and format. The order and spacing of the components are different for the business letter and the personal-business letter. All letters have the following components: date, return address, inside address, salutation, body of the letter, the closing line, and the signature block. In addition, there may be a reference (or subject) line below the salutation and "c" and "enclosure" lines below the closing lines.

The following is the order and spacing for business letters keyed on letterhead stationery.

Date line. The date line begins 15 lines from the top of the page. Be sure to spell out the month completely.

You can now use vertical centering in Word or Word Perfect, and the letter is automatically centered vertically. You do not have to count to line 15.

(QS)

Inside address. The inside address line begins 4 lines below the date line. Include the addressee's title.

Attention. Attention can be keyed in all capitals or the first letter capitalized. Attention is keyed double-spaced after the last line of the address before the salutation.

(DS)

Salutation. The salutation line begins two lines below the final inside address line. Be sure to include the recipient's full name and end the line with a colon. With open punctuation, you will not use anything. (*Example:* Dear Dr. Smith:)

(DS)

Reference line. If there is to be a reference line, begin keying two lines below the salutation line or above the salutation. (Re: Sara Smile Medical Record No.: 52)

(DS)

Body of the letter. The body of the letter begins two lines below the salutation line (or reference line). Key the body of the letter single-spaced (SS) with double-spacing (DS) between paragraphs.

(DS)

Closing lines. The closing lines begin two spaces below the final line of the body of the letter. Key "Sincerely yours," or the close you prefer.

Blind copy notation: The notation "bc" is used when a letter is sent to someone without the knowledge of the addressee. The name of the person receiving the bc is keyed in the left margin double-spaced below the last part of the letter. *Example:* bc Mary Pale, MD

Signature block. The signature block begins (QS) below the closing line. Key the writer's full name and title.

Reference initials. Initials are keyed a (DS) below the keyed signature at the left margin. Do not key initials when you key a letter for your own signature. Use a colon or virgule with reference initials.

Example:
MT:EM or mt:em
MT/EM or mt/em

C and enclosure lines. These lines begin two spaces below the writer's title (or name, if there is no title). Single-space the "c:" line and any others that follow. C stands for copy of the letter. Enclosure means an item is being sent with the letter.

If the letter is more than one page long, begin the second page 1 inch from the top of the paper. Use blank paper for the second and subsequent pages; use letterhead stationery for the first page only. Never divide a word across pages. Always leave at least two lines at the bottom of the first page, and carry at least two keyed lines to the top of the second page. You can now use the widows and orphans feature of software or the "keep text together" feature.

Key the business letter on page 289 in the block style.

Second Page Letters

Example: Horizontal
Re: Judy A. Mast   2   August 5, 200__

Example: Vertical
Re: Judy A. Mast
         Page 2
         August 5, 200__

The patient comes in today for follow-up of recurrent   11
abdominal pain. She is following up the results of a pelvic   22
ultrasound. Overall, she is feeling much better. She has   33
been on Prevacid, 30 mg q.d., and I had also given her some   44
Tagamet, which she has not been using. She says her symptoms   56
only bother her when she eats too much or eats too late at   67
night. She otherwise has no complaints. The patient appears   79
well. Vital signs are stable. A pelvic ultrasound was done   90
on January 21 to evaluate what appeared to be a possible   101
ovarian cyst. The pelvic ultrasound showed a uterine fibroid,   113
and no evidence of any cystic masses. The ovaries were not   124
well visualized on the ultrasound. No free fluid was identi-   136
fied. She had abdominal pain with some weight loss. Her   147
weight has now been stable. Her symptoms are improved on   158
proton pump inhibitors. She will followup with me for any   169
further problems.   172

▢▢▢▢1▢▢▢▢2▢▢▢▢3▢▢▢▢4▢▢▢▢5▢▢▢▢6▢▢▢▢7▢▢▢▢8▢▢▢▢9▢▢▢▢10▢▢▢▢11▢▢▢▢12

Letterhead	Mobile Hospital
	4070 Rock Street
	Mobile, AZ 60000-2000
	(000) 000-0000 FAX: (000) 000-0000
	www.mobilehospital.com
Dateline	June 21, 200__
	QS
Letter	Eliza Malacia, MD
address	Emergency Clinic
	3978 Foley Street
	Mobile, AZ 60000-2000
	DS
Salutation	Dear Dr. Malacia:
	DS
	Re: Excessive Freckling Symposium

Thank you so much for your invitation to the Hyper-melanotic/Excessive Freckling Symposium. This subject is a particular interest of mine, as many of my patients cannot be convinced to stay out of the sun or use proper sunscreens.

DS

The enclosed guidelines outline the subject on Hypermelanotic/Excessive Freckling Symposium.

DS

I will surely be in attendance and look forward to meeting you there.

DS

Complimentary	Sincerely yours,
close	QS
Title	Edward Burns, MD
	Chief of Dermatology
	DS
Reference	EB:ES
initials	DS
Enclosure	Enclosure

Business Letter 2

Instructions:

Key the following letter in block format. Proofread your copy and correct errors.

```
                        current date/Evie W. Wright, MD        11
                        3842 Cactus Lane/Mobile, AZ            21
                        60000-1644/Dear Dr. Wright:            31
                        RE: Mrs. Jean S. Poly                  40
                        Medical Record No.: 49C                49
```

DS

```
Thank you for asking me to see this 52-year-old lady for       60
evaluation of type II diabetes mellitus. Mrs. Jean Poly has a  71
history of hypertension, psoriasis of approximately five years 83
duration, and degenerative joint disease. With these diseases, 94
she developed a gangrenous ulcer of the right foot. Mrs. Poly  105
was treated with antibiotics, but it became necessary for her  116
to have surgery.                                               119
```

DS

```
On September 20, she underwent right foot surgery because of   130
the infection. Enclosed is an operative report. She became     141
febrile and hypertensive. Medications were administered for    152
fever and hypertension. On September 25, she was discharged to 163
home without fever.                                            166
```

DS

```
A follow-up visit showed healing of the right foot, and a      177
prosthesis was provided. She was seen several days later for    188
swelling of the surgical site from the prosthesis. The area was 200
aspirated, yielding 4 ml of bloody serum. Mrs. Poly was advised 211
to call if she had any problems.                               217
```

DS

```
Sincerely,/Matthew T. Sampson, MD                             224
Professor of Infectious Disease                               230
```

```
MS:PD/Enclosure                                               233
```

```
□□□□1□□□□2□□□□3□□□□4□□□□5□□□□6□□□□7□□□□8□□□□9□□□□10□□□□11□□□□12
```

Business Letter 3

Key in block format. Key the letter below in a 3-minute timing. If you finish before time is called, start over. Proofread your copy and corect errors.

```
current date/Judy Cast, MD/4554 Condyle Street               9
San Jose, CA 92017-6203/Dear Dr. Cast:                      16
Re: Kellie Cold/Medical Record No: 4510                     24

DS

Kellie is a 16-month-old baby girl who was admitted to the   35
Children's Center with acute lymphocytic leukemia diagnosed  46
July, XXXX. She is currently in remission. Her fever was 104° 57
and a neutropenia report showed a total white blood count of 68
300. Cultures were obtained, and she was started on antibiotic 80
therapy. Cultures remained negative. She defervesced, then   91
became febrile again for four days and is now afebrile. During 103
this period of time, her blood counts recovered. At the time 114
of discharge, her white blood count was 3,100 with 25 segs, 53 126
bands, platelets were 80,000, hemoglobin 8.5, and hematocrit 137
was 23.8.                                                   138

DS

She developed diaper dermatitis and was treated with nystatin. 150
She was discharged today. I instructed her parents to apply  161
nystatin cream to the diaper area three times a day. She is to 182
return to the Pediatric Clinic in two weeks for blood counts. 193
Thank you for referring this patient to me.                 201

Sincerely yours,/Mary Spine, MD                             207

Director, Children's Center/MS:ES                           213
```

□□□□1□□□□2□□□□3□□□□4□□□□5□□□□6□□□□7□□□□8□□□□9□□□□10□□□□11□□□□12

THE PERSONAL-BUSINESS LETTER

Personal-business letters are keyed on blank paper. Because there is no letterhead to give the return address, it must be added.

Instructions

Key the following letters in the personal-business style. Key the example personal-business letter below.

Example Personal-Business Letter 1—Block Format

```
                        Crystal Tract, MD                          7
                        Orthopedic Clinic                          14
                        2401 Fleet Street                          21
                     Mobile, AZ 60000-6203                         29
                        605-003-0004                               36
DS
Current Date                                                       38

DS
John Supine, MD                                                    41
4258 Curve Street                                                  44
Mobile, AZ 60000-6203                                              48

DS
Dear Dr. Supine:                                                   51

DS
RE: Dawn Bone                                                      54

DS
Thank you for referring this 21-year-old woman to me. She has      66
a history of pseudo-locking of her knee. She is a professional     78
golfer and has had pain with this knee. There has been no          89
effusion of her knee.                                              93

DS
On examination, she complained of pain and popping of her          104
knee. The patient was placed in the supine position. A             114
resector was inserted and part of the plica was incised. The       125
knee was irrigated with 4 liters of saline. The skin was           136
closed with 3-0 Vicryl. Steri-Strips were applied.                 146

DS
She will return to the Orthopedic Clinic in three weeks for a      158
follow-up evaluation. She should be able to return to her          169
normal activities in two months.                                   175

DS
Sincerely,                                                         177

QS
Crystal Tract, MD                                                  180

DS
ev                                                                 181
```

☐☐☐☐1☐☐☐☐2☐☐☐☐3☐☐☐☐4☐☐☐☐5☐☐☐☐6☐☐☐☐7☐☐☐☐8☐☐☐☐9☐☐☐☐10☐☐☐☐11☐☐☐☐12

```
                              current date/Dr. Mary Bands          10
                              4350 Cobb Avenue/Laveen, AZ 61000-1344  22
                              Dear Dr. Bands:/Re: Marci Ileum        33
                              Medical Record No.: 1919               43
```

DS
```
This 12-year-old girl was seen in my office today for not      54
sleeping at night. She has no wheezing. She has been using her  66
inhaler as needed for asthma. Since her last visit, Marci has   78
missed no school.                                               81
```

DS
```
On physical examination, she was alert and cooperative. Head,   92
eyes, ears, nose, and throat examination revealed mild         102
rhinitis and conjunctivitis. Her lungs are clear to            112
auscultation and percussion.                                   117
```

DS
```
Marci is doing well. However, I instructed her parents that    128
she should use the inhaler before exercising. Marci is to      139
return in two months for reevaluation.                         146
```

DS
```
Thank you for allowing me to manage this patient's care.       156
```

DS
```
Sincerely,/Charles Sinus, MD/Children's Health Center          166
```

```
5225 Dust Street                                               169
Mobile, AZ 60000-5555                                          173
605-001-3000/CS:ES                                            176
```
□□□□1□□□□2□□□□3□□□□4□□□□5□□□□6□□□□7□□□□8□□□□9□□□□10□□□□11□□□□12

Instructions

Key the letter in block format. Study the sample letter first. Proofread your document and correct errors.

```
Current date/Mrs. Jane Renal/Attorney at Law/3980 Dry Road/    11
Mobile, AZ 20000-2000/Dear Mrs. Renal/Re: Sore Nelson: /Medical 22
Record No.: 390                                                25
```

DS
```
Miss Sore Nelson was in the office on June 18 and relates the   36
following history. The patient is a 25-year-old woman who was   47
a rear-seat passenger in a minivan proceeding south of          57
Flagstaff on Highway 17, whereupon the vehicle had slowed due   68
to excessive traffic and was rear-ended by another vehicle.     79
The patient was thrown around within the interior of the        90
vehicle. She did not strike her head; however, she was dazed   101
following the accident and developed pain within the cervical  112
and low back area. She also suffered multiple contusions and   123
abrasions. The patient saw her physician, Dr. Cool Summer,     134
who referred her to an orthopedic surgeon by the name of Dr.   145
Bone Flowers. Dr. Flowers examined her and felt that the       156
```
□□□□1□□□□2□□□□3□□□□4□□□□5□□□□6□□□□7□□□□8□□□□9□□□□10□□□□11□□□□12

---

symptoms would subside with time. However, the patient has 167
persisted to have pain within the neck and low back area and 178
presented herself at this facility for evaluation. The patient 190
is right-hand dominant and works as a coder for Mobile Clinic. 201
She has noted great difficulty in carrying out her normal 212
activities. 214
DS

PAST HISTORY: There have been no previous accidents or serious 226
injuries. The patient has not been hospitalized previously nor 238
does she have major medical problems. 245
DS

REVIEW OF SYSTEMS: Within normal limits. 251
DS

FAMILY HISTORY: Noncontributory. 257
DS

PHYSICAL EXAMINATION: The patient is a well-developed, well 268
nourished female who is clear mentally, oriented to time, 279
person, and place. The vital signs reveal a blood pressure of 290
118/70, pulse 80, and respiratory 18. 297
DS

HEAD: Examination of the head does not reveal any evidence of 308
contusions, abrasions, or lacerations. 315
DS

EYES: The pupils are round, equal, and reactive to light and 326
accommodation. The fundoscopic examination is within normal 337
limits. 338
DS

NECK: The trachea is within the midline. The thyroid is 348
palpable without defect. There is no jugular venous 358
distension. The carotid pulsations are 4+ and equal without 369
bruit or thrill. 372
DS

Examination of the cervical paraspinal muscles reveals muscle 383
spasm and tenderness from C1 to T1 with limitation of forward 394
flexion, rotation to the right and left, and bending to the 405
right and left, approximately 15 degrees off the 0 position. 416
DS

UPPER EXTREMITIES: There is no evidence of contusions, 426
abrasions, or lacerations. There is no motor or sensory loss. 437
Deep tendon reflexes are normal, active and equal. 447
DS

CHEST: The chest wall is intact without bony defect. There is 458
no chest wall compression tenderness. Respiratory excursions 469
are full and equal without limitation. There is no evidence of 481
cyanosis. The lungs are clear to percussion and auscultation. 492
DS

HEART: Regular rhythm without murmur or thrill. 501
DS

DORSAL SPINE: The dorsal paraspinal musculature reveals a 512
normal kyphotic curvature being present. There is no 522
percussion tenderness. Full range of motion is experienced. 533

□□□□1□□□□2□□□□3□□□□4□□□□5□□□□6□□□□7□□□□8□□□□9□□□□10□□□□11□□□□12

DS

ABDOMEN: There is no hepatosplenomegaly. There is localized   545
tenderness. Bowel sounds are within normal limits. There are   556
no masses palpable.   559
DS

LUMBAR SPINE: Examination of the lumbar spine reveals muscle   570
spasm and tenderness from the paraspinal muscle from L5 to S1   581
with marked limitation of motion in forward flexion, being   592
able to accomplish only 90 degrees off the vertical and with   603
findings of aggravation of her symptoms and muscle spasm with   614
rotation to the right and left and bending to the right and   625
left. Straight leg raising sign is negative.   634
DS

HERNIA: None present.   638
DS

LOWER EXTREMITIES: There is no pedal edema. There is no   648
evidence of contusions, abrasions, or lacerations. Deep   658
tendon reflexes are normal, active, and equal. The patient   669
has a normal gait and has a normal station.   677
DS

NEUROLOGICAL: The peripheral nerves II-XII are within normal   688
limits.   689
DS

IMPRESSION: 691
1. Musculoligamentous strain of the cervical paraspinal   701
muscles.   702
2. Musculoligamentous strain of the lumbar paraspinal muscles.   713
DS

PLAN: I am requesting x-rays be taken of the cervical and   724
lumbar paraspinal areas and will start the patient on an   735
intensive course of physical therapy supplemented by a course   746
of nonsteroidal anti-inflammatory pain medication. I would   757
like to have the patient evaluated by an orthopedic surgeon   768
and return to see me in one week.   774
DS

If I can be of further help, please contact me at this   784
office.   785
DS

Sincerely,/Sally Lumbar, MD/Director of Pain Medical Group/   796
SL: Typist's initials   800
□□□□1□□□□2□□□□3□□□□4□□□□5□□□□6□□□□7□□□□8□□□□9□□□□10□□□□11□□□□12

Key the letter in block format.

```
Current Date/Hand Sampson, MD/3980 Dust Road/Mobile, AZ        10
20000-2000/Dear Dr. Sampson/Re: Robbie Pain/MR#: 002/          20
```

DS

```
Robbie was diagnosed as having stage II Wilms tumor on         30
November 9. Chemotherapy was started according to the          40
protocol November 10. Radiation therapy was initiated on       51
November 15 but had to be held on November 21 when Robbie      62
was admitted to Mobile Hospital with evisceration. He was      73
transferred to Laveen Hospital on November 28 for intravenous  84
antibiotics and was discharged on December 4. Radiation        94
therapy was again initiated on December 9 and completed on    105
December 24 with 2000 rads given to the left abdomen at the   116
site of the left nephrectomy. A chest film on December 28 was 127
normal. He returned on January 10 for continuation of        137
chemotherapy. Physical examination at that time was within   148
normal limits.                                               150
```

DS

```
Chemotherapy was initiated on January 16 and, in addition, a 161
chest film was obtained, which showed suspicious areas of    172
metastasis. Chemotherapy was continued, and special views of 183
the chest were obtained on January 19, which confirmed new   193
lesions in the chest. There are two lesions on the left and  204
two lesions on the right side of his chest.                  212
```

DS

```
Unfortunately, there has been a recurrence of disease in the 223
chest of this patient. This is not unexpected for the amount 234
of disease Robbie had initially. Chemotherapy should be      244
continued, but consideration should also be given for surgical 256
and radiation therapy intervention at this time. I would like 268
to refer Robbie to Dr. Colic Cobb for a thoracic surgery     279
consultation. My preference is for surgical removal of lung  290
metastasis. Following tumor removal, I feel that radiation    301
therapy to both lungs should be initiated.                   309
```

DS

```
Thanks for allowing me to continue in Robbie's treatment.    320
```

DS

```
Sincerely,/Minnie Heart, MD/Director of Oncology/MH:Typist's 331
initials                                                     332
```

```
□□□□1□□□□2□□□□3□□□□4□□□□5□□□□6□□□□7□□□□8□□□□9□□□□10□□□□11□□□□12
```

Instruction

Key the letter in block format.

```
Current Date/Liver Sampson, MD/3941 Dust Road/Mobile, AZ       11
20000-2000/Dear Dr. Sampson/Re: Jane Foot/Medical Record No.:  21
49 C                                                           22
DS
Thank you for referring Mrs. Foot to the Gastroenterology      33
Clinic for evaluation of her gastroesophageal reflux disease   44
symptoms.                                                      45
DS
Mrs. Foot is a 40-year-old woman with no significant past      56
medical history who has been complaining of abdominal          66
discomfort over the past two to four years; however, it has    77
progressively worsened over the past two to four months.       88
DS
She was started on Tagamet 400 mg p.o. b.i.d., which has       98
provided partial relief of her reflux symptoms; however,      108
despite this medication, she continued to describe midabdom-  119
inal discomfort. She states that this is aggravated by eating 130
and is associated with reflux.                                136
DS
In addition, she states that this has been associated with    147
increased gas, for which over-the-counter simethicone has     158
provided relief. She complained of some bloating, which has   169
been relieved, and she has discontinued taking Metamucil.     180
DS
Currently, she denies any nausea or vomiting, gastrointestinal 192
bleeding, water brash, sore throat, dysphagia, or odnyophagia. 204
During this recent bout of discomfort, she has lost 20 pounds. 215
She also denies taking any aspirin or nonsteroidal anti-      226
inflammatory drugs, and she does not drink alcohol.           236
DS
Therefore, I recommend an esophagogastroduodenoscopy to       247
evaluate her abdominal discomfort.                            254
DS
Sincerely,/Louis Hubbard, MD/Chief of Gastroenterology/LH:    265
Typist's initials                                             268
```

□□□□1 □□□□2 □□□□3 □□□□4 □□□□5 □□□□6 □□□□7 □□□□8 □□□□9 □□□□10 □□□□11 □□□□12

This 90-year-old male had been confined to his home for 11
approximately four years during which time he has gradually 22
deteriorated. He stayed in bed most of the time and had not 33
bathed for several days. His intake of nourishment and fluid 45
had been minimal. He was observed to have a staggering gait, 56
and he fell frequently. 60

The patient was obtunded and seemed to be unaware of his 72
surroundings. Lungs were clear. Abdomen was benign. Neuro- 84
logical examination was not remarkable. There were myotic 95
deformities of the nails. There was a healing abrasion of 106
the scalp; an erythematous path on the left groin. Phosphate 118
was normal. Urinalysis showed white blood cells and was 129
positive for occult blood. Urine culture showed significant 140
growth of yeast. CPK and LDH were elevated as well as SGOT. 151
Serum iron was decreased. X-ray of the chest showed hyperin- 162
flation. The patient responded well to intravenous hydration, 174
but developed a fever that persisted for two days. He also 185
responded well to antibiotic treatment. The patient's BUN and 197
creatinine levels gradually returned to normal. There was 208
satisfactory urinary output. 213

The patient was also given Hydergine and Haldol for 224
agitation. The patient was transferred by ambulance to an 235
assisted living facility. He is to continue all medications 246
as instituted in the hospital. 252

▢▢▢▢1▢▢▢▢2▢▢▢▢3▢▢▢▢4▢▢▢▢5▢▢▢▢6▢▢▢▢7▢▢▢▢8▢▢▢▢9▢▢▢▢10▢▢▢▢11▢▢▢▢12

Modified Block Letter, Five-Minute Timed Writing

Goals

After completing this lesson, you will be able to:

✔ Key a business letter in a modified block format.
✔ Key a personal-business letter in a modified block format.

The modified block format has the same components as does the block format. The difference is in the placement of certain components on the page. In the modified block format, the date line, the closing line, and the signature block begin not at the left margin, but at the horizontal center of the page. For a personal-business letter, the return address is also keyed at the horizontal center of the page.

Instructions

Key the following letters in modified block format. Proofread and mark any errors, then rekey the corrected copy.

Use current date

QS

Linda Fossa, MD

5777 Follicle Drive

San Diego, CA 92111-6304

DS

Dear Dr. Fossa:

DS

Re: Jane Henna

Medical Record No.: 49

DS

Thank you for referring this patient to me. After three sessions with the patient, I have come to the following conclusions.

DS

This patient is a paranoid schizophrenic. She has been having hallucinations of CIA-engineered insects invading her apartment. She claims they ate her cat. She describes these insects as small, hard-shelled creatures that look like cockroaches, but which have cat-like faces, hands, and prehensile tails. She claims that these creatures are intelligent and are possibly in contact with space aliens; she avers that they have taken control of the government.

DS

I will continue to see this patient, prescribing drugs to control the hallucinations and level the patient's mood swings.

DS

I will keep you apprised of her progress.

DS

Sincerely yours,

QS

Alice Hubbard, PhD

Chief of Psychiatry

```
Current date/Paula Cord, MD/3704 Vein Avenue              9
Mobile, AZ 85200-6201/Dear Dr. Cord:                     16
Re: Mrs. Sally Lateral                                   21
Medical Record No.:47                                    25
Mrs. Sally Lateral was seen by me May 15, 200__. The     35
93-year-old white female was having abdominal pain, diarrhea,  46
gastric tenderness, and vomiting.                        52
DS
She had her throat sprayed with a solution and gargled with a  63
gel. She was given Xanax and Demerol to relieve anxiety and    74
to produce a drowsy state.                               79
DS
The endoscope was passed through the pharynx without     89
complications. The esophagus and gastroesophageal mucosa were  101
normal. The rugae appeared hypertrophic. The antrum was  112
scarred,and there was a pyloric spasm. The endoscope was 123
withdrawn, and no other abnormalities were seen. The patient   135
tolerated the procedure well.                            141
DS
Thank you for referring this patient to me.              149
DS
Sincerely yours,/Jeff Bilious, MD/JB:Typist's initials   160
```

□□□□1□□□□2□□□□3□□□□4□□□□5□□□□6□□□□7□□□□8□□□□9□□□□10□□□□11□□□□12

Personal-Business Letter 1

```
Current date/Mable Buccal, MD/2409 Apnea Street            9
Mobile, AZ 85104-6667/Dear Dr. Buccal:                    16

Re: Rosie Basophil                                        19

Medical Record No.: 42                                    23
DS
I was kindly asked to consult on Rosie Basophil, a 32-year-old  35
black female suffering from a urinary tract infection.    45
DS
The patient came to the emergency room with her husband. The   56
patient was complaining of vomiting, diarrhea, headache,  67
nausea, and abdominal pain. She has a history of carcinoma of   78
the cervix. She received radiation and chemotherapy.      88
DS
Her urinalysis showed a 30 white blood count, 1+ bacteria,     99
and pyuria. On examination, pelvic exam was negative. IV  110
antibiotics were given for the urinary tract infection.   121
DS
Thank you for asking me to consult with this patient.     131
DS
Sincerely,/Roosevelt Palate, MD/4567 Bile Drive          140

Mobile, AZ 85104-0000/RP: Typist's initials               149
```

Personal-Business Letter 2

```
Current date/Garden Insulin, MD/5703 Field Avenue         10
Mobile, AZ 85102-6203/Dear Dr. Insulin:.Re: Mr. Charles Hernia/  22

Medical Record No.: 52                                    26
DS
I am writing regarding Mr. Charles Hernia, whom you kindly      37
referred for evaluation of leg pain. He is a 45-year-old  48
Caucasian male.                                           51
DS
PRESENT ILLNESS                                           54
DS
The patient is complaining of back pain that radiates to the   65
lower extremities, more on the right than the left. The pain   76
radiates to the thighs down to his feet. He is also       86
experiencing numbness and weakness in the upper extremities.   97
The pain and weakness are aggravated by standing, sitting, and 109
exertion. He can get relief by lying down and getting into the 121
fetal position.                                           124
```

□□□□1□□□□2□□□□3□□□□4□□□□5□□□□6□□□□7□□□□8□□□□9□□□□10□□□□11□□□□12

DS

PAST HISTORY   126

DS

He had a diskectomy in Alaska several years ago, as well as   137
minor orthopedic surgery; otherwise, he has been healthy.   148

DS

MEDICATION   150

Vicodin.   152

DS

ALLERGIES   154

None.   155

DS

SOCIAL HISTORY   157

DS

The patient is not married. He is an attorney. He used to play   169
basketball professionally.   174

DS

FAMILY HISTORY   177

DS

Both parents are living and well.   183

DS

REVIEW OF SYSTEMS   186

DS

He does not have any complaints referable to the chest, heart,   198
abdomen, head, ears, eyes, nose, and throat.   206

DS

PHYSICAL EXAMINATION   210

DS

This is a 45-year-old male, well developed, and well nourished.   222
He mentioned that he gained about 35 pounds in the last   233
several months. The patient is obese. I have scheduled an   244
appointment for him to meet with a dietitian. His physical   255
exam of the chest, heart, and abdomen are within normal   265
limits.   266

DS

NEUROLOGICAL EXAMINATION   271

DS

He is alert and oriented. Cranial nerves II-XII are intact.   282
Motor—normal.   285

DS

□□□□1□□□□2□□□□3□□□□4□□□□5□□□□6□□□□7□□□□8□□□□9□□□□10□□□□11□□□□12

```
SPINAL EXAMINATION                                            289
DS
There is a well-healed laminectomy incision. Straight leg     300
raising causes back and leg pain.                             306
DS
REVIEW OF X-RAY DATA                                          310
DS
I had the opportunity to review the MRI of the lumbar spine   321
which was done in September. He does have a left L2-L1         332
herniated disk. I think the patient is suffering from         343
radiculopathy. The patient needs diskectomy performed. We are 355
going to proceed with surgery as soon as the insurance company 367
permits the authorization.                                    372
DS
Thank you again for referring him to me. I will keep you      383
informed.                                                     385
DS
Sincerely yours,/Richard M. Carpal, MD/Orthopedic Surgeon    396
2405 Crocker Drive/Mobile, AZ 85102-9000                      404
605-300-0000/RC:Typist's initials                             410
□□□□1□□□□2□□□□3□□□□4□□□□5□□□□6□□□□7□□□□8□□□□9□□□□10□□□□11□□□□12
```

Use current date/Dr. Mary Tricious/2000 Professional Circle	11
Zanzibar, KS 90000-8000	16
Dear Dr. Tricious:	20
I received your letter on December 21. I thank you for the	31
invitation to join the hospital's Christmas party; I will be	43
delighted to attend.	47
DS	
Attending the party will give me an excellent chance to meet	58
your fine staff. I do hope that our contract negotiations	69
work out and that I will be able to become a member of the	80
hospital staff. The varied experience of your staff will	91
surely be of great educational value to me, and perhaps I can	102
add to their knowledge with my own specialty.	110
DS	
Thank you again for the invitation. I will see you on	120
December 24.	122
DS	
Sincerely,/George M. Feelgood, MD/6161 Happy Valley Road	133
Bellview, WA 97979-0000	138
GF: Typist's initials	142

Instruction

Key the letter in modified block format. Proofread your document and correct errors.

Current Date/Darnell Muscle, MD/4250 Dirt Road/Mobile, AZ	11
20000-2000	13
Dear Dr. Darnell Muscle:/Re: Carol Hip/Medical Record No.: 450	24
DS	
Carol returned to the office approximately 3 1/2 weeks after	35
surgery. The wound is perfect. X-rays are perfect. The patient	47
is dong quite well. Her gait is still unsteady, and a walker	58
has been ordered. There is some calcification forming about	69
the hip joint which at this time is causing no problems.	79
DS	
The patient is ready to begin rehabilitation, muscle	89
strengthening, gait training, and careful explanation of all	100
precautions with endoprosthetic replacement.	108
DS	
However, she can be discharged to home, and we have provided	119
Home Health Services to monitor her daily rehabilitation	130
program.	131
DS	
Sincerely,/Jack Costal, MD/Chief of Surgery/JC:Typist's initials	143

```
□□□□1□□□□2□□□□3□□□□4□□□□5□□□□6□□□□7□□□□8□□□□9□□□□10□□□□11□□□□12
```

Key the letter in modified block format. Proofread your document and correct your errors.

```
Current date/Liver Sampson, MD/3941 Dust Road/Mobile. AZ        11
20000-2000                                                      13
Dear Dr. Sampson:/Re: Sara Meatus/Medical Record No.: 45 A      24
DS

Thank you very much for allowing me to see your patient Sara    35
in consultation for a probable Wilms tumor. Following her       46
initial admission to Mobile Hospital on June 22, a large        57
intracapsular left renal tumor was removed on June 29. The      68
tentative diagnosis of Wilms tumor seems appropriate, and since 80
her chest film is within normal limits, she is a stage I        91
patient.                                                        92
DS

I would not be surprised with the history of hematuria, and     103
the large size mass may be more extensive with capsular         114
invasion and vascular invasion, giving this patient a stage     125
II. If our feelings are confirmed, I would suggest initiating   136
chemotherapy July 5 with intravenous Vincristine 50 mcg per     147
kg for five days.                                               150
DS

If radiation therapy is indicated, it should be started July    161
20; final arrangements can be made with Dr. Louis Hubbard.      172
DS

Thanks again for allowing me to help.                           179
DS

Sincerely,/Minnie Heart, MD/Director of Oncology/MH:Typist's    190
initials                                                        191
    □□□□1□□□□2□□□□3□□□□4□□□□5□□□□6□□□□7□□□□8□□□□9□□□□10□□□□11□□□□12
```

Key the letter in modified block format. Proofread your document and correct errors.

```
Current date/Angia Burns, MD/5780 Dust Road/Mobile, AZ        10
20000-2000                                                     12
Dear Dr. Burns:/Re: Ruby Bolus/Medical Record No.: 78 D       22
DS

Thanks for allowing me to see Ruby. I saw her in the outpatient 34
department at Mobile Clinic on May 20. She has had psychiatric  46
consultation on several occasions for multiple problems.        56
DS

Her current somatic complaints are those such as "pain in my   67
back," "my stomach hurts," "my head hurts," and all are        77
unrelated to food or activity. They seem to be minimally       88
intensified by periods of emotional stress.                    96
DS

One month ago, you saw this girl and found her to have a      107
very rapid pulse. On further questioning, the past history is 118
essentially unremarkable except for a divorce between the     129
parents two years ago.                                        133
DS

On physical examination, this is a twitchy girl who talks     144
almost incessantly. She volunteers a great deal of information 156
and asks many questions about her body. She answers most      167
questions about her symptoms before her mother can even begin 178
to consider the questions.                                    183
DS

Her general physical examination is unremarkable except for   194
a moderate amount of dental carries. There are no signs of    205
thyroid hyperfunction on detailed examination.                214
DS

I believe that this child has an emotional disorder as she    225
has apparently had in the past. The most reasonable course to 236
take is one of counseling for both mother and child, and I    247
have taken the liberty of referring this family to the Family 258
Counseling Clinic. Her rapid pulse is a manifestation of her  269
anxiety in the doctor's office.                               275
DS

Sincerely,/Stress Brown, MD/SB:Typist's initials             285
```

□□□□1□□□□2□□□□3□□□□4□□□□5□□□□6□□□□7□□□□8□□□□9□□□□10□□□□11□□□□12

```
        Betty is an 83-year-old widow who lives in an apartment     11
by herself.  She was doing quite well until the past four days.     23
The patient was brought to Mobile Hospital emergency department     34
where she was found to be markedly hypokalemic and febrile.         45
The patient denies any dyspnea, cough, or abdominal pain.           56
She is not able to describe the nature of her illnesses.  She       68
denies any recent diarrhea, abdominal cramps, or urinary            79
symptoms.  She has been on digoxin and ramipril for hyper-          90
tension.                                                            91
        During the last five years, she has been hospitalized      102
several times because of respiratory infections and severe         113
anxiety.  She was last hospitalized here in May of 2000, at         124
which time she was treated for bronchial pneumonia, hyper-          135
tension, and chronic brain syndrome.  She had been on Haldol        146
at one time.                                                       148
        Her temperature on admission was recorded as 100 degrees   160
F in the emergency department with blood pressure of 120/50.       171
She is alert and oriented.  There is arcus senilis bilaterally.    183
The ears are clear.  She has dentures, upper and lower.  The       194
lungs are clear except for a few rales at the left base.  The      206
heart is enlarged on x-ray.  The abdomen is soft.  The kid-        217
neys, spleen, and liver are not palpable.  The extremities         228
show osteoarthritis in the right knee.  There is no edema.         239
The patient is allergic to codeine and penicillin.  Pulses         250
are felt.  The white blood count is elevated.  This appears to     262
be a urinary tract infection, possibly pyelonephritis with         273
leukocytosis.  She is on erythromycin and is improving.            284
□□□□1□□□□2□□□□3□□□□4□□□□5□□□□6□□□□7□□□□8□□□□9□□□□10□□□□11□□□□12
```

Medical Reports

Medical reports are documents that describe an encounter between a health care provider and a patient. They are legal documents that become part of a patient's official medical record. They are also confidential documents; the information they contain should not be discussed or otherwise disclosed to individuals not directly involved with the patient's case. Examples of medical reports include history and physical examination, operative, pathology, consultation, and discharge summary.

Medical transcription is the process of taking dictated or written medical information and producing a permanent, uniform, and legible record of that information in a keyboarded form. Professional medical transcriptionists are medical language specialists who typically work in a hospital, medical office or clinic, or for a medical transcription service. However, smaller medical offices or other ambulatory care settings are often unable to employ full-time medical transcriptionists and medical assistants may then perform medical transcription in addition to their other duties.

This unit provides an overview of the various medical reports that are typically encountered in either a hospital or ambulatory care setting. Each report includes formatting instructions and a sample report, and is followed by exercises for you to key.

The CD-ROM packaged with this text contains reports from this unit and is included to give you the opportunity to practice transcribing dictated material. Be sure to review the entire unit before practicing with the CD-ROM so you are familiar with the proper formatting.

History and Physical Examination Reports, Five-Minute Timed Writing

History. The history part of the report includes chief complaint (CC), history of present illness (PI), past history (PH), family history (FH), social history (SH), that may be pertinent to the present illness, and review of systems (ROS).

Chief complaint is the symptoms that brought the patient to the physician.

Present illness is also called history of chief complaint or history of present illness. Information is sought about the time the symptoms were first noticed.

Past history includes childhood diseases, adult diseases, accidents, surgeries, pregnancies, deliveries, and allergies to medications.

The family history consists of information about family members' diseases that could be hereditary.

Social history is the summary of the patient's environment and life that may be contributing to the disease. The use of drugs, alcohol, and tobacco can affect a person's health as well as marital status and occupation.

Review of systems (ROS) are called systemic review, inventory by systems and functional inquiry. The physician will ask questions and record the presence or absence of symptoms. The following list of subtopics are: Head, Eyes, Ears, Nose, Throat, and Mouth (HEENT), Cardiorespiratory (CR), Gastrointestinal (GI), Genitourinary (GU), Gynecological (GYN), Neuropsychiatric (NP), Musculoskeletal Systems (MS), Hair, and Skin.

Physical Examination. The physical examination (PE) is performed by the physician and usually involves four techniques. (1) observation by sight, (2) palpation by using the hands to touch body parts, (3) percussion using fingertips to tap the body, and (4) auscultation using a stethoscope to listen for bowel sounds, heart and breath tone, and bruits.

The physician makes notes about the appearance of the patient that includes: height, age, nutrition, pulse, weight, respiration, temperature, blood pressure, rectal area, extremities, reflexes, genitalia, heart, lungs, chest, neck, lymph nodes, mouth, nose, ears, eyes, head, and skin.

The physician may order tests as part of an examination. After the physical examination and tests results, the physician will give a diagnosis. When the diagnosis is made, a plan of treatment will follow. Instructions are given to the patient about follow-up treatment.

Medical transcriptionists work in hospitals, medical centers, private clinics, and state health departments.

Rule.   A sentence ends with a period.

Rule.   Periods are not used with acronyms. Example: AIDS

Rule.   Periods are not used within or after most abbreviations, including abbreviated units of measure and brief forms. Example: mg, CMT

Rule.   Unrelated laboratory tests are separated by using a period. Example: Hemoglobin 15.6. Hematocrit 46.2. BUN 9.

Rule. Use a period after each numeral in a vertical list of enumerated items and use a period to close the list.

Example: Diagnoses:

1. Endometriosis.

2. Rheumatoid arthritis.

3. Diabetes, type 2.

Rule. Periods are not used in a list of horizontally enumerated items. Numerals are enclosed in parentheses.

Example: Diagnoses:

(1) Tuberculosis   (2) Rubella   (3) Carditis

Rule. Commas are not used to separate a drug name from doses and instructions.

Example: Take Tagamet 400 mg p.o. q.d. before meals

Rule. Commas are not used to separate a lab value from the test it describes.

Example: potassium 4.3

chloride 105

NOT chloride, 105

Rule. Abbreviations are not used for admission, discharge, preoperative, or postoperative diagnosis; operative title; or consultation conclusion. Spell out all abbreviations.

Example: (T&A) Tonsillectomy and Adenoidectomy

Example: Admission Diagnosis: Diabetes Mellitus

Rule. A numeral is not separated from the unit of measure or abbreviation. Key on the same line.

Rule. Reference initials. Example: JM:EM

Rule. For date of dictation and date of transcription

Use: D: (no space) 08-09-200__

T: (no space) 08-10-200__

Rule. Key the word (continued) in parentheses on the first page and succeeding pages, double-spaced at the last keyed line. The word "continued" is keyed at the left.

Rule. Begin second page and key a header: Physical examination, page 2; patient's name, medical record number.

Goals

After completing this lesson, you will be able to:

✔ Key history and physical examination reports.
✔ Key reports in several formats.

Instructions

Key a history and physical report using a block format. Key the sample report. The title of the report is centered on the page and keyed in all capitals. The main topics are keyed in all capitals and followed by a colon. Begin keying on the same line. Omit the colon after the heading if the information begins on the next line. See the sample report. The subtopics are keyed in capital letters and followed by a colon. Begin keying on the same line. Omit the colon if the information begins on the next line.

Note: This can be used for any medical report. All paragraphs are single-spaced. Double-space between topics. Begin the signature block at the right margin four spaces after the last keyed line. Double-space after the dictator's name. Key reference initials of the dictator followed by your initials. Key date of dictation and date of transcription. Begin transcribing slowly by listening carefully to a few words. Speed will come as you gain knowledge and more experience.

Note: The main topics and subtopics are followed by a colon and two spaces. Leave 1.5-inch top, bottom, left, and right margins.

History and physical examination reports include the patient's name, medical record number, the date, the physician's name, and the reference initials. The report is keyed on letterhead paper or plain paper with 1-inch margins. Key the main topics in all capital letters. Leave 1.5-inch top, bottom, left, and right margins. Double-space between headings; single-space the report body. Key the following reports. Study and key the sample report.

SAMPLE REPORT

HISTORY AND PHYSICAL
DS

Patient Name: Bobbie Chest
Medical Record No.: 52
Physician: Jay Oto, MD
Date: 07/16/200__
DS

CHIEF COMPLAINT
Painful hemorrhoids.
DS

HISTORY OF PRESENT ILLNESS
This is a 50-year-old black female with a 2-week history of
diarrhea and prolapse of internal hemorrhoids.
DS

PAST MEDICAL HISTORY
No previous surgical history. No medical history to speak of. She
is on no medications.
DS

ALLERGIES
She has no known allergies.
DS

PHYSICAL EXAMINATION
DS

VITAL SIGNS: Stable. She is afebrile.
HEENT: Pupils equal, round; extraocular movements intact.
NECK: Adenopathy.
CHEST: Clear to auscultation and percussion.
CARDIOVASCULAR: S1 and S2 are regular. No S3, S4, and no murmur.
ABDOMEN: Soft, nontender. There are no masses or organomegaly.
EXTREMITIES: Within normal limits.
NEUROLOGIC: Within normal limits.
RECTAL: Reveals a thrombosed prolapsed hemorrhoid.
DS

IMPRESSION
The patient has thrombosed internal hemorrhoids.
DS

PLAN
She is going to be brought in for an elective hemorrhoidectomy.
QS (quadruple space)

_____

Jay Oto, MD
DS from signature block

JO:PY
SS

D:07/16/200__
SS

T:07/17/200__

Instructions

Study the report sample before keying. Key report 2 in block format. Proofread your copy and correct errors.

REPORT 2

```
                    HISTORY AND PHYSICAL EXAMINATION              10
Patient Name Tamara Rales/Medical Record No. 57/Date of          20
Admission 08/08/____/Physician: Ruby Cyanosis, MD                30
CHIEF COMPLAINT: Vomiting and right-sided abdominal pain.         41
HISTORY OF PRESENT ILLNESS: This is a 30-year-old white female    53
who was brought to the emergency room with a 4- or 5-hour         64
history of emesis and upper abdominal pain. She denied            74
constipation or diarrhea. She stated that she took some kind      85
of recreational drug two days prior to admission.                 94
PAST MEDICAL HISTORY: The patient is not very cooperative in      105
giving us a history. However, she has leukemia and has been       116
in remission. She had an appendectomy a year ago.                 125
PHYSICAL EXAMINATION                                              129
GENERAL: The patient is lethargic, arousable, and not             139
delusional.                                                       141
VITAL SIGNS: Temperature: 97. Pulse: 69. Respiratory: 22.         151
Blood pressure: 110/80.                                           155
HEENT: Normocephalic. Eyes: Pupils equal. Fundi: Normal. Ears:    166
Tympanic membranes cannot be seen. Nose: No mucus. Oropharynx:    177
Normal appearance of the mucous membranes.                        185
NECK: No masses. No jugular venous distention. No carotid         196
bruits.                                                           197
CHEST: No masses of the chest wall.                               204
LUNGS: Clear to auscultation and percussion.                      212
ABDOMEN: Nondistended. There was tenderness in the right          223
upper and lower quadrants. No masses were felt.                   232
NEUROLOGICAL: Sensory examination was intact.                     240
LABORATORY DATA: The workup in the emergency room indicated       251
dehydration resulting in electrolyte imbalance. An ultrasound     262
was performed and showed gallstones. After examination, the       273
patient was vomiting.                                             277
IMPRESSION: Cholecystitis.                                        282
PLAN: (1) Admit for dehydration and management of abdominal       293
pain and vomiting. (2) Surgical consultation and workup for       304
cholelithiasis and cholecystitis.                                 310
     Ruby Cyanosis, MD, RC:mm, D:08/08/200__ T:08/14/200__        322
```

□□□□1□□□□2□□□□3□□□□4□□□□5□□□□6□□□□7□□□□8□□□□9□□□□10□□□□11□□□□12

Instructions

Key a history and physical report using a modified block format. Key the sample modified block.

1. The title is centered on the page and keyed in all capital letters.
2. The main topics are keyed in capitals at the left margin and followed by a colon. Begin keying on the same line at the left margin.
3. Double-space between topics. Key the paragraph single-spaced.
4. Subtopics are indented five spaces under the main topics. Subtopics are keyed in all capitals followed by a colon. Begin keying on the same line.
5. Begin the signature block at the right margin four spaces after the last keyed line.
6. Double-space after the dictator's name. Key reference initials of the dictator followed by your initials. Key the date of dictation and date of transcription.
7. Tabbing is determined by the longest word in the sample (Review of Systems:). Review of Systems is the longest word plus two tab stops after the colon. Tab over to see where one begins keying Review of Systems.

SAMPLE MODIFIED BLOCK

```
Patient Name: Darnell Chest      Medical Record No.: 01-01-01    11
Physician: Martin Sampson, MD    Date: 08-09-200__               21
                      DS
                      HISTORY                                    27
                      DS
CHIEF COMPLAINT:      Dizziness, nausea, weakness, shortness of  38
                      breath.                                    43
                      DS
PRESENT ILLNESS:      This 58-year-old white male has been treated  54
                      for chronic obstructive pulmonary disease and 66
                      emphysema. However, this morning he developed 78
                      dizziness, shortness of breath, weakness,   89
                      nausea, and was unable to stand.            98
                      DS
PAST HISTORY:         Paget disease of the spine, peptic ulcer. 109
                      Operations: Hemorrhoidectomy, cholecystect- 120
                      omy, appendectomy, and hernia.             129
                      DS
ALLERGIES:            No known allergies.                       136
                      DS
SOCIAL:               He stopped smoking. He drinks alcohol to  147
                      help him sleep. He takes care of his wife  158
                      at home who is an invalid in a wheelchair. 169
                      DS
FAMILY HISTORY:       His father died of kidney failure and mother 181
                      of a stroke.                               187
                      DS
                      REVIEW OF SYSTEMS: Noncontributory         197
                      DS
(continued)
□□□□1□□□□2□□□□3□□□□4□□□□5□□□□6□□□□7□□□□8□□□□9□□□□10□□□□11□□□□12
```

HEENT:	Vision poor. Eyes burn and itch. Hearing is poor. Has earaches.	208 215
	DS	
CR:	Shortness of breath.	222
	DS	
GI:	Weight is stable.	229
	DS	
GU:	Nocturia one time.	236
	DS	
MS:	Has leg cramps. He complains of headaches.	247
	DS	
	PHYSICAL	253
	DS	
GENERAL:	His chest is deformed with kyphosis due to Paget disease. He is cooperative, oriented, and alert. Blood pressure: 180/110. Pulse: 78. Temperature: 95.5.	264 276 287 295
	DS	
HEENT:		296
	DS	
HEAD:	Normal.	301
	DS	
EYES:	PERRLA.	306
	DS	
EARS:	Tympanic membranes intact. Nose and throat clear.	317 322
	DS	
NECK:	Stiff; unable to rotate head or flex head. No adenopathy.	333 339
	DS	
CHEST:		340
	DS	
LUNGS:	Rales both bases, some rhonchi.	350
	DS	
HEART:	Normal sinus rhythm. No murmurs. Heart not enlarged.	361 366
	DS	
ABDOMEN:	Cholecystectomy scar, appendectomy scar, hernia scar. No masses. No tenderness. No enlarged organs.	377 388 395
	DS	
GENITALIA:	Normal male.	401
	DS	
EXTREMITIES:	Reflexes physiological. No edema.	411
	DS	

(continued)

□□□□1□□□□2□□□□3□□□□4□□□□5□□□□6□□□□7□□□□8□□□□9□□□□10□□□□11□□□□12

```
IMPRESSION:          1. Chronic obstructive pulmonary disease,      422
                        emphysema.                                  428
                     2. Arteriosclerotic cardiovascular renal       439
                        disease with hypertension.                  448
                     3. Paget disease.                              455
                           QS


                                    _____

                                         Martin Sampson, MD     466
DS from signature block
MS:EJ                                                            467
SS
D:08/10/200__.                                                   469
SS
T:08/11/200__                                                   471
□□□□1□□□□2□□□□3□□□□4□□□□5□□□□6□□□□7□□□□8□□□□9□□□□10□□□□11□□□□12
```

Instructions

Study the sample modified block before keying. Key report 3 in modified block format. Proofread your copy and correct errors.

REPORT 3

```
              HISTORY AND PHYSICAL EXAMINATION                    9
Patient Name: Sally Foss/Medical Record No. 82/Date of          19
Admission 07/16/_____/Dr. Jeffrey Spleen                        27
CHIEF COMPLAINT: Vomiting and congestive heart failure.         37
HISTORY OF PRESENT ILLNESS: This 90-year-old Indian female      48
with pulmonary disease, tachyarrhythmias, and gastroesophageal  60
reflux and congestive heart failure, was admitted to the        71
emergency department at 2:15 a.m. History was provided by the   82
patient, indicating that she had begun vomiting last night and  94
developed a fever of 104 degrees. The vomitus was food. There  105
was no blood noted. She had abdominal pain. Her last bowel      116
movement was yesterday. She denies symptoms of urinary tract    127
infection. She has a slight cold. Her sputum has not been       138
purulent.                                                       139
She was examined by Dr. Jeffrey Spleen. Blood was cultured.     150
Serum amylase was obtained and was normal. Chest x-ray and      161
ultrasound of the abdomen were obtained. Her temperature was    172
105.8 degrees but dropped to 102.2 degrees after doses of       183
Tylenol. She was given Timentin 2.1 gm intravenously. Since     194
admission to the ICU, her temperature has been 101.2 degrees.   205
She has had one emesis since being admitted to the unit. She    216
continues to complain of feeling weak. Her breathing is good    227
at this time.                                                   229
PAST MEDICAL HISTORY: Previous medical records revealed         240
hospitalization for acute bronchitis and tachyarrhythmias.      251
ALLERGIES: NONE KNOWN.                                          255
(continued)
```

DS

CURRENT MEDICATIONS: Oxygen at one liter by nasal cannula,   266
Theo-Dur 200 mg b.i.d., Micro-K 8 mEq q.d., vitamin B6 50 mg   277
b.i.d., and Ventolin inhaler 2 inhalations four or five times   288
p.r.n.   289
HABITS: The patient does not smoke cigarettes or consume   300
alcohol.   301
REVIEW OF SYSTEMS: The patient had been in satisfactory   312
condition until three days ago.   318
HEENT: She wears glasses with some visual limitations. The   329
ears reveal hearing to be decreased. She wears hearing aids.   340
The nose reveals symptoms of rhinitis and sinusitis.   350
GASTROINTESTINAL: The patient denies difficulty swallowing.   361
She has a history of diverticulosis.   368
CARDIOVASCULAR: No recent palpitations, edema, or orthopnea.   379
RESPIRATORY: The patient is dyspneic with activity. She walks   391
with a walker. No hemoptysis or pleuritic chest.   400
GENITOURINARY: Negative.   404
SOCIAL HISTORY: She lives with her nephew. She tends her roses   415
and watches television.   419

PHYSICAL EXAMINATION   428

VITAL SIGNS: Blood pressure: 120/68. Pulse: 80 and regular.   439
Respirations: 20 per minute. Temperature: 98.7 degrees.   449
Weight: 41.3 kg.   452
GENERAL: She is alert and appears fatigued.   460
HEENT: Within normal limits.   465
NECK: Veins are distended.   470
BREASTS: Not examined.   474
LUNGS: Crackle heard in both lungs without rhonchi or wheezes.   485
No coughing.   487
HEART: Rhythm is regular.   492
ABDOMEN: Quite firm. Nontender.   498
LOWER EXTREMITIES: Without edema.   504
NEUROLOGIC: She appears neurologically intact.   513
CHEST X-RAY: Shows changes of pulmonary disease with   523
cardiomegaly.   525
ADMISSION ELECTROCARDIOGRAM: Shows left anterior hemiblock   536
and consistent with a previous myocardial infarction.   546
LABORATORY: Admission CBC 12,800. Bands 55%, segs 37%.   556
Hematocrit 37. Serum amylase normal. Urinalysis shows 100 mg%   568
proteinuria. Electrolytes normal.   574
IMPRESSION: 576
1. Nausea and vomiting. No evidence of gastrointestinal   587
bleeding.   588
2. High fever.   590
3. Obstructive pulmonary disease, stable.   598
4. Past history of cardiac arrhythmias.   605
Jeffrey Spleen, MD/JS:EM/D:07-20-200__/T:07-21-200__   615

□□□□1□□□□2□□□□3□□□□4□□□□5□□□□6□□□□7□□□□8□□□□9□□□□10□□□□11□□□□12

Key a history and physical report using an indented format. Leave 1.5-inch top, bottom, left, and right margins. Key the sample history and physical report. The title of the report is centered on the page and keyed in all capitals. Main topics are keyed in capitals at the left margin and followed by a colon. Begin keying on the same line. See sample of how first two lines are indented. Subsequent lines are keyed from the left margin. If the outline is brief, use first two lines. Double-space between topics. Subtopics are keyed in capitals followed by a colon. Subtopics are indented one tab below main topics. Begin the signature block at the right margin four spaces after the last keyed line. Double-space after the dictator's name. Key reference initials of the dictator followed by your initials. Key the date for dictation and date of transcription. Proofread your copy and correct errors.

Note: The main topics and subtopics are followed by a colon and two spaces. Tabbing determined by the longest word in the sample (Review of Systems:). Review of Systems is the longest word plus two tab stops after the colon. Tab the longest words and see where the stop is.

SAMPLE INDENTED FORMAT

```
Patient Name: Brown, Tibia                                          5
Medical Record No.: 82-00-00                                       11
Physician: Harry Bone, MD                                          16
Date: 08-16-200__                                                  19
                                    DS
                                HISTORY                            26
                                    DS
CHIEF COMPLAINT:    Visual loss. Shortness of breath, dyspnea,     37
                    wheezing, and a persistent cough for about     48
                    3 months.                                      53
                    DS
HISTORY OF PRESENT ILLNESS:     This patient has been followed     64
                                by me for glaucoma and cataracts.  76
                                His vision has now decreased to     87
                                approximately 20/200 in each eye,  99
                                and he enters for extraction of    110
                                the right eye cataract.            120
                                DS
PAST MEDICAL HISTORY:       Significant in that he has had rather  131
                            severe cardiac disease and emphysema,  142
                            in addition to the glaucoma and        152
                            cataracts. Some time ago he was on     163
                            Phospholine Iodide but this was        173
                            stopped.                               179
                            DS
  ALLERGIES:        No known allergies.                            186
                    DS
  MEDICATION:       Pilocarpine.                                   192
                    DS
  OPERATIONS:       Prostatectomy and appendectomy.                201
                    DS
(continued)
```

□□□□1□□□□2□□□□3□□□□4□□□□5□□□□6□□□□7□□□□8□□□□9□□□□10□□□□11□□□□12

FAMILY HISTORY:	Not remarkable. There are no familial	212
	diseases. His father died at 53 of	222
	alcoholism, the mother at 75 of a stroke.	233

REVIEW OF SYSTEMS: 241

DS

HEENT:	He wears a hearing aid. Cataracts and	251
	glaucoma both eyes.	258
	DS	
CR:	The patient has severe cardiovascular	268
	disease with emphysema and shortness of	279
	breath for which he uses Primatene.	289
	DS	
GI:	Eats low-salt diet. No tarry stools.	299
	DS	
GU:	Had a prostatectomy and since that time	310
	has had difficulty with his sphincter. No	321
	history of deformity other than the	331
	presence of emphysema.	339
	DS	
NEUROLOGIC:	No history of convulsions or strokes.	349
	DS	

PHYSICAL EXAMINATION   353

DS

GENERAL:	The patient is an elderly male who appears	364
	to be in poor health.	371
	DS	
SKIN:	Clear.	376
	DS	
HEENT:	Head is normocephalic. Hearing rather poor	387
	but aided by a hearing aid. Glaucoma and	398
	cataracts are in both eyes. Nose is clear.	409
	Pharynx is clear.	416
	DS	
NECK:	No adenopathy.	422
	DS	
CHEST:	The lungs are clear to auscultation;	432
	however, the chest is emphysematous. The	443
	heart sounds are distant. The rhythm is	454
	irregular. No murmurs are heard.	464
	DS	
ABDOMEN:	Soft, nontender, no palpable masses, but	475
	previous scars are present from surgery.	486
	DS	
GENITALIA:	Normal male without hernia.	495
DS		
MS:	Emphysema.	500
DS		
NEUROLOGIC:	Deep reflexes present and equal bilaterally.	511
DS		

(continued)

□□□□1□□□□2□□□□3□□□□4□□□□5□□□□6□□□□7□□□□8□□□□9□□□□10□□□□11□□□□12

```
IMPRESSION:      1. Cataract O.U.                                518
                 2. Glaucoma O.U.                                525
                 3. Arteriosclerotic heart disease.             535
                 4. Emphysema.                                   541

QS


                                        _____
                                        Harry Bone, MD   553
                                             DS

HB:ES                                                            554
SS
D:08-17-200___                                                   556
SS
T:08-20-200___                                                   558
```

Instructions

Key the following history and physical in an indented format. Study the sample before keying. Proofread your copy and correct errors.

```
Joan Brown. Medical Record No. 82 Harry Stoma, MD. Date      11
05-09-200___. History. CHIEF COMPLAINT: Chronic constipation. 22
Swollen and bleeding hemorrhoids after a bowel movement.      33
PRESENT ILLNESS: This is the first presentation for this      44
51-year-old, white female for hemorrhoids. She states that    55
she was diagnosed with external hemorrhoids approximately two  66
years ago and has had intermittent problems with itching and  77
burning in the rectal area which are relieved by Preparation H. 89
Lately she has noticed that the hemorrhoids are sometimes     100
painful and she occasionally notes bright red blood in the    111
stool and on toilet tissue. PAST MEDICAL HISTORY: Significant 122
for a colon polyp which was classified as benign, diagnosed   133
via colonoscopy a year and a half ago at Mobile Hospital. She 144
is followed by Dr. Brown of gynecology for Pap smears and     155
mammograms. She denies any surgeries. She denies any history  166
of hypertension, diabetes, coronary disease, lung disease, or 178
kidney disease. MEDICATIONS: Include occasional multivitamins 189
and occasional aspirin. ALLERGIES: No known drug allergies.   200
SOCIAL HISTORY: She is an attorney. She is married and has    211
two children. She denies any tobacco or alcohol use. No IV    222
drug abuse. She exercises occasionally by walking. FAMILY     233
HISTORY: Significant for father who died at age 60 of an MI.  244
Mother died at age 91 of old age. She had 7 brothers and 4    255
sisters. One brother died at 71 of prostate cancer. One       266
brother is alive and well at age 74 with a stroke and 3       277
brothers who died as children with pneumonia. REVIEW OF       288
SYSTEMS: As above, otherwise, noncontributory. Her last       299
tetanus immunization was more than 15 years ago. PHYSICAL     310
EXAMINATION: Her examination revealed a young-appearing white 321
female in no apparent distress, well-developed, well-         331
nourished. Pulse: 80. Blood pressure: 100/74. Respirations:   342

(continued)

□□□□1□□□□2□□□□3□□□□4□□□□5□□□□6□□□□7□□□□8□□□□9□□□□10□□□□11□□□□12
```

14. Weight: 141 pounds. Height: 63¹/₄ inches. HEENT: 352
Normocephalic. Atraumatic. Pupils equal, round, and reactive   363
to light and accommodation. Extraocular movements were intact   374
without nystagmus. She had bilateral contacts in place.   384
Examination of the fundi revealed some copper wiring in   394
both eyes, otherwise discs were sharp. Tympanic membranes   405
were gray with a light reflex elicited on the right; the left   415
ear canal was obscured by cerumen. No sinus tenderness. Mucous   427
membranes were moist. No erythema and no exudate. NECK: Supple   439
without lymphadenopathy. No thyromegaly. No jugular venous   450
distension. RESPIRATORY: Clear breath sounds bilaterally to   461
auscultation and percussion. CARDIAC: Regular rate and rhythm   472
with normal S1, S2. No S3, S4, without murmur. Strong   482
peripheral pulses bilaterally. ABDOMEN: Soft, flat, nontender.   493
Normal active bowel sounds. No hepatosplenomegaly. No masses   504
were noted. RECTAL: Revealed one large external hemorrhoid at   515
the 6 o'clock position. Stool was heme occult negative, brown.   526
There were no other masses. BREAST AND PELVIC EXAM: Deferred   537
by the patient as she has an appointment with Dr. Brown in   548
October. EXTREMITIES: Without cyanosis, clubbing, or edema.   559
NEUROLOGICAL: Grossly nonfocal. IMPRESSION: 1. External   570
hemorrhoids. I have discussed with the patient regarding   581
alterations in diet to increase the fiber content. She will   592
also start Metamucil one packet per day followed by a glass   603
of water and increase to three times a day as tolerated. If   614
needed, we can use sitz baths for her hemorrhoids. If she   625
continues to have persistent symptoms, she will consider   635
referral to general surgery for hemorrhoidectomy. 2. She will   646
obtain a tetanus booster immunization today. She will undergo   657
chemistry, CBC, and thyroid-stimulating hormone panel today,   668
the results of which I will forward to her in a letter. I have   679
encouraged the patient to perform monthly breast self-   689
examinations and to exercise regularly. She will follow up   700
with me in the future.   704

    Harry Stoma, MD, HS:em, D:05-10-200__, T:05-11-200__   714

□□□□1□□□□2□□□□3□□□□4□□□□5□□□□6□□□□7□□□□8□□□□9□□□□10□□□□11□□□□12

The patient is a 20-year-old married female who comes in 11
today to follow up a gastrointestinal evaluation. I had last 22
seen her in May with a complaint of persistent abdominal pain 33
and weight loss. I had referred her to Gastroenterology for 44
an evaluation. She underwent upper endoscopy and colonoscopy. 55
She states that her abdominal pain is about the same. It is 66
a diffuse burning pain. I had also switched her from Tagamet 77
to Prilosec. She thinks it has helped but not significantly. 88
Otherwise, she has had no diarrhea, no fevers, no nausea or 99
vomiting. The patient appears well. No further examination 110
was performed. Her upper endoscopy showed some diffuse 121
gastritis. There were no biopsies done. Her colonoscopy 132
revealed a hyperplastic polyp at 17 cm; otherwise normal. 143
Dr. Creme recommended a CT scan of the abdomen. She did have 154
gastritis on her upper endoscopy. She had not responded to 165
proton pump inhibitors. I will go ahead and check a serum 176
titer of H. pylori and have her take Tagamet 800 mg p.o. at 187
bedtime. I will refer her to Radiology for the abdominal CT 198
scan. I will have her get a chemistry panel with liver 209
function tests, complete blood count, and urinalysis. She 220
will follow up with me after the CT scan has been completed. 231
□□□□1□□□□2□□□□3□□□□4□□□□5□□□□6□□□□7□□□□8□□□□9□□□□10□□□□11□□□□12

Operative Reports, Five-Minute Timed Writing

Goals

After completing this lesson, you will be able to:

✔ Key operative reports in block format.

An operative report is produced on all patients who have an operative or surgical procedure. It details why a surgery was done, how it was performed, what the surgeon discovered during the procedure, and the final diagnosis.

Operative reports are keyed with 1.5-inch margins on the top, left, and right, and a 1-inch margin at the bottom. Double-space between sections, and single-space within sections. Operative report formats vary, but the following headings are required: PREOPERATIVE DIAGNOSIS, POSTOPERATIVE DIAGNOSIS, PRIMARY PROCEDURE (or OPERATION PERFORMED), and PROCEDURE. The wording of these headings may vary. The surgeon's and assistant surgeon's signature lines are typed at the bottom of the report, followed by the typist's initials, "d" and date for "dictated by," and "t" for transcribed and the date.

Instructions

Study and key the sample operative report on page 325. Proofread your copy and correct errors.

```
         Patient Name:  Louise Hernia                          6
         DS
         Medical Record No.:  45                               11
         DS
         Hospital No.:  2409                                   15
         DS
         Date of Surgery:  07/20/200__                         21
         DS
         Admitting Physician:  Paula Catheter, MD              29
         DS
         Surgeon:  Jean Mass, MD                               34
         DS
         Anesthesiologist:  Darnell Quadrant, MD               42
         DS
         Preoperative Diagnosis:  Salpingitis                  49
         DS
         Postoperative Diagnosis:  Salpingitis                 56
         DS
         Operative Procedure:  Salpingostomy                   63
         DS
         Anesthesia:  General                                  67
         DS
         PREPARATION:  With stable vital signs and normal laboratory   78
         studies, the patient was taken to the operating room.         88
         DS
         Description: After satisfactory monitoring, general          98
         inhalation anesthesia was administered. Under anesthesia,    109
         the patient was placed in a dorsal sacral position.          119
         The abdomen was scrubbed, and the area was draped. The bladder 131
         was emptied with a catheter. Examination revealed a small    142
         amount of dark blood in the cervix. The uterus was increased 153
         in size. There were no masses present. A subumbilical incision 165
         was made. Inspection was carried out without elevation of the 177
         uterus. There was a large clot on the fimbriated portion of  188
         the right uterine tube. A salpingostomy was then made on the 199
         uterine tube. The pelvic cavity was irrigated, aspirating    210
         several clots. Inspection of the uterine tube revealed       220
         adequate hemostasis. The uterine tube was identified and     231
         elevated, and the fimbriated end was dilated. There were some 243
         adhesions on the ovary. The appendix was normal. The liver   254
         and gallbladder were normal. The incision was closed with 4-0 266
         Vicryl sutures. Needle, sponge, and instrument counts were   277
         reported correct. The patient was transported to the recovery 289
         room in good condition with stable vital signs and response. 300
         QS                              QS


         _____     _____
         Paula Catheter, MD      Jean Mass, MD                 307
         DS
         ES                                                    308
         D:07/20/200__                                         310
         T:07/20/200__                                         312
```

Key the following operative report. Proofread your copy and correct errors.

OPERATIVE REPORT 2

```
Patient Name: Evelyn Back                                    5
DS
Hospital No.: 2401                                           9
DS
Date of Surgery: April 3, 200__                             16
DS
Surgeon: Robbie Calculi, MD                                 22
DS
Assistant Surgeon: Jason Cannula, MD                        29
DS
Anesthesiologist: Patsy Trocar, MD                          36
DS
Anesthesia: General.                                        40
DS
Preoperative Diagnosis: Cholelithiasis.                     48
DS
Postoperative Diagnosis: Cholelithiasis.                    56
DS
Operative Procedure: Cholecystectomy.                       63
DS
Indications: The patient is a 55-year-old Caucasian female  74
who presents with recurrent episodes of pain in the epigastric  86
region. The pain is triggered by foods such as onion rings and  98
chili. Ultrasound examination revealed calculi in the gall- 109
bladder, which is mildly inflamed.                          116
DS
Description of Procedure: The procedure, alternatives, and  127
risks were explained to the patient. After a signed and     138
witnessed operative consent was obtained, the patient was   149
brought to the operating room and placed under general      159
anesthesia. She was prepared and draped in the usual manner. 170
We cut down the epigastric region about 3/4 of an inch across. 181
We cut into the abdomen. A forceps was used to grasp the    192
gallbladder. We completed the dissections and removed the   203
gallbladder from the liver. The gallbladder was removed     214
without difficulty. We used two #1-0 Vicryl sutures to close 225
the epigastric area.
DS
The patient tolerated the procedure well. Estimated blood   236
loss was 20 cc. She was taken to the recovery room in good  247
condition.                                                  249
QS                              QS
```

_____   _____

□□□□1□□□□2□□□□3□□□□4□□□□5□□□□6□□□□7□□□□8□□□□9□□□□10□□□□11□□□□12

```
Robbie Calculi, MD        Jason Cannula, MD                                257
DS
ejs                                                                        258
d:04/03/200__                                                              261
t:04/05/200__                                                              263
```

Instructions

Key the following operative report. Proofread your copy and correct errors.

OPERATIVE REPORT 3

```
        Patient Name:Georgie Corneal                                       6
        DS
        Hospital No.: 2402                                                10
        DS
        Date of Surgery: 02/25/200__                                     16
        DS
        Surgeon: Charlie Eye, MD                                         21
        DS
        Assistant Surgeon: Sharon Retina, MD                            28
        DS
        Anesthesiologist: Sarah Anterior, MD                            35
        DS
        Anesthesia: Local anesthetic agents                             42
        DS
        Preoperative Diagnosis: Cataract, left eye.                     50
        DS
        Postoperative Diagnosis: Cataract, left eye.                    59
        DS
        Operative Procedure: Lens implantation of the left eye.         70
        DS
        Description: The patient's operative eye received drops. The    81
        patient was transferred to the operating room. The patient     92
        was given intravenous sedation and local anesthetic injections. 104
        The eye was prepped and draped in the usual manner. The        115
        conjunctiva was opened. A capsulotomy was performed using a    126
        continuous tear technique. The wound was enlarged with a 3.0   137
        mm keratome. Remnants were removed using irrigation and        147
        aspiration. The lens was placed in the left eye. The wound was 159
        closed with a single suture. The suture was tied and cut.      170
        Topical drops of medicated ointment were placed in the eye.    181
        It was covered with a patch and a shield. The patient is       192
        returning to the same-day surgery area in excellent condition. 204
        Complications: None.                                           208
        QS                              QS

        _____             _____

        Charlie Eye, MD                 Sharon Retina, MD              216
        DS
        es                                                             217
        d:02/25/200__                                                  219
        t:02/25/200__                                                  221
```

□□□□1□□□□2□□□□3□□□□4□□□□5□□□□6□□□□7□□□□8□□□□9□□□□10□□□□11□□□□12

Instructions

Key the following operative report. Proofread your copy and correct errors.

OPERATIVE REPORT 4

```
Patient Name: Patsy Suture Medical Record No. 80        10
DS
Hospital No.: 2403                                       14
DS
Date of Surgery: 12/01/200__                             20
DS
Surgeon: Ruby Fascia, MD                                 25
DS
Assistant Surgeon: Blanch Rectus, MD                    32
DS
Anesthesiologist: Walter Rectus, MD                     39
DS
Anesthesia: General.                                    43
DS
Preoperative Diagnosis: 1. Uterine prolapse 2. Cystocele.   54
DS
Postoperative Diagnosis: Uterine prolapse; cystocele.   64
DS
Operation: Abdominal hysterectomy, salpingo-oophorectomy.   75
DS
Description of Procedure: The patient was taken to the   85
operating room where she was placed in the supine position and   96
given a general anesthetic. She was then prepared and draped in 107
the usual fashion. A Pfannenstiel skin incision was made across 118
the abdomen. Abdominal and pelvic explorations were carried out 129
with all findings being normal. The ligament was clamped, cut, 140
and ligated. The uterus was cut and ligated with a #1 chromic 151
suture. The uterus, fallopian tubes, and ovaries were then 162
excised, and #1 chromic sutures were placed. Irrigation with 173
normal saline was carried out. The sponge and needle counts 184
were correct. The sponges were removed, and the abdomen was 195
closed with 2-0 chromic sutures. The patient was taken to the 206
recovery room in satisfactory condition.                214
DS
Findings: Normal-appearing uterus, fallopian tubes, and ovaries.225
Cystocele was present.                                  228
DS
Estimated blood loss: 200 cc.                           235
DS
Complications: None.                                    239
DS
  □□□□1□□□□2□□□□3□□□□4□□□□5□□□□6□□□□7□□□□8□□□□9□□□□10□□□□11□□□□12
```

```
Condition: The patient was in stable condition in the recovery        250
room.                                                                 251
QS                              QS


_____          _____

Blanch Rectus, MD            Ruby Fascia, MD                          259
DS
qb                                                                    260
d:12/02/_____                                                         262
t:12/02/_____                                                         264
```

FIVE-MINUTE TIMING—DOUBLE SPACE

```
        She is a 16-year-old female, well known to Mobile         11
Hospital, with metastatic Wilms tumor identified in the lungs,    23
liver, and the brain.  She just completed chemotherapy and        34
radiation for her brain metastases.  Her lung metastases          45
seemed to have diminished in size.  During the  week after        56
discharge, she had an upper respiratory tract infection.          67
Chest x-ray revealed an effusion.  Her CBC and platelet counts    79
were all in good shape.  Physical examination was remarkable      90
for decreased breath sounds in the left lung.  Otherwise, she     101
has symptoms of an upper respiratory tract infection.  The        112
patient received a thoracentesis the next day and bloody fluid    124
was removed from the chest.  Culture of the thoracentesis         135
did not reveal any bacteria but many pus cells.  Other            146
studies on the thoracentesis are pending, including cytology.     158
After the thoracentesis procedure, she became distressed,         169
but toward the evening when the side effects of sedation          180
began to wear off, she began to have pain in the left side of     192
her chest.  Chest x-ray after the thoracentesis showed no         203
evidence of pneumonia; however, metastasis was seen in the        214
left lung.  She did not respond at this time to Tylenol with      225
Codeine.                                                          226
    □□□□1□□□□2□□□□3□□□□4□□□□5□□□□6□□□□7□□□□8□□□□9□□□□10□□□□11□□□□12
```

Pathology Reports, Five-Minute Timed Writing

Goals

After completing this lesson, you will be able to:

✔ Key pathology reports.

Instructions

Pathology is the branch of medicine that studies the causes of diseases and the outcome of the specimen. Pathology reports are keyed in different formats. Space before and after the lowercased x. Single-space body of report. Double-space after headings.

Example:

The tissue measured 5.5 x 3.0 x 0.9 cm.

Instructions

Key the sample pathology report on page 331. Proofread your copy and correct errors.

Instruction

Key the following pathology report. Proofread your copy and correct errors.

Pathology Report	3
DS	
Patient Name: June Cele	8
DS	
Date of Birth: 11/9/1970	13
DS	
Medical Record No.: 11-11	18
DS	
Sex: F	20
DS	
Laboratory No.: 93-V	24
DS	
Physician: Tamara Cystic, MD	30
DS	
Date Collected: 10/14/200__	36
DS	
Date Received: 10/14/200__	41
DS	
Date Completed: 10/14/200__	46
DS	
Specimen Submitted: Gallbladder.	52
DS	

Gross Description: The specimen consists of an 11.5 x 3 x 4 cm   63
organ. In areas where it is intact, the surface is smooth   74
and a purple-tan color. The specimens are four calculi, each   85
measuring 1.5 cm in diameter with a dark green color.   95
DS

Microscopic Description: Sections of the gallbladder show   106
fibrosis with hemorrhagic necrosis. No malignancy is seen.   117
DS

Microscopic Diagnosis: Hemorrhagic cholecystitis with   127
cholelithiasis.   130
QS

_____

Jody Lumbar, MD	133
DS	
Director of Pathology	137
DS	
TC:EJ	139
SS	
D:10/14/200__	141
SS	
T:10/15/200__	143

□□□□1□□□□2□□□□3□□□□4□□□□5□□□□6□□□□7□□□□8□□□□9□□□□10□□□□11□□□□12

Instructions

Study the sample before keying. Key in block format. Proofread and correct errors.

```
Medical Clinic and Hospital Mobile, AZ 67899-6666         10
DS
Department of Pathology                                   15
DS
Cyst, Jean/Date of Birth: 01/01/XX/Medical Record No.: 11G/    26
Sex: F Lab. No.: 95-C/Physician: Charles Poly, MD/Date        36
Collected: 12/09/XX/Date Received: 12/10/XX/Date Completed:    47
12/15/XX                                                      49
DS
Specimen Submitted: Polyp.                                54
DS
Gross Description: The specimen is submitted as a polyp. The   65
specimen consists of 2 biopsies measuring 3 to 4 mm each.      76
DS
Microscopic Description: The section of the polyp revealed     87
adenomatous polyp. These sections are composed of adenomatous  98
glands. No evidence of malignancy.                            105
Microscopic Diagnosis: Benign polyp.                          112
_____/Jody Lumbar, MD/Director of Pathology/  123
                JL:EJS/D:12/16/200__/T:12/16/200__           134
```
▫▫▫▫1▫▫▫▫2▫▫▫▫3▫▫▫▫4▫▫▫▫5▫▫▫▫6▫▫▫▫7▫▫▫▫8▫▫▫▫9▫▫▫▫10▫▫▫▫11▫▫▫▫12

Instructions

Study the sample before keying. Key the following report in block format. Proofread your copy and correct errors.

```
                                      SS
                        SURGICAL PATHOLOGY REPORT                          9
                                      SS
Patient: Femur, Jodie              Unit No.: 60-0                         19
SS                                 SS
DOB: September 29, 1953            Sex: F                                 27
SS                                 SS
Surgeon: Ann Foot, MD             Accession No.: S190                     38
SS                                 SS
Date of Surgery: December 27, ____    Date Received: December 27, ___50
SPECIMEN SUBMITTED: A: Rectal polyp.                                      57
SS
PREOPERATIVE FINDINGS: Three to 4 mm polyp in rectum.                     67
SS
POSTOPERATIVE DIAGNOSIS: Not stated.                                      74
SS
GROSS DESCRIPTION: A: Received in formalin, labeled "rectal               85
                      polyp," are 2 irregular pieces of tan soft          96
                      tissue, measuring 0.2 and 0.3 cm in                106
                      greatest dimension respectively. Totally           117
                      submitted in cassette A1.                          125
                      SS
AF:AS                                                                    126
SS
MICROSCOPIC DIAGNOSIS: A: Large intestine, rectum, biopsy.              137
Tubular adenoma.                                                        140
SS
AF:AS                                                                    141
SS


                                        _____
                                        Ann Fox, MD                    151
                                        Attending Surgical             162
                                        Pathologist                    172
                                        SS
AF:AS                                                                   173
D:12-27-200__                                                           175
T:12-28-200__                                                           178
```

□□□□1□□□□2□□□□3□□□□4□□□□5□□□□6□□□□7□□□□8□□□□9□□□□10□□□□11□□□□12

The patient is a 32-year-old woman who comes in today for   12
follow-up of her abdominal pain. The last time I saw her, I   23
had placed her on a course of Prevpac. She completed the full   35
14-day course about a week ago. She says "she is feeling   46
better," but still has to very careful about what she eats or   57
she will get epigastric retrosternal pain and discomfort.   68
She also describes a burning abdominal pain that seems to   79
correlate with eating spicy foods. She is eating bland food   90
and avoids eating late at night. She takes Tagamet 800 mg   101
p.o. q.h.s. She came today for follow-up of the results of   112
the abdominal CT scan. The abdominal/pelvic CT scan that was   123
done on December 5, 2001, showed a low-density lesion adjacent   135
to the uterus that represents an ovarian cyst. Ultrasound is   146
recommended. Her liver, gallbladder, and pancreas all   156
appeared normal on CT scan. Her weight has been stable over   167
the past month. I had treated her with Prevpac because of   178
the presence of gastritis on her endoscopy and positive   189
H. pylori serology. I will have her start taking Prevacid   200
30 mg p.o. q.a.m., and she may also continue the Tagamet at   211
bedtime, as needed. I was not able to palpate any masses on   222
examination today. I will refer her for a pelvic ultrasound   233
to evaluate an ovarian mass seen on CT scan.   242

▢▢▢▢1▢▢▢▢2▢▢▢▢3▢▢▢▢4▢▢▢▢5▢▢▢▢6▢▢▢▢7▢▢▢▢8▢▢▢▢9▢▢▢▢10▢▢▢▢11▢▢▢▢12

Consultation Reports, Five-Minute Timed Writing

Goals

After completing this lesson, you will be able to:

✔ Key consultation reports.

Consultation reports are used when a physician consults with another physician to manage a patient's care. The format is similar to the History and Physical Examination Report.

Instructions

Study and key consultation reports in block format. Key the sample consultation first. Leave 1.5-inch top, bottom, left, and right margins. Add "continued" if there is a continuing page. Proofread your copy and correct errors.

CONSULTATION REPORT 1 SAMPLE

```
Patient Name: Nodes, Peaches                             6
Medical Record No.: 54                                  10
Requesting Physician:Matthew T. Sampson, MD             19
Date: October 10, 200__                                 24
DS

CONSULTATION REPORT TO                                  28
DS

John F. Gastric, MD                                     32
DS

HISTORY OF PRESENT ILLNESS                              37
DS

This 22-year-old black female presented to the emergency    48
department with abdominal pain. The patient was known to have    59
gallstones. She thought she had her gallbladder removed;    69
however, an abdominal exploration for perforated appendicitis    80
revealed that a gallbladder was present. The patient has had    91
pain in the right upper quadrant which is quite severe.     101
DS

PAST MEDICAL HISTORY                                    105
SS

Positive for asthma as well as multiple sclerosis. She takes    116
no medications and has no known drug allergies. Examination    127
showed right upper quadrant tenderness.                 134
DS

(continued)
```

☐☐☐☐1☐☐☐☐2☐☐☐☐3☐☐☐☐4☐☐☐☐5☐☐☐☐6☐☐☐☐7☐☐☐☐8☐☐☐☐9☐☐☐☐10☐☐☐☐11☐☐☐☐12

```
Initial laboratory studies showed a normal white blood cell        145
count. An ultrasound was obtained which showed cholelithiasis.      156
DS

The patient has remained afebrile with normal vital signs.         167
Her abdominal tenderness has remained. On the date of              177
consultation, the patient again complained of right upper           188
quadrant tenderness. Physical examination shows marked right       199
upper quadrant tenderness.                                         204
DS

DIAGNOSIS                                                          206
1. Cholelithiasis.                                                 209
2. Asthma, inactive at this time.                                 215
3. Multiple sclerosis stable, at this time.                      223
QS


Matthew T. Sampson, MD                                            227
MS:ES/D:10/10/200__/T:10/11/200__                                 233
```

Instructions

Key the following consultation report. Study the sample first. Proofread your copy and correct errors.

CONSULTATION REPORT 2

```
Requesting Physician: Matthew T. Sampson, MD                       9
Consultation Report to Marvin Downs, MD                           17
Date: December 5, 200__                                           21
Medical Record No.: 55                                            25
Patient Name: Leslie Fundus                                       30
History of present illness: This 42-year-old white male was        41
admitted to Mobile Hospital with jaundice and a tentative         52
diagnosis of cholelithiasis and choledocholithiasis. The          62
patient was admitted by Dr. Mable Apex. The patient had           72
experienced a history of gallbladder problems, which were         83
diagnosed several days ago. CT scan of the abdomen revealed        94
the presence of cholelithiasis and choledocholithiasis. The       105
patient had developed severe upper abdominal pain, back pain,     116
and jaundice. In addition, his past medical history revealed      127
he had an ulcer for which he had been taking Zantac. He also      138
had a history of passing kidney stones. At the time of            148
admission to Mobile Hospital, his white count was 12,900,         159
bilirubin elevated at 10.8, AST 400, alkaline phosphatase 600.    170

Physical Examination: On physical examination, the patient had    182
been febrile. He was jaundiced. There was abdominal tenderness    194
in the right upper quadrant. The patient's urine was dark.        205
Impression:                                                       207
1. Cholelithiasis and choledocholithiasis.                        215
2. Kidney stones.                                                 218
3. Ulcer.                                                         219
```
□□□□1□□□□2□□□□3□□□□4□□□□5□□□□6□□□□7□□□□8□□□□9□□□□10□□□□11□□□□12

```
At the time of surgery, the incision was made and there were      230
pus and stones. His condition improved. He did develop rales     241
and atelectasis. He had low-grade fevers. Cultures taken of      252
blood, urine, and sputum were negative. His urine returned to    264
normal color.                                                    266
Medication: Zantac.                                              269
The patient is to make an appointment in my office in one        280
week.The patient was asymptomatic at the time of discharge.      291
Thank you for referring this patient to me.                      299
```

Matthew Sampson, MD/MS:ES/D:12/05/200___/T:12/07/200___   309

FIVE-MINUTE TIMING—DOUBLE SPACE

```
        The patient is a 45-year-old woman who noticed a tender    11
lump in the upper right breast about two weeks ago.  She           22
denies previous problems with her breasts.  There has been         33
no nipple discharge or nipple inversion.  The breasts are          44
average size without any abnormality.  Palpation finds a           55
movable nontender mass in the upper right breast.  Aspiration      67
was negative.  The left breast is negative and both axillary       78
areas are normal.  She remembers having mastitis with her          89
first child.  She possibly injured her breast a month ago         100
when she fell on the floor.  She takes no medications or          111
hormones.  Her health seems excellent.  She does not smoke but    123
drinks alcoholic beverages socially.  She has not had any         134
major illnesses requiring hospitalization.  Operations include    146
tonsillectomy, appendectomy, and removal of the right ovary.      157
Her father died of cancer of the larynx and pancreas; the         168
mother is in good health.  There is cancer involving the          179
maternal grandfather, but no breast disease.  She is an only      190
child.  She has no headaches, problems with sinuses, eyes,        201
ears, nose, or throat.  No chest symptoms such as coughing,       212
wheezing, chest pain, or shortness of breath.  No gastrointes-    224
tinal complaints such as heartburn, fatty food intolerance,       235
constipation, diarrhea, or hemorrhoids.  No urinary symptoms      246
such as stress incontinence, dysuria, or frequency of urina-      257
tion.  She has had no seizures or fainting episodes.  She is      268
alert, cooperative, and oriented to time and place.              278
□□□□1□□□□2□□□□3□□□□4□□□□5□□□□6□□□□7□□□□8□□□□9□□□□10□□□□11□□□□12
```

Discharge Summaries/Discharge Instructions, Five-Minute Timed Writing

Goals

After completing this lesson, you will be able to:

✔ Key discharge summaries.

Discharge summaries can be keyed in different formats. Each patient who is discharged from the hospital has a discharge summary. Single-space the body of the report. Double-space between headings. Leave 1.5-inch top, bottom, left, and right margins.

Instructions

Key the discharge summary example and other discharge summaries in the same format. Use a header if needed for the reports. Proofread your copy and correct your errors.

DISCHARGE SUMMARY 1 EXAMPLE

```
DISCHARGE SUMMARY                                      4
DS
PAIENT NAME: Palsy, Betty                              9
DS
Medical Record No.: 475                               14
DS
PHYSICIAN NAME: Doris Nausea, MD                      20
DS
DATE: February 15, 200__                              25
DS
DATE OF ADMISSION                                     28
DS
February 15, 200__                                    31
DS
DATE OF DISCHARGE                                     34
DS
February 15, 200__                                    37
DS
ADMITTING DIAGNOSIS                                   41
DS
Ileitis                                               42
DS
DISCHARGE DIAGNOSIS                                   46
(continued)
```

□□□□1□□□□2□□□□3□□□□4□□□□5□□□□6□□□□7□□□□8□□□□9□□□□10□□□□11□□□□12

DS

Ileitis   47
DS

HISTORY OF PRESENT ILLNESS   52
DS

The patient is a 42-year-old female who presents with crampy   63
abdominal pain in her left lower quadrant associated with   74
nausea and vomiting. This started on the day of admission.   85
She was taken to the emergency department at Mobile Hospital   96
and found to have abdominal pain and ileitis.   105
DS

PHYSICAL EXAMINATION   109
DS

The examination revealed a patient who was alert, oriented,   120
and cooperative. Her abdomen is soft and nontender.   129
DS

LABORATORY DATA   132
DS

Potassium 3.9. Hemoglobin 10.8. White blood count 20,000.   143
DS

HOSPITAL COURSE   146
DS

The patient was treated with an antibiotic and had improvement   158
in her symptoms. Cultures of her blood were negative. It   169
is felt that the patient responded to the intravenous   179
antibiotics. She feels much better, is eating, has no   189
abdominal pain, and is ready for discharge providing that   200
she takes her oral antibiotics.   206
DS

DISCHARGE PLAN   209
DS

She will be discharged to home and will come to the office in   221
one week for reevaluation.   226
QS

_____

Doris Nausea, MD   229
DS

DN:EJ   230
SS

D:02/16/200__   232
SS

T:02/16/200__   234

□□□□1□□□□2□□□□3□□□□4□□□□5□□□□6□□□□7□□□□8□□□□9□□□□10□□□□11□□□□12

Key the following discharge summary. Study the sample first. Add "continue" if the discharge report is longer than one page. Proofread your copy and correct errors.

DISCHARGE SUMMARY 2

```
          DISCHARGE SUMMARY                                          3
          PATIENT NAME: Homer Cocci                                  8
          DS
          MEDICAL RECORD NO.: 474                                   13
          DS
          PHYSICIAN NAME: Paul Organic, MD                          20
          DS
          DATE OF ADMISSION: 09/09/200__                            26
          DS
          DATE OF DISCHARGE: 09/11/200__                            32
          DS
          ADMITTING DIAGNOSIS: Pneumonia.                           38
          DS
          DISCHARGE DIAGNOSIS: Pneumonia.                           44
          DS
          HISTORY OF PRESENT ILLNESS: This patient is a 92-year-old  55
          white male who is disoriented. He took a walk and was found 66
          to be looking for his house. He is known to have organic brain 77
          syndrome and has problems with his memory. He was admitted to 88
          the SOCARE Unit for depression and pneumonia.             97
          DS
          PAST MEDICAL HISTORY: He has a history of hypertension, which 108
          has been controlled by blood pressure medication.        117
          DS
          PHYSICAL EXAMINATION: The examination revealed a lethargic 128
          male in no apparent distress. His lungs are inflamed. Blood 139
          pressure: 160/80. Pulse: 80. Respirations: 12. Temperature: 150
          102. Skin reveals ecchymosis on the left side of his face. 161
          Chest: Clear. Abdomen: Soft without organomegaly.        170
          DS
          LABORATORY DATA: Potassium 2.1. Hemoglobin 14.0. Hematocrit 181
          38.                                                      182
          SS
          X-RAYS: CT scan of the head revealed cerebral atrophy.   192
          DS
          HOSPITAL COURSE: The patient was admitted to the hospital 203
          and started on intravenous fluids. Urinalysis results were 214
          obtained, which showed pyuria. He is taking intravenous  224
          antibiotics for pneumonitis and urinary tract infection. 235
          DS
          (continued)

          □□□□1□□□□2□□□□3□□□□4□□□□5□□□□6□□□□7□□□□8□□□□9□□□□10□□□□11□□□□12
```

```
                    DISCHARGE PLAN: The patient will be discharged to home with      246
                    medications.                                                     248
                    QS


                    _____
                    Paul Organic, MD                                                 251
                    DS
                    PO:es                                                            252
                    SS
                    D:09/12/200__                                                    254
                    SS
                    T:09/14/200__                                                    256
```

Instructions

Key the following discharge summary. Study the sample and then key. Proofread and correct your errors.

DISCHARGE SUMMARY 3

```
                    DISCHARGE SUMMARY                                                  3
                    DS
                    Patient Name: Jasmine Polyp                                        9
                    DS
                    Medical Record No.: 473                                           14
                    DS
                    Physician Name: Evan Scan, MD                                     20
                    DS
                    Date of Admission: 12/01/200__                                    26
                    DS
                    Date of Discharge: 12/01/200__                                    32
                    DS
                    Admitting Diagnosis: Polyp of the larynx.                         40
                    DS
                    Discharge Diagnosis: Polyp of the larynx.                         48
                    DS
                    Operative Procedure: Polypectomy.                                 54
                    DS
                    History: The patient is a 57-year-old white female with           65
                    heart disease who is on a calcium blocker. She has mild           76
                    hypertension. Her general health is good.                         84
                    DS
                    Physical examination: The examination revealed polyps in the      95
                    larynx. Biopsies were taken of the polyps. The CT scan showed    106
                    a mass in the larynx. There was no lymphadenopathy, and no       117
                    nodes were seen in the neck. Neck palpation: Negative. Lungs:    128
                    Clear to auscultation and percussion. Heart: No murmurs. No      139
                    cardiomegaly.                                                    141
                    DS

          □□□□1□□□□2□□□□3□□□□4□□□□5□□□□6□□□□7□□□□8□□□□9□□□□10□□□□11□□□□12
```

```
Abdomen: Soft and nontender. Laboratory: Hemoglobin: 9.3.     152
Hematocrit: 27. Cholesterol: 150. Phosphorus: 4.3. Albumin:   163
4.1. Calcium: 9.4. Glucose: 97. BUN: 18.                      171
DS

Hospital Course: On the first hospital day, in the Outpatient 182
Surgical Unit, the patient underwent laryngoscopy for polyps.  193
The polyps were benign. The patient was taken to the recovery  204
room in satisfactory condition.                               210
DS

Discharge Plan: She was discharged to home in good condition.  221
Tylenol was prescribed for pain. She is to come to my office   232
Wednesday for a follow-up.                                    237
QS

_____

Evan Scan, MD                                                 239
DS
ES:EM                                                         240
SS
D:12/02/XX                                                    242
SS
T:12/02/XX                                                    244
```

DISCHARGE INSTRUCTIONS

Goals

After completing this lesson, you will be able to:

✔ Key discharge instructions report.
✔ Define discharge instructions report.

Discharge instructions are for patients who have received treatment. The patient and staff member are required to sign the discharge instructions. Key the main topics in all capital letters. Double-space between headings; single-space the report body. Key the following report. Proofread your copy and correct errors.

```
                DISCHARGE INSTRUCTIONS                     8
DS
Patient Name: Flowers, Beulah                             14
Patient No.: 6289                                         19
Physician Name: Matthew T. Sampson, MD                    26
Medical Record No.: 000-001-0000                          31
Date: May 16, 200__                                       35
DS

TENSION HEADACHE
A tension headache may be triggered by emotional stress,  45
overeating, alcohol use, certain foods, lack of sleep,    55
oversleeping, or a busy environment.                      62
DS

□□□□1□□□□2□□□□3□□□□4□□□□5□□□□6□□□□7□□□□8□□□□9□□□□10□□□□11□□□□12
```

This causes strain on the face, neck, and scalp due to   72
tension. This may last from hours to days.   80
DS

PREVENTING FUTURE HEADACHES   85
Pay attention to those factors that seem to trigger your   95
headache and try to avoid these when possible. If you feel   106
that stress is a factor in your headaches, identify the   116
sources of stress in your life and find ways to release   126
those stresses by walking, relaxation methods, or taking time   137
out for yourself. If you have been prescribed a medicine to   148
stop a tension headache, follow instructions for the best   159
results.   160
DS

MEDICATION   162
Fioricet. You have been prescribed a medicine for tension   173
headaches called Fioricet.   178
DS

DIRECTION FOR USE   181
Take Fioricet as prescribed by the physician. Fioricet may be   192
taken with food or milk to prevent stomach upset. Avoid   202
caffeine and alcohol.   206
DS

WHAT TO WATCH FOR   209
Possible side effects include nausea and lightheadedness.   220
Report to the physician blurred vision, drowsiness, dizziness, 231
and breathing problems.   235
DS

RETURN PROMPTLY   238
1. Worsening of your headache.   244
2. Weakness in the muscles of the face, arms, or legs.   254
3. Fainting, drowsiness, confusion, or difficulty with   264
vision, speech, or walking.   269
DS

I have received and understand the above instructions.   279
QS

_____   _____   _____

Patient Signature   Staff Signature   Date   289
□□□□1□□□□2□□□□3□□□□4□□□□5□□□□6□□□□7□□□□8□□□□9□□□□10□□□□11□□□□12

This is a 78-year-old single woman who was admitted to   11
Mobile Hospital with edema of both ankles, mild dyspnea, and   22
fecal incontinence. She has had heart disease for many years   34
without obvious congestive heart failure. In January of 2002,   46
she was started on Motrin for osteoarthritis. A week ago,   57
she moved into an assisted living facility. She is not sure   68
of the duration of her edema, but it appears to have developed   80
over the past few weeks, at least since December when she was   91
last seen in the office. She is chronically depressed. She   102
has mild dyspnea on exertion. She denies recent chest pain.   113
A few days ago, she had a syncopal episode on rising from a   124
chair. She is sedentary. She has occasional fecal incon-   135
tinence without abdominal pain. She denies urinary symptoms   146
and vaginal discharge. She has severe osteoarthritis of both   158
knees and the right hip that cause her considerable pain. On   170
February of 1999, she was hospitalized with abdominal pain   181
and diarrhea. Gastrointestinal evaluation included abdominal   193
ultrasonography, which showed cholelithiasis in her right   204
upper quadrant. The stools were negative for occult blood.   215

□□□□1□□□□2□□□□3□□□□4□□□□5□□□□6□□□□7□□□□8□□□□9□□□□10□□□□11□□□□12

Autopsy Reports, Five-Minute Timed Writing

Goals

After completing this lesson, you will be able to:

✔ Key autopsy report.

An autopsy is done to discover the cause of death. Specimens are examined by a pathologist. The pathologist examines the body for external and internal evidence and reports on his or her findings.

Autopsy report includes various headings: external exam, internal exam, body systems, dissections, microscopic exam, cause of death, and comments.

Instructions

Key the following autopsy report. Add "(continued)" if the autopsy report is longer than one page. Proofread your copy and correct errors.

AUTOPSY REPORT EXAMPLE 1

```
Jane Spur                                                          2
File No. 843A                                                      4
June 10, 200__                                                     6
Aladrianne E. Young, MD                                           11
DS

GROSS DESCRIPTION                                                 14
Upon external examination of the abdomen, neck, and thorax,       25
there is no evidence of injury other than the recent surgery.     36
DS

EXTERNAL EXAMINATION                                              40
The body is that of a well-developed, well-nourished Asian        51
female, age 35. The body measures 60 inches in length and         62
weighs 190 pounds. The head is of normal size and shows no        73
abnormalities. The eyes, ears, nose, and mouth show no            83
abnormalities. The neck has a tracheostomy incision, in which     94
the tracheostomy tube is in place, in the midline of the neck    105
and a chest tube incision, with chest tube in place. No other    116
scars or marks are noted. On examination of the external         127
surface of the body, the chest is normal except for the          138
previously described scars. The breasts are normal. The          149
abdomen is normal. The back, external genitalia, and             159
extremities show no other abnormalities.                         167
DS

INITIAL INCISION                                                 170
The subcutaneous fat measures 2 cm over the abdomen and 2.2      181
cm over the chest. The left pleural cavity contains no lung      192
DS
```

▫▫▫▫1▫▫▫▫2▫▫▫▫3▫▫▫▫4▫▫▫▫5▫▫▫▫6▫▫▫▫7▫▫▫▫8▫▫▫▫9▫▫▫▫10▫▫▫▫11▫▫▫▫12

and shows evidence of a left radical pneumonectomy with strip- 204
ping of the lymph nodes. The left pleural cavity contains 215
approximately 3 liters of hemorrhagic fluid. The right pleural 227
cavity contains 2 liters of serous clear fluid. The 237
mediastinum shows a stripping of the lymph nodes. The peri- 248
cardial cavity is clear. The liver and spleen are subcostal. 259
The thoracic and abdominal cavities are normal. 268
DS

CARDIOVASCULAR SYSTEM 272
The heart weighs 200 g. Right ventricular thickness is 0.2 cm, 290
length 6 cm. Left ventricular thickness is 1.1 cm, length 7 cm.302
The epicardium contains the usual amount of fat. The chambers 314
are the usual size. The myocardium is firm and red brown. The 325
endocardium is translucent. The valves are thin. The coronary 336
arteries show severe atherosclerosis and narrow, tiny coronary 347
arteries. The left anterior is 85 percent occluded with fatty 358
athersclerosis. The aorta has atherosclerosis. 367
DS

RESPIRATORY SYSTEM 370
The pharynx and larynx are clear. The trachea shows a 380
tracheostomy incision with hemorrhagic discoloration to the 391
trachea. The left lung is not present. A section of the lung 402
shows bronchopneumonia. The bronchi are not remarkable. The 413
pulmonary arteries are clear. A few lymph nodes are noted and 414
these are not involved with the tumor. 421
DS

DIGESTIVE SYSTEM 424
The salivary glands are not examined. The esophagus is clear. 435
The stomach shows 15 cc of clear brown fluid but shows no 445
abnormalities. The bowel contents are normal. The appendix is 456
normal. The liver is normal. 461
DS

PANCREAS 462
The gland is the usual size, shape, consistency, and color. 473
DS

RESPIRATORY SYSTEM 476
Multiple sections of the left lung show pulmonary edema and 487
congestion with bronchopneumonia and acute inflammatory cells. 498
Examination of the right and left lymph nodes reveal no 509
residual or metastatic carcinoma. 515
DS

CARDIOVASCULAR SYSTEM 519
Sections of the heart are normal. 525
DS

URINARY SYSTEM 528
Sections of the kidney are normal. Sections of the myometrium 539
are normal. Sections of the ovary shows a hemorrhagic corpus 550
luteum but no other abnormalities. 556
(continued)

□□□□1□□□□2□□□□3□□□□4□□□□5□□□□6□□□□7□□□□8□□□□9□□□□10□□□□11□□□□12

```
DS
```
ENDOCRINE SYSTEM   559
Sections of the adrenal glands are normal.   567
```
DS
```
LYMPHATIC SYSTEM   570
The spleen and lymph nodes show no evidence of metastatic   581
disease.   582
```
DS
```
COMMENT   583
This 35-year-old female has squamous cell carcinoma of the   594
left lung which was removed two days prior to her death, and   605
the procedure was a left radical pneumonectomy.   614
```
DS
```
CAUSE OF DEATH   617
The cause of death is congestive heart failure with   627
pulmonary edema and bronchopneumonia.   634
```
QS
```
_____

Matthew T. Sampson, MD/Pathologist/MTS:EJS/D:06/12/200__/   645
T:06/12/200__   647

FIVE-MINUTE TIMING—DOUBLE SPACE

        Mary Dystocia is a white female with a previous cesarean   11
delivery who presents for induction of labor at term secondary   23
to gestational diabetes. The patient has had a previous   34
delivery, and she desired an attempt for trial labor. The   45
patient was contracting irregularly every 10 to 15 minutes.   56
As the developing labor ensued, she was taken to the operating   68
room for a cesarean delivery. After epidural anesthesia was   79
induced, the patient was placed in the supine position and   90
prepped for an abdominal procedure. A Pfannenstiel skin   101
incision was made through the previous incision. A uterine   112
incision was made with bandage scissors. The lovely female   123
baby was delivered. The placenta was removed. The uterus   134
was cleaned of all amniotic fluid and blood clots; the uterus   146
was closed with a single layer of chromic suture. The skin   157
was closed with skin staples. A sterile dressing was applied.   169
There were no complications. All sponge, needle, and instru-   181
ment counts were correct. The patient was taken to the   192
recovery suite in satisfactory condition. The baby was taken   204
to the nursery.   207
□□□□1□□□□2□□□□3□□□□4□□□□5□□□□6□□□□7□□□□8□□□□9□□□□10□□□□11□□□□12

Radiology Reports, Five-Minute Timed Writing

Goals

After completing this lesson, you will be able to:

✔ Key radiology reports.

Instructions

Key the radiology report on page 349. Double-space between the headings. Key headings in upper-case letters. Single-space the report. Study and key the sample radiology report first.

FIVE-MINUTE TIMING—DOUBLE SPACE

```
        Patricia was seen in my office complaining of a severe       11
low back pain.  It was almost impossible to examine her              22
because any motion would send her into a muscular spasm.  She        34
entered the Brown's Pain Clinic to control this extreme pain.        46
The patient had a tubal ligation some years ago and vein            57
stripping of varicose veins in both legs.  Aside from the back       69
pain, she has had no other injuries.  She has Parkinson              80
disease, chronic cardiac disease, and hypothyroidism.  The          91
patient has two adult children.  Her husband died of gastric        102
carcinoma.  Blood pressure and urinalysis are within normal         113
limits.  Since her last visit, she has gained 11 pounds.  She       125
works as a schoolteacher at the high school where she teaches       137
math.  She was instructed to follow up with Dr. Pain every          148
week for pain therapy.                                              152
```
▢▢▢▢1▢▢▢▢2▢▢▢▢3▢▢▢▢4▢▢▢▢5▢▢▢▢6▢▢▢▢7▢▢▢▢8▢▢▢▢9▢▢▢▢10▢▢▢▢11▢▢▢▢12

```
Radiology Report
DS
Patient Name: Ruby Chronic
DS
X-ray No.: 32ZY
DS
Physician: Robert Duct, MD
DS
Proceudre: Chest x-ray.
DS
Date: 04/10/200__
DS
CHEST: No films are available for comparison. The lungs are clear.
DS
No abnormalities of the spine or rib cage are identified.
DS
IMPRESSION: Normal chest examination.
DS
ABDOMEN: Flat and upright views of the abdomen are normal without
DS
evidence of obstruction. There are no abnormal masses.
DS
IMPRESSION: Negative study.
DS
LUMBOSACRAL SPINE: There is no evidence of scoliosis or kyphosis.
No lesions.
DS
IMPRESSION: Normal lumbosacral spine. No evidence of metastatic
disease.
DS
LEFT KNEE: No bony or soft tissue abnormalities.
DS
IMPRESSION: Normal study.
QS

_____

Robert Duct, MD
SS
Chief Radiologist
DS
RB:ES
SS
D:04/10/200__
SS
T:04/10/200__
```

RADIOLOGY REPORT 2

Instructions

Study the sample first and then key. Proofread your copy and correct errors.

```
RADIOLOGY REPORT                                              3
EXAMINATION DATE: 08/02/200__/DATE REPORTED: 08/09/200__     14
PHYSICIAN: Susie Bony, MD/PATIENT: Carla Section             23
X-RAY NO.: 33XY/AGE: 27                                      27
DS

HISTORY: Abdominal pain. Chest pain.                         34
DS

CHEST: The heart and pulmonary vessels are normal. The lungs 45
are clear. The bony thorax is normal.                        52
DS

IMPRESSION: Chest is normal.                                 57
DS

GALLBLADDER ULTRASOUND: Multiple images through the          67
gallbladder were obtained. Multiple gallstones were noted.   78
The gallbladder wall showed thickening but no other          88
abnormalities.                                               90
DS

IMPRESSION:  Cholelithiasis.                                 95
DS

Susie Bony, MD/Director of Radiology/JB:SB                  103
D:04/10/200__/T:04/10/200__                                 108
```

RADIOLOGY REPORT 3

Instructions

Key the following report. Proofread your copy and correct errors.

```
                    Radiology Report
Valve, Andrea       Examination Date: July 12, 200_
X-ray No.: 5954     Technologist: Cardia Jones
Thomas Barium, MD   Age: 51
DS
PROCEDURE: Barium enema with air contrast.
DS
COMPARISON: None.
DS
FINDINGS: The preliminary film shows a large amount of gas
throughout the bowel likely related to a prior endoscopic proce-
dure. The bowel is noted to be tortuous, but no significant
extrinsic abnormalities are identified. The ileocecal valve area
is normal.
DS
```

```
□□□□1□□□□2□□□□3□□□□4□□□□5□□□□6□□□□7□□□□8□□□□9□□□□10□□□□11□□□□12
```

```
CONCLUSION: Normal air contrast barium enema.
DS
Thank you for referring this patient.
Charles Gag, MD/Radiologist/CG:EH
D:07/12/200__/T:07/14/200__
```

RADIOLOGY REPORT 4

Instructions

Key the following report. Proofread your copy and correct errors.

```
                   RADIOLOGY REPORT                        8
Patient: Duct, Lee              Room No.: OR              17
DOB: October 10, 1963           X-ray No.: 41             27
Jane Cyst, MD                   MR No.: 10                36
Examination: Cholangiogram      Date: August 12, 200__    47

HISTORY: Rule out stones.                                 52
There are four round calcifications in the right upper    62
quadrant in the area consistent with gallstones.          71
There is a catheter entering the cystic duct and filling the  82
cystic duct and the common bile duct with contrast media. They  93
both appear to be normal in size and no filling defects are  104
identified. There was some minimal reflux of the pancreatic  115
duct.                                                     116
DS

IMPRESSION: 1. Gallstones with normal appearing common bile  127
duct and cystic duct.                                     131
DS

Charles Gag, MD/Radiologist/CG:EH                        137
D:08/12/200__/T:08/13/200__                              142
```

RADIOLOGY REPORT 5

Instructions

Key the following report. Proofread your copy and correct errors.

```
                   RADIOLOGY REPORT
Patient: Gall, Jean             Room No.: 30
DOB: September 10, 1963         X-ray No.: 419
Jane Mass, MD                   MR No.: 157
Examination: Portable KUB       Date: August 10, 200__
HISTORY: 1. Status post cholecystectomy.
         2. Postoperative ileus.
```

□□□□1□□□□2□□□□3□□□□4□□□□5□□□□6□□□□7□□□□8□□□□9□□□□10□□□□11□□□□12

Surgical clips and a drain are noted in the right upper quadrant from a previous cholecystectomy. A single surgical clip is noted adjacent to the transverse process of L4 on the right. An ileus is present with air noted within both the large and small bowel. No mass is identified.

DS

IMPRESSION: 1. Postoperative ileus.
              2. Surgical clips and a drain noted in the right upper quadrant from a recent cholecystectomy.

Thomas G. Gas, MD/Radiologist/TG:NB

D:08/13/200___/T:08/16/200___

RADIOLOGY REPORT 6

Instructions

Study the sample report first. Key the following report. Proofread your copy and circle errors.

```
                RADIOLOGY REPORT                              7
DS
Patient: Orange, Jean/        Sex: F                         14
DS                            DS
DOB: 10/1/1960/               MR No.: 676                    22
DS                            DS
Requested by: Laurie Muscle, MD/    Attending Physician:    33
                                    Lyn Rad, MD              41
DS                                  DS
Examination: Lumbar spine complete  Date: August 4, ____    52
DS
HISTORY: Right thigh pain, probable radiculopathy.          62
DS
REFERENCE FILMS: None.                                      66
DS
FINDINGS: Five lumbar-type vertebral bodies were visualized. 77
The lumbar vertebral bodies appeared normally aligned. There 88
is no evidence of spondylolysis or spondylolisthesis. Facet  99
joint degenerative changes are visualized bilaterally in the 110
lower lumbar spine, predominantly at the L5-S1 level.        120
DS
IMPRESSION: Degenerative changes in the lower lumbar spine,  131
as described.                                                133
DS
Vincent Spine, MD/Radiologist/VS:MA                          140
D:08/07/200___/T:/08/09/200___                               145
```
□□□□1□□□□2□□□□3□□□□4□□□□5□□□□6□□□□7□□□□8□□□□9□□□□10□□□□11□□□□12

Special Procedures—Sample, Five-Minute Timed Writing

SPECIAL PROCEDURES—SAMPLE REPORTS

Instructions

Key the following reports. Proofread your copy and correct errors.

```
MAGNETIC RESONANCE IMAGING REPORT 1
DS

Patient Name: Paul, Jane                                        5
MR No.: 89056                                                   7
Physician: Jane Sykes, MD                                      12
Date: May 13, 200__                                            15
DS

PROCEDURE                                                      17
MRI of the Cervical Spine                                      22
DS

COMPARISON                                                     24
None.                                                          25
DS

TECHNIQUES                                                     27
1. A preliminary series of sagittal T1 weighted scans were    38
   obtained of the cervical spine.                             44
2. Axial T1 weighted scans were obtained through the          54
   cervical cord.                                              57
3. Axial T2 echo images were obtained of the cervical cord.   68
DS

FINDINGS                                                       70
There is no intrinsic abnormality arising from the            79
craniocervical junction or cervical cord.                     87
DS

At C3-4, the disc is narrowed in height. There are minimal    98
anterior osteophytes projecting forward from the inferior C3  109
vertebral body endplate.                                      113
DS

At C4-5, there is moderately advanced degenerative disc       123
disease and spondylosis with disc height narrowing.           133
DS
```

□□□□1□□□□2□□□□3□□□□4□□□□5□□□□6□□□□7□□□□8□□□□9□□□□10□□□□11□□□□12

```
CONCLUSION                                                        135
There is extensive midcervical degenerative disc disease          146
and spondylosis.                                                  149
QS


_____

Jane Sykes, MD                                                    152
Radiologist                                                       154
DS

JS:ES                                                             155
SS

D:05/13/200__                                                     157
T:05/14/200__                                                     159
```

SPECIAL PROCEDURES

Instructions

Study the sample, then key. Proofread your copy and correct errors.

```
RADIOLOGY REPORT 2
DS
MAMMOGRAPHY REPORT/Sara Walker/MR.# 29945/                          9
Bilateral Exam                                                    12
Physician Jane Sykes, MD/August 14, 200__                         20
DS

REASON FOR EXAM                                                   23
Ten years since last mammogram. There is a lump in the upper      34
outer quadrant of the right breast.                               41
DS

FINDINGS                                                          43
There is a cluster of pleomorphic calcifications in the upper     54
outer quadrant of the right breast. Left breast demonstrates      65
a cluster of calcifications in the lower outer quadrant.          75
DS

IMPRESSION                                                        77
Cluster of pleomorphic calcifications of upper outer quadrant     88
right breast which is suspicious for malignancy. Biopsy is        99
recommended. Left breast calcifications addressed on separate    110
report.                                                          111
DS

RECOMMENDATION                                                   114
Evaluate with right breast biopsy of calcifications and          125
palpable lump. The patient is referred to surgery today.         136
QS


_____

Jane Sykes, MD/JS:ES/D:08/14/200__/T:08/15/200__                 146
```
□□□□1□□□□2□□□□3□□□□4□□□□5□□□□6□□□□7□□□□8□□□□9□□□□10□□□□11□□□□12

SPECIAL PROCEDURES

Instructions

Study the sample first, then key. Proofread your copy and correct errors.

```
COLONOSCOPY REPORT 3                                              4
DS

Jean Burns/MR.# 57680/Physician: Jane Sykes, MD/May 15, 200__    15
DS

INSTRUMENT                                                        17
CF-100L 506                                                       19
DS

MEDICATIONS                                                       21
1. Versed 5 mg IV                                                24
2. Demerol 50 mg IV                                              28
DS

PROCEDURE                                                         30
After placing the patient in the left lateral decubitus          41
position, the colonoscope was inserted into the rectum. The      52
quality of the prep was good. There were no complications.       63
DS

FINDINGS                                                          65
There was a sessile polyp in the rectum. The forceps was used    77
to remove the polyp, and the tissue was retrieved.              87
DS

IMPRESSION                                                        89
A 4 mm sessile polyp was removed by biopsy forceps.             99
DS

RECOMMENDATION                                                  102
Colonoscopy within one year.                                    108
QS
_____

Jane Sykes, MD/JS:ES/D:05/15/200__/T:05/16/200__               118
□□□□1□□□□2□□□□3□□□□4□□□□5□□□□6□□□□7□□□□8□□□□9□□□□10□□□□11□□□□12
```

Gloria is a 50-year-old woman who reported having had   11
bleeding from the right nostril for a period of approximately   23
one hour. She presented in the emergency department of this   34
hospital where she was found to have a tissue pack in her   45
right nostril and no evidence of active bleeding. Laboratory   57
studies showed no significant drop in hemoglobin or hemato-   68
crit. However, her blood pressure was markedly elevated with   80
readings of 220/160. She denies any previous bleeding from   91
the nose and any recent symptoms of hypertension. She has   102
had labile hypertension for several years and in recent   113
months has shown adequate control of her blood pressure by   124
taking only lisinopril.   128

She was hospitalized here in 2002 for treatment of a   139
laceration of the right eye followed by complications   149
requiring removal of a cataract from the right eye. She   160
denies any hospitalization for any other serious illnesses or   172
surgery. After overnight observation, there was no recurrence   184
of epistaxis, and the blood pressure remained labile with   195
several readings in a normotensive range.   203

The patient was discharged in improved condition and   214
advised to continue her lisinopril.   221

□□□□1□□□□2□□□□3□□□□4□□□□5□□□□6□□□□7□□□□8□□□□9□□□□10□□□□11□□□□12

SOAP Notes/Chart Notes, Five Minute Timed Writing

Goals

After completing this lesson, you will be able to:

✔ Key SOAP notes in the correct format.
✔ Define SOAP notes.

The letters of the acronym SOAP come from the following words. *S* is from *subject:* what the patient is complaining about. *O* is from *objective:* this states the physician's diagnosis. *A* is from *assessment:* the physician's assessment of the patient's current condition (this sometimes includes past medical history information). *P* is from *plan:* how the physician decides to manage the patient's care.

Insert those abbreviations vertically.

S:

O:

A:

P:

SOAP notes include the patient's name, the medical record number, the date of the examination, each of the SOAP categories, the doctor's name, the reference initials, and the D: and T: lines.

The words of the categories may be spelled out or not. Type the patient's name, medical record number, and the date on one line. Double-space and begin typing the SOAP categories, double-spacing between each. Leave four spaces to the physician's signature line, and double-space to the final three lines. Leave two spaces after the colon.

Instructions

Key the SOAP notes in the correct format on page 358. Study and key the sample SOAP note.

FIVE-MINUTE TIMING—DOUBLE SPACE

```
        The patient is a 65-year-old Caucasian female with severe    12
chronic arthritis admitted from home with a right lobar             23
pneumonia and dehydration.  The patient suffered a cardiac          34
arrest early this morning and was resuscitated successfully.        45
She was placed on the respirator, and her blood pressure has        57
been maintained on high amounts of dopamine and Isuprel.  The       69
patient has no significant cardiac history according to the         80
medical records.  She has had transient ischemic attacks in         91
the past.  She had a history of moderately severe rheumatoid       103
arthritis and degenerative arthritis.                              110
```
□□□□1□□□□2□□□□3□□□□4□□□□5□□□□6□□□□7□□□□8□□□□9□□□□10□□□□11□□□□12

Key the following SOAP note in correct format. Proofread your copy and correct errors.

SOAP NOTES 1 SAMPLE

```
Patient Name: Pap, Mary
DS
Medical Record No.: 78
DS
Date:  03/23/200__
DS
S:  She comes in for a routine examination. She had been placed on
    Megace 40 mg three times a day. She complains of gaining
    weight on Megace.
    DS
O:  BREASTS: No masses or tenderness.
    DS
    ABDOMEN: Soft and nontender.
    DS
    PELVIC EXAM: Within normal limits. Uterus slightly enlarged.
DS
A:  1. History of endometrial hyperplasia.
    SS
    2. Fibroid of uterus, asymptomatic at the current time.
    SS
P:  1. Pap test.
    SS
    2. Routine screening mammogram performed.
    TS
    _____
SS
Henry Algia, MD
DS
HA:ES
SS
D:03/23/200__
SS
T:03/24/200__
```

Instructions

Study the sample, then key. Proofread your copy and correct errors.

```
Laser, Jessica                                                    3
Medical Record No. 54                                            7
09/05/200__                                                      9
SS
SUBJECTIVE                                                       11
The patient comes in for a routine examination complaining of   22
a sore throat and sneezing for several days.                    31
SS
OBJECTIVE                                                        33
BREASTS: No mass or tenderness. ABDOMEN: Soft and nontender.    44
PELVIC EXAM: Within normal limits.                              51
SS
ASSESSMENT                                                      53
1. History of squamous atypia, now resolved.                   61
2. Premenopausal.                                              64
SS
PLAN                                                            65
Pap smear and mammogram.                                       70
SS


_____

Shirley Lamb, MD                                               73
RL:JA/D:09/05/200__/T:09/06/200__                             80
```
□□□□1 □□□□2 □□□□3 □□□□4 □□□□5 □□□□6 □□□□7 □□□□8 □□□□9 □□□□10 □□□□11 □□□□12

CHART NOTES

Goals

After completing this lesson, you will be able to:

✔ Key chart notes.

Chart notes are also called progress notes. Chart notes are written by the physician or other personnel on all patients who come to the office. Even telephone calls are recorded on chart notes. The style and content vary widely.

Chart notes are keyed so that they are easy to read. Chart notes include the patient's name, date, medical record number, diagnosis, physician's signature, and reference initials. "D:" means dictated and is followed by the date; "T:" means transcribed and is also followed by the date. Chart notes may be typed on a plain sheet of paper, on lined paper, or on preprinted forms. Chart notes are keyed single-spaced.

Instructions

Key the following chart notes in the correct format. Study and key the example first. Proofread your copy and correct errors.

CHART NOTES 1 EXAMPLE

```
Shirley Anterior, Medical No.: 48, August 9, 200__          10

This 57-year-old female is in excellent spirits. She had a    21
laminectomy several days ago. The CT scan report revealed     32
evidence of a disc herniation in the nerve root. Lumbar spine 43
at L4-L5 appears normal. Blood pressure: 120/80. Weight: 72 kg. 55



_____

Shana Diplopia, MD                                           58

SD:EJ                                                        59
D:08/08/200__                                               61
T:09/09/200__                                               63
```

Instructions

Key the following chart notes. Study the sample first. Proofread your copy and correct errors.

CHART NOTES 2

```
Homer Chest Medical Record No. 47 July 5, 200__             10

This patient came to the clinic today for a checkup. Previous 21
records were reviewed with him. Blood chemistries were normal. 32
Cholesterol is 190. Electrocardiogram shows no significant   43
changes. The test for AIDS was negative.                     51

Chest x-ray showed that fluid on left side of the heart has  62
resolved. Prostatic specific antigen was normal at 1.5.      73



_____

John Megaly, MD                                              76

JM:ej                                                       77
D:06/07/200__                                               79
T:06/10/200__                                               81
```
□□□□1□□□□2□□□□3□□□□4□□□□5□□□□6□□□□7□□□□8□□□□9□□□□10□□□□11□□□□12

Study the sample first, then key. Key the following SOAP notes. Proofread your copy and correct errors.

SOAP NOTE 3

Mary Bone, Medical No: 55, October 1, 200__		9
S:	She is here to review blood test results; generally feels	21
	tired all the time, is having intermittent symptoms of	32
	crying spells.	35
O:	Exam revealed blood tests were completely nonfocal and	46
	unremarkable.	49
A:	Separation anxiety, depression, and fatigue.	58
P:	Trial of Paxil 20 mg q.d. Risks and benefits and	68
	alternatives to treatments discussed with the patient.	79
	Additional home care is outlined; follow up in two to	90
	four weeks or p.r.n. symptoms.	97

_____

Henry J. Algia, MD/HA:ES/D:10/03/200__/T:10/04/200__	108

SOAP NOTE 4

Mary Bone, Medical No.: 55, October 9, 200__		9
S:	She complains of sharp pain in the lower back and right	20
	flank. She also has complained of urinary incontinence,	31
	primarily with coughing or sneezing. The patient relates	42
	that she has been having difficulty with this at her	53
	karate class.	56
O:	Examination shows palpatory tenderness in the paravertebral	68
	musculature, right side greater than left of the lower	79
	lumbar spine. She also has some flank tenderness. SLR	90
	however, is negative. DTR are symmetric. Urinalysis shows	102
	1 to 3 WBCs and RBCs and trace bacteriuria.	111
A:	Thoracolumbar strain and mild urinary tract infection.	122
P:	Septra DS 1 p.o. b.i.d., Soma compound, 1 q6h p.r.n. pain	134
	and spasm. Additional home care is outlined for the	145
	patient. I have asked the patient to follow up for	156
	complete physical to further evaluate her incontinence.	167

_____

Henry J. Algia, MD/HA:ES/D:10/08/200__/T:10/10/200__	178

□□□□1□□□□2□□□□3□□□□4□□□□5□□□□6□□□□7□□□□8□□□□9□□□□10□□□□11□□□□12

Key the following progress report in block format. Proofread your document and correct errors.

PROGRESS RECORD 2

```
Date: November 4, 200__                                    4
Colon, Sara                                               6
MR No.: 49-A                                              8
Chris Lipoma, MD                                         11
DS

This is a 42-year-old, African-American female, previously    22
seen August 10. Please see dictated note from that date for   33
further information. In the interim, she followed up with Dr.  44
Blue at Mobile Hospital for a recheck regarding a benign       55
adenomatous polyp found on colonoscopy in July, 200__.        65
Apparently Dr. Blue performed a flexible sigmoidoscopy on      76
October 10, 200__ which apparently revealed another polyp. It  88
was not removed at that time and she was told that she would   99
need a full colonoscopy. She presents here for a second       110
opinion. She has tolerated the Metamucil taking it twice a    121
day, once after breakfast and once before bedtime, without any 133
further problems with her hemorrhoids.                        140

DS


She also underwent breast, pelvic, and Pap smear examinations  151
with Dr. Cyte in October. She has not yet received a postcard  162
regarding her Pap smear. Dr. Cyte apparently discussed        172
hormonal therapy with the patient and instructed her that if  183
she starts noticing her periods getting longer in duration    194
associated with menopause symptoms to return for consideration 205
of hormonal replacement therapy. He has scheduled her for a   216
mammogram this month.                                         220
DS

MEDICATIONS: Metamucil 1 packet twice a day.                  229
DS

ALLERGIES: None known to medications.                         236
DS

PHYSICAL EXAMINATION: Deferred.                               242
DS

IMPRESSION: 1. History of benign adenomatous polyp on         252
               colonoscopy in July, 200__ with polyp found on 263
               flexible sigmoidoscopy in October 200__. We    274
               will obtain the records from Dr. Blue regarding 286
               the nature of this polyp. She agrees to proceed 298
               with colonoscopy, but she wishes to have this   309
               procedure done here at Memorial Hospital.      319
```

□□□□1□□□□2□□□□3□□□□4□□□□5□□□□6□□□□7□□□□8□□□□9□□□□10□□□□11□□□□12

                    2. External hemorrhoids, improved. She has   329
                       tolerated the Metamucil well as noted above and 340
                       will continue with this fiber supplement.   351

         DS
         She will follow up with me in January for evaluation of the   362
         above problem or sooner if problems arise in the interim.   373

                                              _____

                                              Chris Lipoma, MD/   384
                                              CL:MB/D: 11/04/200__   396
                                              T: 11/05/200__   407

CHART NOTE: 3

         March 10, 2002 - Patient: Smear Jana, ID 56789   9

         Jana comes for a routine examination. She is currently having 21
         no problems and had decided not to use hormone replacement   32
         therapy. Her last Pap smear was performed April 2001 and was   43
         negative. She has no complaints at the current time. Review of 55
         systems negative. Examination: Breasts and axillae negative.   66
         Neck without thyromegaly. Abdomen soft and nontender. Pelvic   77
         exam: External genitalia, the vagina, and cervix normal. Uterus 89
         small, nontender. Adnexa negative. Rectovaginal examination   100
         negative. Guaiac negative. Impression: Normal examination.   111
         Plan: Pap smear, mammogram.   116

         _____

         Jodie Guaiac, MD/JG:MP/D:03/11/02/T:03/11/02   125

SOAP NOTE 5

Instructions

         Study the sample SOAP note first before keying. Proofread your document and correct errors.

         Pap, Mary/Medical Record No.: 45/09/09/200__   9

         SUBJECTIVE: Mary was seen today with complaints of fatigue,   20
         intermittent mid-cycle spotting, and change in her periods.   31
         She had menarche at age 10. She relates that her mother went   42
         through menopause at a very early age. OBJECTIVE: Examination   53
         is limited to the abdomen and showed soft abdomen with   64
         diffuse suprapubic tenderness. Pelvic examination will be   75
         deferred to the patient's annual physical scheduled next week. 87
         Today, I will have her get a CBC, SMAC, FSH, and thyroid   98
         function tests. ASSESSMENT: Menopausal symptoms. PLAN: 108
         Comprehensive physical examination.   115

         _____

         Shirley Lamb, MD/RL:PM:/D:09/10/200__/T:09/10/200__   125

         □□□□1□□□□2□□□□3□□□□4□□□□5□□□□6□□□□7□□□□8□□□□9□□□□10□□□□11□□□□12

Key the following chart note. Proofread your document and correct errors.

PROGRESS RECORD —MOBILE CLINIC NOTE 3

```
Julie Face/07/17/200__/Medical Record No.: 7788          10
MEDICAL HISTORY: The patient is a 40-year-old lady who comes  21
in for a checkup. The patient has no new complaints at this  32
time. She continues to take Prilosec for some reflux symptoms  43
for which I had evaluated her previously. A few weeks ago, she  55
switched from Metamucil to Citrucel, and that seemed to      65
alleviate some of her gastrointestinal symptoms. She has not  76
been having any other reflux recently. PAST MEDICAL HISTORY:  87
Otherwise unremarkable. She does have a history of colon     98
polyps. She does continue to have sporadic periods, last one  109
was in May. She has never experienced hot flashes or other   120
significant signs of menopause. SOCIAL HISTORY: She is an    131
attorney. PHYSICAL EXAMINATION: VITAL SIGNS: Stable, blood   142
pressure 110/74, pulse 60. NECK: Supple with no thyroid      153
enlargement or masses. LUNGS: Clear to auscultation          163
bilaterally. CARDIAC: Regular rate and rhythm with no murmurs  174
or gallops. ABDOMEN: Soft, nontender, active bowel sounds.   185
EXTREMITIES: Warm and dry with no peripheral edema or joint  196
deformities. SKIN: No significant lesions noted. ASSESSMENT &  207
PLAN: 1. HISTORY OF PREVIOUS GASTROESOPHAGEAL REFLUX DISEASE.  218
She is currently doing well with no symptoms. I gave her a   229
prescription for Tagamet 400 mg b.i.d. p.r.n. 2. ROUTINE     240
HEALTH MAINTENANCE: She is, otherwise, current on her Pap    251
smear and mammogram, and I will have her obtain some routine  262
screening labs today, including a lipid panel and glucose. I  273
also discussed with her obtaining a baseline bone density    284
study, which she is agreeable to, so I will give her a referral  296
to see Dr. Bone. 3. The patient will follow up with me in one  307
year. or p.r.n.                                              310


Lillie Oral, MD,/LO:FC/D:07/18/200__/T:07/18/200__          320
□□□□1□□□□2□□□□3□□□□4□□□□5□□□□6□□□□7□□□□8□□□□9□□□□10□□□□11□□□□12
```

Worker's Compensation Letters, Five-Minute Timed Writing

Goals

After completing this lesson, you will be able to:

✔ Key worker's compensation letters.

Worker's Compensation letters are for employees who are injured on the job.

Instructions

Key the following letters in block format. Use 1-inch margins. Proofread your document and correct errors. Use "(continued)" if there is more than one page.

WORKER'S COMPENSATION LETTER 1

```
Charles Sole, MD                                              3
5345 Lobe Street                                             6
Mobile, AZ 62034-6203                                       10
605-279-2211  FAX 605-279-2222                              16
DS

November 21, 200__                                          20
DS

Mr. Nash Thumb                                              23
BUN Insurance Company                                       27
940 Nitrogen Lane                                           30
Mobile, AZ 62222-6204                                       34
DS

RE: Injured: Calvin J. Mellitus                            40
Date of Injury: October 20, 2000                           46
Employer: Mobile Chemical                                  51
File No.: 530I                                              54
DS

Dear Mr. Thumb:                                            57
DS

HISTORY OF PRESENT ILLNESS: This is a 30-year-old male who  68
sustained an industrial injury to his left knee on October 20,  79
200__. He had pain, locking, and swelling in his knee which  90
caused him to fall to the floor. Treatment consists of physical 112
therapy and an anti-inflammatory medication. His symptoms are 123
not improving. He will undergo diagnostic arthroscopy.      133
DS

(cntinued)
```

▯▯▯▯1▯▯▯▯2▯▯▯▯3▯▯▯▯4▯▯▯▯5▯▯▯▯6▯▯▯▯7▯▯▯▯8▯▯▯▯9▯▯▯▯10▯▯▯▯11▯▯▯▯12

PAST MEDICAL HISTORY: None.   138
SS

ALLERGIES: NONE.   141
SS

MEDICATIONS: Naprosyn as needed.   147
SS

PAST SURGICAL HISTORY: None.   152
DS

FAMILY HISTORY: His father and mother are in excellent health. 163
SS

SOCIAL HISTORY: The patient is single and employed as an   174
electrical engineer. He had played golf and tennis twice a   185
week.   186
SS

REVIEW OF SYSTEMS: Healthy-appearing male who is afebrile.   197
Pulse: 90 and regular. Blood pressure: 120/80. Respiratory   208
rate: 17. HEENT: Unremarkable. Neck: Carotids are normal.   219
Lungs: Clear. Heart: Regular rate and rhythm without murmurs. 230
Abdomen: No masses.   234
SS

ORTHOPEDIC EXAMINATION: Patient walks with one crutch. He has 245
swelling in the left knee. He has an effusion with redness on 256
the knee. He has tenderness over the lateral joint line.   267
SS

X-RAYS: X-rays for the knee show an effusion.   276
SS

IMPRESSION: This knee injury is intra-articular. Arthroscopy 287
of the left knee is recommended. He understands there are   298
risks which include bleeding, infection, stiffness in the knee, 310
vein thrombosis, and failure to relieve pain. He wishes to   321
proceed with surgery.   325
Sincerely,   327
QS

Charles Sole, MD   330
Orthopedic Surgeon   333
CS:em   334
☐☐☐☐1☐☐☐☐2☐☐☐☐3☐☐☐☐4☐☐☐☐5☐☐☐☐6☐☐☐☐7☐☐☐☐8☐☐☐☐9☐☐☐☐10☐☐☐☐11☐☐☐12

Key the following letter in block format. Study the example first on page 365. Proofread your document and correct errors.

WORKER'S COMPENSATION LETTER 2

```
Andrew Disc, MD                                          3
3040 Palsy Lane                                          6
Mobile, AZ 72000-7200                                   10
605-299-0000 FAX 605-299-0000                           16
SS
August 10, 200__                                        19
SS
Mrs. Minnie Joint                                       22
MRI Insurance Company                                   26
320 Bicep Drive                                         29
Mobile, AZ 62030-6200                                   33
SS
RE: Injured: Lorene Membrane                            39
Employer: Heart Supply                                  43
Date of Injury: 05/05/200__                             48
File No.: 4780Z                                         51
Dear Mrs. Joint:                                        54
DS
HISTORY: Mrs. Lorene Membrane, a 32-year-old white female,    65
sustained injury to her fingers and wrist on May 5, XXXX. She 76
was evaluated today for numbness in her right fingers and     87
swollen right wrist. She is permanent and stationary and      97
medical care is necessary. The patient has problems in the   108
right upper extremity of her fingers, wrist, right arm, and  119
nerve compression in the hand. She is being treated with anti-131
inflammatory medication and splints. Surgery is a possibility.143
The patient continues to have problems with the metacarpal   154
joint. Surgery performed on her left wrist has worked out    165
quite well. She complains of wrist swelling, numbness, and   176
weakness of the right thumb.                                 181
DS
PHYSICAL EXAMINATION: The patient's strength in her right    192
wrist and fingers is weak. The patient's left wrist is well  203
healed. There is tenderness in the right wrist and metacarpal 214
joints. The right upper extremity of her wrist is swollen. Her 226
nerve is tender at the elbow. There is no dislocation, but   237
there is muscle atrophy in the wrist.                        244
DS
X-RAYS: The x-rays show a fusion in the wrist joint. There   255
are 6 screws that are fused in her wrist. X-ray revealed loss 266
of motion in the right wrist which is tender.                275
DS
(continued)
□□□□1□□□□2□□□□3□□□□4□□□□5□□□□6□□□□7□□□□8□□□□9□□□□10□□□□11□□□□12
```

ASSESSMENT: The patient is permanent and stationary. She is an 287
injured worker and cannot return to her previous occupation. 298
The patient cannot do repetitive work with both hands. Her 309
grip is not strong. I recommend no heavy lifting over five 320
pounds and vocational rehabilitation training. 329
DS

Sincerely,/Andrew Disc, MD/Orthopedic Surgeon 338
          AD:EJ 341

FIVE-MINUTE TIMING—DOUBLE SPACE

The physical examination revealed a well-developed, well- 12
nourished white female in no acute distress. I attempted to 23
get her to remember objects after 4 minutes, but she could 34
not retain any information for longer than the initial 44
repetition. She was able to name simple objects, such as a 55
watch and a book. 58
Her head and neck revealed no evidence of trauma. The 69
patient denies headaches. Cranial nerves II-XII were normal. 81
Motor examination revealed good grip strength and normal 92
finger-to-nose in the upper extremities; rapid alternate 103
movement was also within normal limits. Deep tendon reflexes 115
are physiological but feet withdrew markedly from plantar 126
stimulation. Sensory examination is normal to light touch, 137
pin, vibration, but double simultaneous stimulation was 148
impossible to assess. 152
The patient appears to have advanced dementia probably 163
of the Alzheimer type. Apparently, this patient was totally 174
independent, able to care for herself, and lived in Utah 185
until December when she suffered a heart attack. 194
On discharge from the hospital, she was independent and 205
arrived in Scottsdale in January. She was intermittently 216
confused but seemed to be able to carry on a conversation and 228
converse with neighbors, although her daughter wonders 239
whether she actually knew the date. 246
The patient, on the morning she broke her arm, was 257
leaning against her walker and fell on the floor. Attempts 268
to keep her in bed after her arm injury were impossible 279
because she was very agitated. She has been disoriented, and 291
this is clearly a distinct change. I recommend that we 302
proceed with a workup for causes of her dementia. Appropriate 314
orders have been initiated. 319
□□□□1□□□□2□□□□3□□□□4□□□□5□□□□6□□□□7□□□□8□□□□9□□□□10□□□□11□□□□12

Marketing Your Skills

Know Your Skills, Five-Minute Timed Writing

Goals

After completing this lesson, you will be able to:

✔ Recognize and list your skills.

Skills are abilities learned via coursework or other instruction. Skills are often listed in a résumé and sometimes used in job applications.

Instructions

Key the following skills list then think about your own skills and create a similarly formatted list. Proofread your document and correct all errors.

Skills List

1. Medical Keyboarding 72/0 wpm
2. Medical Billing
3. Medical Terminology
4. Anatomy and Physiology
5. Business Communication
6. Medical Transcription
7. Ten-Key by Touch
8. Word Software
9. Proofreading
10. Electronic Medical Record System
11. Organizational Skills
12. Biology
13. Medical Ethics
14. Medical Record Coder
15. 3M Coding Software

Common Interview Questions

1. Tell me about yourself.
2. What did you like least about your last place of employment?
3. What is your strength?
4. What is your weakness?
5. When were you employed last?
6. What kind of people do you enjoy working with?
7. What skills do you have for this position?
8. Will you be able to be on time for work?
9. What is your salary range for this position?
10. Do you plan to further your education?

Questions That Cannot Be Legally Asked

1. How old are you?
2. Are you married?
3. What is your religious status?
4. Do you have children?
5. How many children do you have?
6. What is the status of your health?

Obtain a List of References for Employment from the:

1. Teacher
2. Externship Supervisor
3. Employer

FIVE-MINUTE TIMING—DOUBLE SPACE

```
        On physical examination, the patient is a well-developed,     12
adequately nourished, elderly female who is presently in no           23
acute distress.  The patient has a hacking cough that is not          34
productive of mucus.  The sclerae are clear.  The conjunctivae        46
are perfused.  The patient wears thick glasses, but iridecto-         57
mies are not evident.  The pupils are equal, round, and               68
reactive to light.  Head, eyes, ears, nose, and throat are            79
otherwise negative.  The nasal passages are patent.  The              90
patient is edentulous.  There is a weak gag reflex bilaterally.      102
There is drooping and weakness of the left side of the mouth.        113
In attempting to protrude her tongue, the tongue deviates to         124
the left side of her mouth.  Carotid bruits are not heard on         135
auscultation.  There are no palpable neck masses.  The patient       147
is unable to sit up by herself.                                      153
        Examination of the chest is remarkable for rales and         164
rhonchi at the right lung base.  The left lung is clear.  The        175
heart sounds are heard at the lower left sternal border where        186
there is a grade II-VI systolic ejection type of murmur.  The        197
abdomen is soft, slightly protuberant, and nontender to palpa-       209
tion.  There are healed surgical incisions of the abdomen.           220
The peripheral pulses are in a symmetrical fashion, although         231
slightly diminished.  There is a trace of pitting edema of           242
the ankle bilaterally.  Gram stain of the sputum shows gram-         253
positive cocci in clusters, yeast, inflammatory cells.  Sodium,      265
potassium, and BUN are normal.                                       271
        The patient has been placed on intravenous hydration.        282
Ampicillin has been initiated on the gram-positive organisms         293
noted on the sputum culture.  It would be good to keep the           304
patient's head higher than her stomach in case she is                314
experiencing gastroesophageal reflux.                                321
```

□□□□1□□□□2□□□□3□□□□4□□□□5□□□□6□□□□7□□□□8□□□□9□□□□10□□□□11□□□□12

Job Application, Five-Minute Timed Writing

Goals

After completing this lesson, you will be able to:

✔ Complete a job application.

Answer every question on the application. Do not leave questions unanswered; use N/A (means "not applicable") if the question does not apply to you. Key the application or print legibly. Use black ink. Proofread the application carefully and correct all errors.

Instructions

Complete the following application.

JOB APPLICATION

<u>Application for Employment</u>

Answer every question. (write legibly)

Name of position for which you are applying: _____ Date ____

1. Print name in full   2. Social Security # _____

Last name   First name   Middle name

3. Home Phone   Message Phone

4. Address   City   State   Zip Code

<u>Circle Yes or No</u>

5. Will you accept part-time work?   Yes   No

6. Will you accept full-time work?   Yes   No

7. Education: Circle last grade completed: 1 2 3 4 5 6 7 8 9 10 11 12

High School: _____ Did you graduate? _____

Address   City   State

                                        Years
8. Jr. College _____ Major   Completed Degrees

College or _____ _____ _____ _____

University _____ _____ _____ _____
            Address   City   State

Technical _____ Currently taking courses   Circle
                                                        Yes or No

                                                        Yes   No

Vocational _____

School   Address   City   State

Other experience or training. Include other information on
education programs

School _____ Course _____

Degrees or Certificate _____

School _____ Course _____

Degrees or Certificate _____

9. Do you have any physical condition(s) which may limit your
ability to perform the jobs for which you have applied?   No   Yes
If yes, explain:
_____

_____

10. Person to notify in case of an emergency

_____
Name

_____
Address   City   State

_____
(Area Code) Telephone

11. Skills, talents, volunteer work
Tell us about yourself. What is your occupational goal? What
skills or talents do you have?
_____

_____

_____

_____

Employment Record

12. List the most recent employment first. Include any volunteer experience that relates to the job for which you are applying.

Dates   Employers   Duties

From (Mo. & Yr.)   Name of Employer   Your title _____

To (Mo. & Yr.)   _____   Duties _____

_____   _____

Total months   Address   _____

worked _____   _____   _____

                    City   State   Zip

Hours per   _____   _____

week _____   Supervisor's Name   Reason for leaving

From (Mo. & Yr.)   Name of Employer   Your title _____

To (Mo. & Yr.)   _____   Duties _____

_____   _____

Total months   Address   _____

worked _____   _____   _____

                    City   State   Zip

Hours per   _____   _____

week _____   Supervisor's Name   Reason for leaving

From (Mo. & Yr.)   Name of Employer   Your title _____

To (Mo. & Yr.)   _____   Duties _____

_____   _____

Total months   Address   _____

worked _____   _____   _____

                    City   State   Zip

Hours per   _____   _____

week _____   Supervisor's Name   Reason for leaving

Signature _____ Date _____

I understand that any false statements on this application are cause for refusal of employment or termination of employment if already employed.

        I have been asked to evaluate this 90-year-old woman who   12
was admitted to the hospital for insertion of a Rush rod   23
because of a fractured humerus. Review of the patient's   34
history and physical examination indicates the patient moved   45
to Arizona from Florida three months ago. It became apparent   57
to the family that she required care, and she has been having   69
trouble walking. There is also note of a myocardial infarc-   80
tion in December, although there is also reference to a   91
seizure. The patient has had her arm fixed, and it has been   102
determined that she will require nursing home placement. She   114
is unable to give meaningful information and is quite dis-   125
oriented and believes she is still in Florida. I have   135
attempted to call the family for other history of her past   146
medical evaluations, particularly as regards to dementia, but   158
I am not able to get through at this time and will try again.   170
        The patient is somewhat suspicious and believes that the   182
staff thinks she is crazy. She would like to go home. When   193
asked where that home would be, she indicates, "Where do you   204
think? My home is in Florida."   210
        Review of the admission chemistry panel and hematological 222
profile is normal. Albumin is low, suggesting inadequate   233
nutrition. BUN is normal. The patient's chest x-ray showed   244
hypoventilation without evidence of congestive heart failure,   256
and the EKG does not reveal evidence of myocardial infarction.   268
        Review of the nursing notes indicates that the patient is 280
completely disoriented. She is incontinent of urine.   290
☐☐☐☐1☐☐☐☐2☐☐☐☐3☐☐☐☐4☐☐☐☐5☐☐☐☐6☐☐☐☐7☐☐☐☐8☐☐☐☐9☐☐☐☐10☐☐☐☐11☐☐☐☐12

Résumé Outline and Résumé, Five-Minute Timed Writing

Goals

After completing this lesson, you will be able to:

✔ Key a résumé outline.
✔ Key a résumé.

The résumé outline is written to prepare information for writing the résumé. A résumé is used to obtain a job interview. The job objective is a statement about the job you are seeking. A résumé is written for each job objective. Résumés are written in many different styles and formats; to explore further, check your library or bookstore.

Instructions

Key the résumé outline using the skills you have identified. Then, key the résumé following. Finally, write and key a résumé of your own. Proofread your document and correct errors.

RÉSUMÉ OUTLINE

1. Personal Information
   A. Your name
   B. Address
   C. City, State, and Zip Code information
   D. Area code and telephone number
2. Job Objective
   A. Name your job objective. For example, to obtain a position as a medical keyboarding secretary
3. Education
   A. Name of school attended
   B. Date of attendance
   C. Location of school
4. Work Experience
   A. Name of company
   B. Job title
   C. Work responsibilities
   D. Dates of employment
5. Membership

  A. Names of professional organizations

6. Honors

  A. List grade point average at graduation

  B. Certificates

  C. Achievement awards.

7. Special Skills

  A. Name special skills

8. References

  A. Names of three references

<u>Dorothy Scan</u>
2409 Cell Street
Mobile, AZ 62011-2204
602-291-0000
FAX: 602-111-1111

<u>JOB OBJECTIVE:</u> A position as a Medical Coder/Analyst that will utilize my skills and offer opportunities and growth.

<u>EDUCATION:</u> <u>2003-Present Mobile College, Mobile, AZ</u>
COURSES:

Medical Keyboarding 1 & 2	Medical Terminology
Business English 1, 2, 3	Medical Insurance
Business Math	Medical Transcription
Pharmacology	Anatomy
Biology	Word Processing 1, 2, 3
Medical Coding 1, 2	Health Information Technology

<u>1989-1993 Nelson High School, Mobile, AZ</u>
COURSES:

Keyboarding 1 & 2	Speed and Accuracy
English 1 & 2	Math
Public Speaking	Biology
Lotus 1-2-3	Word Processing 1 & 2
Chemistry	Algebra 1

<u>EXPERIENCE:</u> 1989-Present, MRI Clinic, Mobile, AZ
Receptionist. Answer telephone, schedule patients' appointments, wordprocess correspondence.

<u>INTERNSHIP:</u> 120 Hours, Urgent Care Clinic, Mobile, AZ
Medical Coder/Analyst

<u>HONORS:</u> Certificate of Appreciation—Radiology Division
Keyboarding Certificate 72/0 wpm

<u>SPECIAL SKILLS:</u> Excellent speller, organized, self-motivator, attentive to detail, patient, and work well with people.

<u>CONTINUING EDUCATION:</u> Health Insurance Portability Accountability Act (HIPAA)

The patient is a 40-year-old Latino female with palpa- 11
tions, nausea, and weakness. The patient was noted to be in 22
a supraventricular tachycardia when placed on the monitor in 33
the emergency department. The rhythm slowed to atrial 43
fibrillation when she was given intravenous digoxin and 54
verapamil. A heart murmur was noted at that time, and the 65
patient gives a history of having this heart murmur since her 76
teens. Her physical examination revealed a grade III harsh 87
systolic ejection murmur, heard in the base, radiating up 98
the left sternal border to the apex and also up into the neck. 110
Her EKG revealed atrial fibrillation with an increased 121
ventricular response. Her chest x-ray revealed borderline 132
cardiomegaly. 134

The patient was admitted to the intensive care unit for 145
observation and monitoring. A repeat dose of digoxin intra- 156
venously converted the patient back to a normal sinus rhythm. 168
Echocardiogram revealed a noncritical aortic stenosis. The 179
patient has done well since her hospitalization. She was 190
transferred to the telemetry unit for progressive ambulation. 202

The patient is discharged to home and will be followed 213
by her physician in Arkansas. 219

□□□□1□□□□2□□□□3□□□□4□□□□5□□□□6□□□□7□□□□8□□□□9□□□□10□□□□11□□□□12

Curriculum Vitae, Five-Minute Timed Writing

Goals

After completing this lesson, you will be able to:

✔ Key a curriculum vitae.

A curriculum vitae is a summary of qualifications submitted for physicians and academic personnel. The curriculum vitae can be several pages in length.

Instructions

Key the following curriculum vitae. The headings should be keyed in uppercase letters. Begin keying 1.5 inches from the top of the paper. Use 1-inch margins. Center the title "curriculum vitae" keyed in uppercase letters. Double-space between the headings. Single-space within each section. Proofread your document and correct errors.

CURRICULUM VITAE
Matthew T. Cardia, MD

BUSINESS ADDRESS	3409 Cactus Drive Mobile, AZ 62011-6203
TELEPHONE	602-279-0000, FAX 602-279-0001
EDUCATION 1960 1965	University of California, San Diego, CA B.S. in Chemistry McGill University, Montreal, Canada M.D. Degree
RESIDENCY 1966-1970	Montreal General Hospital, Montreal, Canada Internal Medicine
FELLOWSHIP 1970-1971	University of Pennsylvania Gastroenterology
INTERNSHIP 1966-1970 1965-1966	Montreal General Hospital, Montreal, Canada Internal Medicine
BOARD CERTIFICATION 1971	Royal College of Physicians and Surgeons Gastroenterology
HONORS 1970	Best Resident/Intern of the Year in the emergency room, Montreal, Canada
MEDICAL LICENSURE	State of Arizona (A123456) May 1971
MEDICAL SPECIALTY 1971-Present	Gastroenterology

PROFESSIONAL AFFILIATIONS

1971-Present	Fellow, Royal College of Physicians and Surgeons
1971-Present	Member, Arizona Medical Association
1980-Present	Council of the Arizona Medical Association

STAFF APPOINTMENTS

1971-Present	Chief of Staff, Memorial Hospital, Phoenix, AZ
1971-Present	Attending Physician, Mobile Hospital, Mobile, AZ

TEACHING EXPERIENCE 1980-Present	Guest Lecturer-Gastroenterology Howard University Medical School Washington, D.C.
COMMITTEE	Chair of Bioethics Committee

This 97-year-old Caucasian female was admitted to Mobile   11
Hospital because of shortness of breath, generalized weakness,   23
chest congestion, and coughing up yellowish mucus. She had   34
not been feeling well, and has not been eating or drinking   45
water for at least two days. A chest x-ray showed a right   56
apical lung nodule.   60

Past medical history includes appendectomy, splenectomy,   71
hysterectomy, cholecystectomy, and cystocele repair. She   82
fractured her right hip four years ago and underwent surgical   93
fixation. A year ago, she had a cerebrovascular accident,   104
manifested by weakness, drooping of the mouth, and difficulty   115
forming words. She seems to understand everything said to   126
her but has difficulty expressing herself.   134

Father died from pneumonia. Mother died from ovarian   145
cancer. There is a family history of diabetes, but no history   157
of tuberculosis.   160

The patient does complain of headaches. She wears thick   172
glasses and has not had cataract surgery. The patient has   183
mouth pain and difficulty swallowing food and ambulating since   195
the cerebrovascular accident. There is no history of food   206
regurgitation or vomiting.   211

□□□□1□□□□2□□□□3□□□□4□□□□5□□□□6□□□□7□□□□8□□□□9□□□□10□□□□11□□□□12

Cover Letter, Five-Minute Timed Writing

Goals

After completing this lesson, you will be able to:

✔ Key a cover letter.

A cover letter is always sent with a résumé or application. In the first paragraph of the cover letter, name the position that you are applying for and how you heard about it. The second paragraph should summarize your background, education, training, work experience, and how your qualifications will make you the best person for the position. In the last paragraph, request an interview.

Instructions

Key the following cover letter in block format. Proofread your document and correct errors.

COVER LETTER

```
3943 Scleral Avenue                                         4
San Diego, CA 92111-6203                                    9
619-279-0000                                               11
Current date                                               14

Jane A. Cortex, MD                                         17
Health Care Foundation Center                              23
3940 Buccal Avenue                                         26
San Diego, CA 92111-6100                                   31

Dear Dr. Cortex:                                           34

I have the necessary education and skills to qualify me for    45
the Medical Coder/Analyst position advertised in the Star on   56
July 2, 200__.                                             59

My training, education, internship, and work experience have   70
given me the qualifications to succeed with the Health Care    81
Foundation Center as a Medical Coder/Analyst.              90
Skills that I have obtained are: medical keyboarding at 72/0   101
wpm, medical terminology, medical insurance, business      111
communication, medical transcription, medical coding,      121
proofreading, math, and word processing.                   129

Enclosed is my résumé for you to review. I will telephone you  140
soon to arrange for an interview at your convenience.       150

Sincerely yours,/Mrs. Jessica J. Costal/Enclosure          160
```

☐☐☐☐1☐☐☐☐2☐☐☐☐3☐☐☐☐4☐☐☐☐5☐☐☐☐6☐☐☐☐7☐☐☐☐8☐☐☐☐9☐☐☐☐10☐☐☐☐11☐☐☐☐12

The patient is a 65-year-old female, visiting from   11
Chicago, who was en route by train to visit her daughter in   22
Gila Bend, Arizona when she developed palpitations, weakness, 33
nausea, and vomiting. She has had these symptoms inter-   44
mittently for the past five years. The train stopped at the   55
service station and let her off. She was transported by   66
ambulance to Gila Bend Hospital emergency department where   77
she was noted to be in supraventricular tachycardia. This   88
slowed down to atrial fibrillation with a slightly increased   99
ventricular response with intravenous digoxin and Calan. The 110
patient gives a history of having rheumatic fever as a child. 121

The patient was told several years ago that she had   132
gallstones. She was seen at the Green Clinic for an inguinal 143
hernia and a hiatal hernia. She had an appendectomy at the   154
age of 10. She has had multiple ulcers of the ankles secon-   165
dary to poor circulation.   170

The patient's mother had a myocardial infarction, a   181
brother had bypass surgery, and another brother died of   192
prostate cancer.   194

The patient is presently visiting her daughter here in   205
Gila Bend. She and her husband travelled from Chicago and   216
were en route from their daughter in Buckeye to their   226
daughter in Maricopa by train. She denies drinking alcoholic 238
beverages or smoking.   242

□□□□1□□□□2□□□□3□□□□4□□□□5□□□□6□□□□7□□□□8□□□□9□□□□10□□□□11□□□□12

Thank-You Letter, Five-Minute Timed Writing

Goals

After completing this lesson, you will be able to:

✔ Key a thank-you letter.

A thank-you letter is typed after the interview. Before you leave the interview, get the name of the person who interviewed you.

The first paragraph will thank the interviewer for the interview. State the position you interviewed for. The second paragraph should show that you are interested in the position and should remind the interviewer of your qualifications. The last paragraph should show that you are willing to work for the company.

Instructions

Key the following letter in modified block format. Proofread your document and correct errors.

THANK-YOU LETTER

```
Current date                                                    3

Health Care Foundation Center                                   9
3940 Buccal Avenue                                             12
San Diego, CA 92111-6100                                       17

Dear Dr. Cortex:                                               20

Thank you for taking your valuable time to interview me on     31
Wednesday for the Medical Coder/Analyst position. The interview 42
was very informative, and I enjoyed meeting you and the staff. 53
DS

My skills and education as a Medical Coder/Analyst will be an  64
asset to your division. For the past five years I have         74
demonstrated my abilities as a competent and successful medical 86
secretary.                                                     87
DS

If hired, you will find me to be diplomatic, dependable, and   98
a competent Medical Coder/Analyst.                            104
DS

Sincerely yours,/Jessica J. Costal/3943 Scleral Avenue/San    115
Diego, CA 92111-6345/619-500-0000                             121
```

□□□□1□□□□2□□□□3□□□□4□□□□5□□□□6□□□□7□□□□8□□□□9□□□□10□□□□11□□□□12

```
      This 34-year-old female was evaluated by Dr. Gastro for      11
abdominal pain and was found to have colitis and choleli-          22
thiasis.  The pain has been primarily in the upper right           33
quadrant.                                                          35
      She was seen in consultation regarding a cholecystectomy,    47
and the pros and cons were discussed with her husband.            57
      Her past medical history includes the usual childhood       68
diseases.  No rheumatic fever.  She had a heart murmur as a        79
child. She is sensitive to codeine, which causes nausea.           90
      Previous surgery includes tonsillectomy and adenoidectomy  102
as a child, a tubal ligation, and surgery twice on the left      113
foot for warts.                                                  116
      She takes Bentyl as needed for abdominal pain.  She        127
smoked two packs of cigarettes every day, but only at work       138
because her family does not approve.  She drinks two to four     149
glasses of wine every evening.  She had hepatitis mono-          160
nucleosis last year.  She also had occasional dyspnea and        171
cough if she smokes too much.                                    177
      Her father and mother are alive and well.  No diabetes     188
or tuberculosis.  She is a thin, well-developed, alert female    200
in no distress.  Pupils are round, equal, and react to light     211
and accommodation.  Lungs are clear to auscultation and          222
percussion.  The uterus is retroflexed and slightly enlarged.   234
Rectal examination was not done because she had a sigmoid-       245
oscopy two weeks ago, which was normal.                          253
```

□□□□1□□□□2□□□□3□□□□4□□□□5□□□□6□□□□7□□□□8□□□□9□□□□10□□□□11□□□□12

Answers to Review Questions

LESSON 39

1. 22-year-old
2. 70-year-old

1. 10 1/2-year-old
2. 4 1/2-year-old
3. 8 1/2-year-old

1. 42-year-old
2. 10-year-old
3. 9 1/2-year-old

LESSON 40

1. 5 feet 4 inches
2. 5 feet 3 inches

LESSON 41

1. 220 pounds
2. 130 pounds

LESSON 42

1. 128/98
2. 124/74

LESSON 43

1. 50
2. 62

LESSON 44

1. 24
2. 40

LESSON 45

1. 100.6
2. 99.3

LESSON 46

1. 35 mL (or ml)
2. 20 ml (or mL)
3. 50 ml, 70 ml

1. 40 mg t.i.d.
2. b.i.d. 20 mg

1. 25 mEq
2. 2.8 mEq

1. 1.3 × 0.4 cm
2. 2 × 2 cm

LESSON 49

1. 5%
2. 3%
3. 0.5%

1. 1:100,000
2. 1:14
3. 1:112
4. 1:6,000

LESSON 51

1. 39-year-old
2. 130/80
3. 98.6 degrees Fahrenheit

LESSON 53

1. #2-0
2. #2, #3-0
3. #2-0

LESSON 54

1. 1:20 p.m.
2. 10 a.m.
3. 11 a.m.
4. 12:00 o'clock, 6:00 o'clock

LESSON 55

1. 2+
2. 2+
3. 2+

LESSON 56

1. January 5, 2001
2. July 5, 2003
3. August 5, 2003

1. 06 November 19XX
2. 11 November 200__
3. 12 September 200__

LESSON 57

1. 0.75%
2. 0.50%
3. 1.75%

LESSON 58

1. TP-40, Pentam 300, Theo-24, Oxy 5, Ovcon 50.
2. Demulen 1/35, D.H.E. 45
3. Humulin 70/30
4. Obetrol 20
5. VP 16

LESSON 60

1. 2.5 million
2. $3.6 million
3. $1.8 million

LESSON 61

1. thirty 2-room
2. twelve 1-cup
3. sixteen 31-year-olds
4. 210-page

1. 7 physicians, 20 pathologists
2. 50 residents, 7 interns
3. 5 drains, 17 Band-Aids, 1 package, 20 swabs
4. 5 trucks, 8 gurneys, 30 walkers, 70 crutches
5. Thirty-four surgeons, 10 residents, 3 interns, 6 externs

LESSON 62

1. 130,000s
2. 1970s, mid-1970s
3. 1960s, mid-1970s

LESSON 65

1. addiction
2. postpartum
3. coroner
4. Camalox
5. coma
6. Valium
7. gait
8. cancerous
9. lipoma
10. hirsute
11. psychosis
12. cirrhosis
13. cholectomy
14. plain
15. oral
16. Cytoxan
17. graft
18. gavage
19. Perls'
20. Ball's valve

21. moles
22. Excedrin
23. cerumen
24. pharynx
25. faint
26. vein
27. liter
28. liver
29. bruit
30. nephrosis
31. dysphagia
32. wound
33. venous
34. scar
35. sight
36. palpation
37. variceal
38. enervation
39. vesicle
40. carpal

1. agony, comfort
2. excite, calm
3. faint, revive
4. unconscious, alert
5. tell, conceal
6. strife, harmony
7. comfort, blame
8. fantasy, reality
9. gloom, joy
10. expire, live
11. feeling, apathy
12. black out, revive
13. heat, afebrile
14. sadness, joy
15. exclude, unit
16. mad, sane
17. cut, suture
18. illness, health
19. bare, clothed
20. stupid, sensitive
21. false, genuine
22. calm, lively
23. clear, turbid
24. pressing, unimportant
25. image, blindness

LESSON 66

1. postoperative
2. all right
3. calendar

4. preoperative
5. anxious
6. weak
7. somebody
8. personal
9. here
10. fewer
11. continuously
12. accepted
13. assured
14. proceed
15. effect
16. bone scan
17. herpes virus
18. bacteria
19. venipuncture, EKG
20. remission
21. dust cells
22. double vision
23. concussion
24. mouthwash
25. iliofemoral

1. ability
2. believe
3. desert
4. patient
5. neighbors
6. review
7. unfortunately
8. hospital
9. doctor
10. asthma
11. emphysema
12. heparin
13. parcel
14. xiphoid
15. callus
16. pyoderma
17. polyp
18. seize
19. relief
20. separate
21. pancreas
22. malignant
23. rely
24. expense
25. success
26. scleroderma
27. lipocyte
28. coccygeal
29. ganglion
30. thalassemia
31. edema

32. dysuria
33. postoperative
34. abscess
35. nitrogenous
36. preoperative
37. nephrosclerosis
38. hysterectomy
39. adnexa
40. areola
41. nephropathy
42. keratosis
43. pulmonary edema
44. postmature
45. fallopian tube
46. ovarian
47. purulent
48. prostate gland
49. leukocyte
50. cytotoxic cells

1. apha/sia
2. ath/er/o/ma
3. ceph/a/lal/gia
4. en/ceph/a/lo/ma
5. hy/per/eme/sis
6. deaf
7. cir/cum/scribed
8. os/si/fy
9. psy/chi/a/trist
10. gin/gi/vi/tis
11. ure/mia
12. post/par/tum
13. fe/brile
14. scle/rec/to/my
15. pre/can/cer/ous
16. ul/tra/vi/o/let
17. sym/pa/thec/to/my
18. mes/en/tery
19. eu/pho/ria
20. ova
21. ne/cro/sis
22. claus/tro/pho/bia
23. para/ne/phri/tis
24. phar/yn/gi/tis
25. irid/algia
26. plas/ma/pher/e/sis
27. bron/chi/ec/ta/sis
28. leu/ko/phe/re/sis
29. ret/ro/per/i/to/ne/al
30. ure/thri/tis

1. 2409 Fleetwood / Street
2. 2056 Bush / Avenue

3. Do not divide contractions
   Spell out. Example:
   can / not, would / not
4. Do not divide
5. Do not divide
6. Do not divide
7. Do not divide
8. Do not divide
9. Do not divide
10. Do not divide
11. Do not divide
12. Do not divide
13. Do not divide
14. Do not divide

LESSON 67

1. Foley
2. Alzheimer, Bell
3. Chamberlen
4. MRI
5. ZDV

LESSON 68

1. N. meningitidis
2. S. enteritidis
3. H. influenzae
4. M. tuberculosis

LESSON 69

1. Australian X disease
2. Roux-en-Y
3. Cytosar-U
4. Micro-K, Pen-Vee K
5. Slow-K, Vira A, Wyamine E

LESSON 70

1. Bailey-Morse
2. Bard-Parker
3. Wolf-Schindler
4. Calhoun-Merz
5. Glisson

LESSON 71

1. She is ^sick.

2. to together
3. receive
4. put on the floor
5. medications e
6. Hemoglobin
7. Her appointment is at
   2:15 p.m.
8. He is an excellent
   physician for dermatology.
9. 101° temperature
10. Goiter enlarged.
11. ¶Suture class is at 6 p.m.
12. hiv positive
13. The patient who had
    surgery is named George.
14. Please buy towels; lotion;
    and bandages.
15. The hyphen is a word-
    dividing mark.
16. He's gone.
17. You should have given this
    patient the medication!
18. Did he say, "All is well?"
19. Refer to Section 426 of the
    manual.
20. She's graduated; therefore,
    she's working now.
21. B/P
22. Proofreading—Paragraph
    Hispanic, weakness,
    dizziness, tingling,
    weakness, cleared, patient,
    trauma, chronic, migraine,
    gait, CT, spine, EEG,
    Electrolytes, TIA
23. Capitalization
    1. I, EMG
    2. Caucasian
    3. October
    4. VA Hospital, Phoenix,
       Arizona
    5. The, IV
    6. CT, Mary's
    7. Mrs. Smith, Nanci
    8. Behavioral, Dr. Moss
    9. Mobile, BUN
    10. pH

LESSON 72

1. The father has heart disease.
2. The thyroid was enlarged.

3. Child with diabetes.
4. <u>Bertie</u> takes <u>nitroglycerin daily</u>.
5. This female developed acute <u>bronchitis</u> associated with <u>dry cough</u> and <u>back pain</u>.

1. During the <u>winter</u>, <u>Ruth</u> worked on her research <u>study</u>.
2. The <u>physician</u> lectured on <u>AIDS</u> at <u>Columbia University</u>.
3. The <u>doctors</u> flew to <u>California</u> for the <u>symposium</u>.
4. <u>Kim</u> was promoted to radiology <u>secretary</u>.
5. After a <u>trip</u> to <u>Atlanta University</u>, <u>Roosevelt</u> accepted the otolaryngology residency <u>position</u>.
6. <u>Parry</u> showed his medical <u>card</u> to the <u>receptionist</u>.
7. <u>Karen</u> was admitted to <u>Mobile Medical Clinic</u> for a diagnostic <u>test</u>.
8. The temporal bone <u>class</u> will be in <u>Brown Hall</u> on Saturday <u>morning</u>.
9. This young <u>female</u> with <u>Tourette syndrome</u> was admitted today after an <u>episode</u> of hemoptysis.

1. <u>Dr. Jean Sampson</u> teaches at <u>Mobile University</u>, but <u>she</u> is a research <u>assistant</u> in the afternoon.
2. <u>Mrs. Mary Leukocyte</u> purchased a new <u>CT scan</u> for the <u>clinic</u>.
3. <u>Dr. Beach</u> recommended <u>Mary</u> because of her honesty and excellent attendance.
4. The <u>patient</u>, <u>Bob</u>, lives in <u>Yuma, Arizona</u>.
5. <u>Mrs. James Rubin</u> has a history of <u>hypertension</u> and <u>diabetes</u>.
6. <u>Mary</u> and <u>Sheree</u> went to the medical <u>library</u> on <u>Bush Street</u> in <u>San Francisco</u>.
7. The <u>secretary</u> wrote a <u>letter</u> of congratulations to the <u>president</u> of the medical society in <u>Chicago, Illinois</u>.

8. The <u>Dodson Radiology Medical Group</u> is moving to <u>Arizona</u> in the spring.
9. The <u>dietitian</u> spoke at a meeting of the <u>Red Cross</u> in <u>New York</u>.
10. <u>Dr. Frank</u> and <u>Dr. Berger</u> will join the medical <u>staff</u> for a <u>luncheon</u>.

LESSON 73

1. The patient had <u>her</u> throat sprayed with Cetacaine.
2. <u>Her</u> rugal folds were normal.
3. The physician prepared <u>his</u> manuscript on AIDS in the United States.
4. <u>We</u> prepared the patient for the endoscopy.
5. <u>Her</u> esophagus was examined, and <u>its</u> entire length was normal.
6. <u>They</u> drove the patient and <u>his</u> mother to the emergency room.
7. <u>We</u> received <u>their</u> x-rays yesterday.
8. The physician showed <u>them</u> how to administer <u>her</u> anesthetic.
9. <u>You</u> may have hemorrhoids, and <u>he</u> may recommend surgery.
10. The doctor may prescribe pain medication; <u>she</u> will instruct <u>you</u> how to care for <u>yourself</u>.

1. The <u>nurse</u> took <u>your</u> temperature to check for fever.
2. The <u>endoscope</u> was withdrawn and no abnormalities were seen.
3. <u>Her</u> <u>throat</u> is sore, and <u>she</u> feels groggy from the <u>anesthesia</u>.
4. <u>He</u> will assume <u>his</u> official duties next week.
5. <u>Antibiotics</u> are given to control a viral infection.

6. <u>She</u> canceled <u>her</u> <u>mammogram</u> appointment until next week.
7. <u>She</u> said, "<u>You</u> are at risk for <u>pneumonia</u>."
8. <u>They</u> released the <u>medical records</u> without authorization.
9. <u>Gila Clinic</u> provided many services for <u>his</u> bypass <u>operation</u>.
10. <u>We</u> reviewed <u>their</u> diagnostic <u>tests</u> and medical history.

1. us
2. her
3. you
4. me
5. her
6. I
7. him
8. them
9. them
10. me

LESSON 74

1. A myelogram <u>is</u> an x-ray of the spinal cord.
2. She <u>took</u> large doses of penicillin for infection.
3. The patient <u>was</u> distressed and febrile for several days.
4. Initial evaluation <u>revealed</u> cardiomegaly.
5. The patient's blood pressure <u>was</u> elevated, and she <u>was</u> treated with antihypertensive medication.
6. She <u>has had</u> dyspnea and migraine headaches.
7. The patient <u>underwent</u> a biopsy for a lesion that <u>was</u> removed from the left breast.
8. He <u>is</u> currently on chemotherapy.
9. Physical examination of her bladder <u>was</u> within normal limits.
10. Sally <u>will receive</u> methotrexate treatment today.

1. This <u>boy</u> <u>is</u> very quiet, but <u>he</u> <u>is</u> not depressed.
2. <u>She</u> <u>is</u> in a special education class and <u>enjoys</u> jogging and working on her computer.
3. The <u>boy</u> <u>is</u> experiencing more weakness and <u>has</u> increasing difficulty with self-feeding.
4. <u>She</u> <u>has</u> a rash on her arms and <u>is being treated</u> with Keri lotion.
5. The <u>patient</u> <u>is taking</u> no medication and <u>reports</u> occasional constipation.
6. <u>Ultrasound</u> <u>showed</u> multiple gallstones.
7. <u>Cholangiograms</u> <u>were taken</u> and no <u>cholelithiasis</u> <u>was found</u>.
8. The <u>patient</u> <u>is</u> not very cooperative in giving a history.
9. The <u>patient</u> <u>is</u> lethargic, subdued, and not delusional.
10. <u>She</u> <u>denied</u> vomiting, fever, and constipation.

1. was
2. are
3. are
4. were
5. was
6. show
7. was
8. was seen
9. have
10. were
1. fallen
2. discharged
3. placed
4. negative
5. heard

LESSON 75

1. arteriosclerotic
2. duodenal
3. intravenous
4. endoscopic
5. vaginal
6. hypertensive
7. cachectic
8. metastatic

9. congestive
10. myocardial

1. The <u>arthroscopic</u> procedure is used to diagnose <u>knee</u> problems.
2. The patient has <u>one chest</u> x-ray taken <u>last</u> Tuesday.
3. <u>Those radiology</u> books are located in the library.
4. An <u>interested</u> doctor will provide treatment for her <u>serious</u> problem.
5. <u>Several</u> residents assisted the surgeon with a <u>radial</u> keratotomy.
6. The information you requested on <u>musculofascial</u> disease can be found in the bookcase.
7. Dr. David Rad will be the <u>graduation</u> speaker for Mobile University School of Medicine.
8. All the <u>medical</u> transcriptionists met to learn about the <u>new</u> computer.
9. The patient is an <u>obese</u> female who was admitted to the hospital with <u>severe abdominal</u> pain.
10. The evaluation failed to show any evidence of a <u>malignant</u> lesion.

1. The patient was admitted with carcinoma of the brain, liver, spine, and left shoulder.
2. The ganglion is in the carotid artery.
3. The patient is suffering from encephalitis of the cerebrum.
4. After surgery, the patient's crises were depression and insomnia.
5. The physician examined his left naris and there was a tumor.
6. The delirium was caused by exhaustion.
7. The x-ray of the knee joints showed bursae.
8. The swollen left epididymis caused pain.

9. The septa of the heart cavities are blocked.
10. The left and right bronchi were found to be infected.

1. He has many ganglia in the brainstem.
2. Two ilia bones were - rayed yesterday.
3. The iris of the left eye is green.
4. The lunula of her fingernail is sore.
5. Her maxilla bone of the upper jaw was fractured in an automobile accident.
6. The meninx of the spinal cord has become inflamed.
7. His nares are filled with a discharge.
8. The patient has nephritis of the left kidney as well as hypertension.
9. Several patients have neuritis that affect the eyeball.
10. Russell Sampson, the dermatologist, plans to remove three nevi from her neck.

LESSON 76

1. The dietitian <u>carefully</u> prepared the menu for the diabetic.
2. Mrs. Weddington <u>humbly</u> accepted the award for working with disabled children.
3. The Radiology Clinic <u>quickly</u> moved to the third floor.
4. Ship the vaccine <u>immediately</u>.
5. The audit of the medical office <u>clearly</u> revealed it to be financially independent.
6. We <u>rarely</u> have time to volunteer in the pharmacy.
7. Our medical staff is working <u>efficiently</u> on the cholesterol project.
8. Please return the patients' charts <u>immediately</u>.

9. She was <u>soon</u> in satisfactory condition after the chondrectomy.
10. As you key the medical reports you must <u>carefully</u> analyze your data.

1. Her operation was successful; <u>however</u>, she will not be discharged.
2. The medical assistants' meeting was not over until 3:30 p.m.; <u>consequently</u>, we missed the demonstration.
3. You may take the book on pregnancy; <u>however</u>, please return it next week.
4. The doctor presented a lecture on anemia; <u>further</u>, she agreed to discuss it with our staff.
5. The presentation on hearing will be at 10 a.m.; <u>undoubtedly</u>, we will attend.
6. Many nurses were angry that the rules on use of radioactive materials were not being followed; <u>accordingly</u>, we will have another meeting with the technician.
7. Inoculation is ultimately far cheaper than caring for a sick child; <u>nevertheless</u>, many people cannot afford vaccinations.
8. She broke her right arm; <u>furthermore</u>, she fractured her left leg.
9. We will have to run the tests; <u>otherwise</u>, we may be sued.
10. He did not go to the physician; he went to the acupuncturist <u>instead</u>.

LESSON 77

1. Tuberculosis is not likely <u>because of</u> the negative skin test results.
2. The bleeding seems to be <u>from</u> an artery.
3. The patient needs to be examined <u>for</u> these lesions.

4. The patient had pneumonia while <u>in</u> the hospital <u>for</u> an appendectomy.
5. This patient has a history <u>of</u> locking <u>of</u> her left knee.
6. She had surgery <u>on</u> her left knee and is <u>in</u> pain.
7. He will return <u>to</u> the clinic <u>in</u> two weeks <u>for</u> evaluation <u>of</u> his hand.
8. I suspect that she will be able to work <u>within</u> six weeks <u>after</u> surgery.
9. <u>On</u> examination he was weak, and he could stand only <u>with</u> support.
10. The patient has no tenderness <u>about</u> the right wrist.

LESSON 78

1. The patient was seen for a hip problem, <u>and</u> the surgeon recommended a hip replacement.
2. Dr. Jeffey placed ventilation tubes in the ear, <u>so</u> Jerry is feeling better.
3. The diagnosis is severe otitis media, <u>yet</u> the clerk scheduled no appointment.
4. <u>Because of</u> the patient's dizziness, she has been seen by a neurologist.
5. Mary is using a nasal saline solution <u>and</u> will return to the clinic tomorrow.
6. Her left ear revealed inflammation of the tympanic membrane, <u>but</u> the ear canal is also swollen.
7. Rhinoplasty will be performed, <u>but</u> the insurance company has to give authorization before surgery.
8. <u>After</u> the patient had a chest x-ray, his blood tests came back negative.
9. <u>When</u> Charles came to the emergency room with epistaxis, thrombi were removed from his nose.

10. <u>Now that</u> he is on antibiotics, pain medications, and oxygen, the physician will see him tomorrow.

LESSON 79

1. <u>Oh</u>! I broke my arm!
2. <u>Well</u>, take the specimen to pathology immediately.
3. <u>Now</u>, your surgery is scheduled for Tuesday.
4. <u>Oh</u>, please hurry!
5. <u>Ah</u>! I understand now!
6. <u>Oh</u>, call a doctor now!
7. <u>Well</u>, you've had a remarkable recovery!
8. <u>Dear me</u>! The emergency room is on fire!
9. <u>Oh</u>, it can be done.
10. <u>Yea</u>! We won!

LESSON 80

1. confirmed,
2. indicated,
3. as you know,
4. none
5. week,

1. <u>Because he suffers from claudication, he will have an examination</u>.
2. <u>Before the patient's aneurysmectomy, he had an infection</u>.
3. <u>Return to the Trauma Service when he is stable</u>.
4. <u>Whose decision was it that he should undergo surgery?</u>
5. <u>After an injection of radiopaque substance, an x-ray is used to locate the tumor</u>.
6. <u>So that you are aware, we plan to use Haldol</u>.
7. <u>Even though Jean is under observation for a rare disorder, she's chipper</u>.
8. <u>After the experimental drug is approved, we'll prescribe it</u>.

9. <u>When this is done, let's go to lunch</u>.
10. <u>Though he had been a heavy smoker, he quit</u>.

1. After they cleared him for surgery, <u>he was taken to be shaved</u>.
2. Until the motorcycle accident, <u>he'd never sustained a fracture</u>.
3. Now that the patient has had prostate surgery, <u>he is doing well</u>.
4. If the doctor's diagnosis is atherosclerosis, <u>why won't he help her</u>?
5. Because of swollen and twisted veins in the legs, <u>she cannot walk</u>.
6. Although the patient is suffering from emotional stress, <u>she handles it well</u>.
7. Since developing pericarditis, <u>she is not feeling well</u>.
8. When the physician ordered an MRI for her heart, <u>she passed out</u>.
9. <u>The patient is having coronary bypass surgery</u> so that he can feel better.
10. <u>Sammie enjoyed jogging on the treadmill</u>, though it made her tired.

1. , and
2. , and
3. , or
4. , for
5. , but

LESSON 81

1. There were no gallstones <u>in the gallbladder</u>.
2. There are several masses <u>within the lung fields</u>.
3. She no longer had carpal tunnel syndrome <u>after the operation</u>.
4. The heart and pulmonary vessels are <u>within normal limits</u>.

5. The patient underwent removal <u>of a polyp</u> several months ago.
6. <u>After satisfactory reduction</u>, the limb was put <u>in a cast</u>.
7. He has been started <u>on</u> Demerol <u>for pain</u>.
8. The patient lives <u>at home with his daughter</u>.
9. He went into congestive heart failure <u>at the office</u>.
10. The patient had carcinoma <u>of the lungs</u> attributable to fifteen years <u>of smoking</u>.

1. George Dwon, <u>our first patient</u>, was born <u>in Mobile Hospital</u>.
2. The four patients <u>who were given blood transfusions</u> are doing fine.
3. Seven of the medical students <u>who graduated from West Bridge Academy</u> were female.
4. William Bilirubin died, twenty days <u>after his heart transplant</u>, surrounded by his family.
5. The intern <u>in the Radiology Room</u> read x-rays <u>of the spine</u>.
6. Which physician <u>of those on call</u> will be <u>in the emergency room</u> this weekend?
7. Dr. John Leuk, <u>acting as secretary</u>, answered the phone.
8. Those patients flew <u>from San Diego to New York</u> <u>for a study on AIDS</u>.
9. The patient sat, <u>looking very irritated</u>, by the nurse.
10. Bruce wanted the poster <u>about autotransfusion</u> displayed <u>across the street</u>.

LESSON 82

1. drowsiness, tremors,
2. dehydration, loss of skin turgor, sunken eyes,
3. pain, nausea,

4. Headaches, diarrhea, stomach pain, vomiting,
5. hematuria, habits,

1. The patient has been treated for a malignant tumor, and he is asymptomatic.
2. She has mononucleosis, and her baby has a sore throat.
3. Because she has a malignant tumor, she will go to the hospital.
4. This doctor, who examined him yesterday, diagnosed a Wilms tumor and hyperemesis.
5. Her moles reappeared, but she had them removed.
6. The baby, whose mother is blind, was born with hyaline membrane disease.
7. There is some fungus, but we see no evidence of pruritus.
8. Mary has rheumatoid arthritis, and her joints are inflamed and painful.
9. He had no chest pain, but his blood results are elevated.
10. The doctor ordered myelograms, and the procedure revealed pressure on the nerve and spinal cord.

1. , who graduated from Stanford University,
2. , Mary Burns,
3. , the coder,
4. , James Buccal,
5. , a research associate at Mobile Natioanl Laboratory,

LESSON 83

1. The child previously had leukemia; unfortunately, he had a relapse.
2. The medical center has offices in Phoenix, Arizona; San Diego, California; Mobile, Arizona; and Miami, Florida.
3. Dr. Holsy Sampson is an otologist; he retired in 1992.

4. Temporal bone labs were held in Chula Vista, California; Gila Bend, Arizona; Dallas, Texas; and San Diego, California.
5. Jean is transferring to the Surgery Department in San Diego; she will be a medical receptionist.
6. The Pulmonary Department has six openings for technician positions; therefore, they will be hiring six technicians.
7. The department head recommended the following: in-service training; purchase of the current procedure terminology book; and a subscription to the medical insurance newsletter.
8. The Radiology Clinic invited Dr. Charles Leuko, director of radiology; Dr. Mary Bun, president of surgery; and Dr. Jake Endo, a chemist, to attend the conference.
9. The patient was admitted to surgery; it will take two hours.
10. The physical medicine conference is at Brown Clinic; will you come?

LESSON 84

1. The medical staff meeting will be at 7:45 a.m.
2. Two patients are scheduled for lab work at 11:45 and 10:50 a.m.
3. Vital signs: Blood pressure 120/70; Weight 140; Respirations 70; Pulse 78.
4. Preoperative diagnosis: Hysterectomy and appendectomy.
5. Several residents were recommended: Mary Smith, Bob Moss, Donald Sampson, and Anita Young.
6. Grayelin Young will speak at the 6:30 p.m. meeting.

7. Two nurses attended the Oncology Meeting: Billi Jo and Janie Wing.
8. The doctor gave her diagnosis: Keloids.
9. She feels strongly about alternative medicine: it gives patients choices.
10. The patient requested only one doctor: you.

1. The progress notes are not signed; therefore, leave a note for the doctor.
2. The otorhinolaryngology residents plan to arrive at 8:15 a.m.; we intend to finish at 6:15 p.m.
3. The surgery grand rounds begin at 7:15; we should be prompt.
4. The surgeon will be completing the operation, and the anesthesiologist will administer the local anesthesia.
5. Dr. John Sully, a pediatrics professor at the University of Mobile Medical School, will speak on immunization.
6. He answered the questions; he received many responses.
7. The physician ordered the following tests: sodium, potassium, SGOT, glucose, and hemoglobin.
8. Postoperative diagnosis: Appendectomy.
9. He said the following: "She is having respiratory difficulty. She will be admitted to the clinic."
10. Allergies: none. Smoking: none. Alcohol: none.

LESSON 85

1. The patient lives on 25 Home Avenue (he's the one who's depressed).
2. The following books were sent: (1) a medical dictionary, (2) a medical typing book, and (3) a surgery book.

3. A group of physicians will be traveling to Washington (they have their tickets).
4. The patient in Room B (the one who asked for ice cream) will have surgery tomorrow.
5. The doctor subscribed to the *Radiology Journal*.
6. Read the *Work Magazine*.
7. Please return both magazines: *The Surgery Word* and *Tumor Journal*.

LESSON 86

1. The patient's doctor did not prescribe Valium.
2. The patient's daughter could not be reached by telephone.
3. This 15-year-old female patient has Tourette syndrome and was admitted to the Children's Medical Center.
4. Due to the patient's symptoms, a cholesterol test was ordered.
5. Because the patient's cholesterol had increased, he was placed on a special diet.
6. This isn't the first visit at the Children's Medical Center for the baby.
7. The baby's mother has been studied and has negative test results based upon her evaluation.
8. Mrs. Brown's father did not die of pneumonia.
9. The family history was updated with information obtained on sickle cell anemia studies in Mrs. Champion's relatives.
10. The mutation of the genes came from Mrs. Cyte's mother's side of the family.

TIMED WRITINGS PROGRESS RECORD

Page of Timed Writing	Minutes	Words per Minute	Errors	Minutes	Words per Minute	Errors	Date of Timed Writing

BIBLIOGRAPHY

Keyboarding

Mitchell, W. M., Mach, K. A., Rutkosky, N. H., & LaBarre, J. E. (1993). *Keyboarding with WordPerfect*. St. Paul, MN: Paradigm.

Peters, C. (1987). *Championship typing drills* (2nd ed.). New York: Gregg Division of McGraw-Hill.

Peters, C. (1992). *Championship keyboarding, skillbuilding, and applications*. New York: Glencoe Division of Macmillan/McGraw-Hill.

Richardson, N. K. (1959). *Type with one hand* (2nd ed.). Cincinnati, OH: South-Western.

Van Huss, S. H., Duncan, C. H., Forde, C. M., & Woo, D. L. (2000). *College keyboarding*. Cincinnati, OH: South-Western Publishing Keyboarding Course.

Merck Manual

Beers, M. H. (1999). *The Merck manual of diagnosis and therapy. Centennial edition* (17th ed.). White-house Station, NJ: Merck Research Laboratories.

Medical Terminology

Chabner, D.-A. (2001). *The language of medicine* (6th ed.). Philadelphia: W. B. Saunders.

Dirckx, J. H. (1991). *H & P: A nonphysician's guide to the medical history and physical examination*. Modesto, CA: Health Professions Institute.

Dirckx, J. H. (1991). *Laboratory medicine: Essentials of anatomic and clinical pathology*. Modesto, CA: Health Professions Institute.

Frazier, M. S., Drzymkowski, J. A., & Doty, S. J. (1996). *Essentials of human diseases and conditions*. Philadelphia: W. B. Saunders.

Jones, B. D. *Delmar's comprehensive medical terminology: A competency-based approach*. Clifton Park, NY: Delmar Cengage Learning.

Lindh, W. Q., Pooler, M., Tamparo, C., & Cerrato, J. (2002). *Delmar's comprehensive medical assisting: Administrative and clinical competencies* (2nd ed.). Clifton Park, NY: Delmar Cengage Learning.

Pyle, V. (1985). *Current medical terminology*. Modesto, CA: Prima Vera.

Sloane, S. (1991). *The medical word book* (3rd ed). Philadelphia: W. B. Saunders.

Smith, G. L., Davis, P. E., & Dennerll, J. F. (1999). *Medical terminology: A programmed text* (8th ed.). Clifton Park, NY: Delmar Cengage Learning.

Sormunen, C. (1999). *Terminology for allied health professionals*. Clifton Park, NY: Delmar Cengage Learning.

Medical Transcription

Blake, R. (1998). *Delmar's medical transcription handbook* (2nd ed.). Clifton Park, NY: Delmar Cengage Learning.

Diehl, M. O. (2002). *Medical transcription techniques and procedures* (5th ed.). Philadelphia: W. B. Saunders.

Fordney, M. T. & Diehl, M. O. (1990). *Medical transcription guide do's and don'ts*. Philadelphia: W. B. Saunders.

Maloney, F. C., & Burns, L. M. (1997). *Medical transcription and terminology: An integrated approach*. Clifton Park, NY: Delmar Cengage Learning.

Novak, M., & Ireland, P. (1999). *Hillcrest Medical Center: Beginning medical transcription course* (5th Ed.). Clifton Park, NY: Delmar Cengage Learning.

Stewart, D. L. C., & Lott, W. L. (1998). *Forrest General Medical Center advanced medical terminology and transcription* (2nd ed.). Clifton Park, NY: Delmar Cengage Learning.

Tessier, C. (1995). *The AAMT book of style for medical transcription*. Modesto, CA: American Association for Medical Transcription.

Pharmaceutical

Billups, N. F. (1993). *American drug index*. Philadelphia: J. B. Lippincott.
Physician's Desk Reference (54th ed.). (2000). Montvale, NJ: Medical Economics Data.
Rice, J. (1999). *Principles on pharmacology for medical assisting* (3rd ed.). Clifton Park, NY: Delmar Cengage Learning.

Style Manuals

American Medical Association. (1998). *Manual of style* (9th ed.). Chicago, IL: Williams & Wilkins.
Fowler, H. R. (1992). *The Little, Brown handbook* (5th ed.). New York: HarperCollins.
Humphrey, D. (1996). *Medical office procedures* (2nd ed.). Clifton Park, NY: Delmar Cengage Learning.
The Chicago manual of style (14th ed.). (1993). Chicago: University of Chicago Press.

Medical Dictionaries

Dorland's illustrated medical dictionary (28th ed.). (1994). Philadelphia: W. B. Saunders.
Stedman's medical dictionary (26th ed.). (1997). Baltimore, MD: Williams and Wilkins.
Taber's cyclopedic medical dictionary (19th ed.). (2001). Philadelphia: F.A. Davis.
Webster's new explorer dictionary. (1999). Springfield, MA: Federal Street Press.

Business Communications

Schacter, N., & Clark, A. T. (1993). *Basic English review* (4th ed.). Cincinnati, OH: South-Western.
Smith, L. (2002). *English for careers, business, professional, and technical* (8th ed.). Upper Saddle River, NJ: Prentice Hall.
Thompson, M. H., & Keithley, E. M. (1991). *English for modern business* (6th ed.). Homewood, IL: Richard D. Irwin.

WORDS THAT HAVE SIMILAR SOUNDS

accept—to take

except—to exclude

advice—recommendation (noun)

advise—to recommend (verb)

all ready—completely ready

already—previously; so soon

altar—platform in a church

alter—to change

affect—a noun that means a state of mind or mood, countenance

effect—a verb meaning to influence, to produce an effect upon

effect—a noun meaning a result, impression

effect—a verb meaning to result in, bring about, to accomplish

afferent—conducting toward a center or specific site, as afferent nerve that transmits impulses from the periphery toward the central nervous system

efferent—conducting or progressing away from a center or specific site, as an efferent nerve that carries impulses from central nervous system to periphery

aid—a verb meaning to help

aide—a noun meaning a worker who is an assistant to another

ante—a prefix meaning before, in front of, earlier

anti—a prefix meaning against, opposite, over

arteriosclerosis—a group of diseases characterized by thickening and loss of elasticity of arterial walls (hardening of arteries)

atherosclerosis—an extremely common form of arteriosclerosis in which deposits of yellowing plaque (atheromas) containing cholesterol and other lipoid material are formed within the intima of large and medium-sized arteries

bile—a fluid secreted by the liver

bowel—intestine

breadth—expanse

breath—air inhaled and exhaled (noun)

breathe—to inhale or exhale (verb)

breach—a break

breech—the buttocks

caliber—the diameter of a hollow, tubular structure (like a bullet)

caliper—an instrument used for measuring diameters (like pelvic diameters)

callous—an adjective meaning hard or bony

callus—a noun meaning bone

celiac—pertaining to the abdomen

cilia—the eyelashes

chorda (pl. chordae)—a cord or sinew

chordee—the downward deflection of the penis due to a congenital anomaly (hypospadias) or to urethral infection

chorea—the ceaseless occurrence of rapid, jerky involuntary movement

Korea—a country in E. Asia

cirrhosal—an adjective describing a diseased liver

serosal—an adjective describing a membrane covering certain cavities of the body

coarse—rough

course—a route, plan

chafe—to rub

chaff—worthless matter

cite—to quote

sight—the power of seeing

site—a place

cue—a hint

queue—a line

complement—something that completes or balances

compliment—praise

defer—to put off or delay, as in "exam was deferred"

differ—to be different

discreet—showing good judgment, prudent

discrete—made up of separate parts, not blended

diagnosis—a medical analysis

prognosis—a medical prediction

effect—to influence

effect—to accomplish; result

---

efflux—outward flow

reflux—backward or return flow

emanates—to flow out, issue, or proceed as from an origin

eminent—high in station or rank

perineum—genital area (between anus and scrotum or vulva)

peritoneum—covering of viscera (internal organs of abdomen), lining of abdominopelvic wall

peroneal—pertaining to the fibula, lateral side of the leg, or to the tissues present there

perineal—pertaining to the perineum

pleural—referring to the pleural cavity

plural—more than one

prostate—the male gland surrounding the urethra

prostrate—overcome, as prostrate with grief; lying in a horizontal position

principal—chief, head person

principle—rule

precede—to go before

proceed—to continue

quite—very

quiet—still

radicle—smallest branches

radical—going to root or source of disease, as in radical dissection at surgery

retroperitoneal—adverb meaning behind the peritoneum (a direction)

reperitonealize—verb meaning to cover again with peritoneum (peritoneum—the serous membrane lining of the walls of the abdominal and pelvic cavities and investing contained viscera)

shoddy—inferior, hastily or poorly done

shotty—like shot, lead pellets used in shotguns (usually used in reference to lymph nodes, e.g., shotty nodes)

sulfa—pertaining to the sulfonamides, or sulfa drugs

sulphur—brimstone, an element, symbol for which is S

tenia (pl. teniae)—any anatomical band-like structure

tinea—ringworm, which is a fungus

ureter—tube from kidney to bladder; there is a left and a right ureter

urethra—tube carrying urine out of the body (we only have one of these)

valgus—an adjective meaning bent outward, twisted, deformed

varus—an adjective meaning bent inward, denoting a deformity in which the angulation of a part is toward the midline of the body

vesicle—little blister or sac

vesical—urinary bladder only

villus (pl. villi)—a noun meaning little protrusion

villous—an adjective meaning shaggy with soft hairs

weather—state of the atmosphere with respect to wind, temperature, cloudiness, etc.

whether—a word introducing the first of two alternatives; example: It matters little whether we stay or go

week—a period of seven days

weak—liable to yield, break, or collapse under pressure

```
                    Mobile Medical Clinic
                     2945 Desert Drive
                    Mobile, AZ 90000-0000
                       700-300-0010
                     (FAX) 700-300-0000
```

August 31, 200__

Mrs. Jean Bone
3900 Cactus Drive
Mobile, AZ 60000-2000

Dear Mrs. Bone:

It was a pleasure seeing you on August 20, 200__. I have received the blood test results from that day and your blood work was normal. You had a normal chemistry including a cholesterol of 152. We usually like to see this less than 200, so your level is quite good in fact. Your blood count and your thyroid hormones were normal.

If you have any questions regarding the above test results, please do not hesitate to contact my office. I look forward to seeing you on your next visit.

Sincerely,

Dawn Liver, MD

Personal-Business Letter: Block

MOBILE MEDICAL CLINIC

MEMORANDUM

TO: Staff

FROM: Matthew T. Sampson, MD
           Chief of Medical Services

DATE: June 8, XXXX

SUBJECT: ABOUT STANDARD PRECAUTIONS

The attached *About Standard Precautions* booklet is intended for use by physicians and staff when reporting incidents on standard precautions and transmission-based precautions in the workplace. Please refer to the attached *About Standard Precautions* when filing an incident report.

Additional copies of the *About Standard Precautions* can be obtained from Bonnie Foot, in the Medical Services Office (x5329).

EF

Attachments

Distribution List:
  Robbie Leg, Health Information
  Joyce Pain, Chemistry
  Jodie Foot, Volunteer Services

```
                    Mobile Medical Clinic
                      2945 Desert Drive
                    Mobile, AZ 90000-0000
                       700-300-0000
                    (FAX) 700-300-0010
```

August 31, XXXX

Mrs. Jean Bone
3900 Cactus Drive
Mobile, AZ 60000-2000

Dear Mrs. Bone:

It was a pleasure seeing you on August 20, XXXX. I have received the blood test results from that day and your blood work was normal. You had a normal chemistry including a cholesterol of 152. We usually like to see this less than 200, so your level is quite good in fact. Your blood count and your thyroid hormones were normal.

If you have any questions regarding the above test results, please do not hesitate to contact my office. I look forward to seeing you on your next visit.

Sincerely,

Dawn Liver, MD

DL:SA

Block Letter

```
                        Mobile Medical Clinic
                          2945 Desert Drive
                        Mobile, AZ 90000-0000
                           700-300-0000
                         (FAX) 700-300-0010

                                                    August 31, XXXX

Mrs. Jean Bone
3900 Cactus Drive
Mobile, AZ 60000-2000

Dear Mrs. Bone:

It was a pleasure seeing you on August 20, XXXX. I have received the blood test
results from that day and your blood work was normal. You had a normal
chemistry including a cholesterol of 152. We usually like to see this less than
200, so your level is quite good in fact. Your blood count and your thyroid
hormones were normal.

If you have any questions regarding the above test results, please do not hes-
itate to contact my office. I look forward to seeing you on your next visit.
                                                    Sincerely,


                                                    Dawn Liver, MD

DL:SA


Modified Block Letter
```

Letter placement table

Length	Dateline position	Margins
Short: 1-2 ¶	Center page or $3^1/_2''$	Default
Average: 3-4 ¶	Center page or 2.5	Default
Long: 4+ ¶	2.3″ (default + 8 hard returns)	Default

Letter Parts

Letterhead: Company name and address

Date: Date letter is mailed

Inside address: Person who will receive the letter. This includes personal title, name, professional title, address, and company.

Salutation/Greeting: Includes name and title. Dear Dr. Sampson:

Body/Message. Single space paragraphs. Double space between paragraphs.

Complimentary close: Such as Sincerely

Signature block: Type the writer's full name and title

Enclosure: Copy is enclosed with the document

Copy notation: Copy being sent to a person, or persons

Audio CD to Accompany *Basic Keyboarding for the Medical Office Assistant,* Third Edition
ISBN 1-4018-1189-2

Computer CD Player Instructions

1. Insert the disk into the CD-ROM player of your computer.
2. The media player should automatically start and bring up track 1.
3. Use the media player as directed by the manufacturer.

For Windows: If the media player does not start automatically:

1. From the Start Menu, choose Programs, then Accessories.
2. Choose Entertainment or Multimedia, then a media player such as Windows® Media Player.

3. Browse to your CD-ROM drive and open the audio file you wish to play.

For Macintosh: If the media player does not start automatically:

1. Start the Apple CD Player.
2. Browse to your CD-ROM drive and open the audio file you wish to play.

System Requirements

- Audio CD player **or**
- Computer with double-spin CD-ROM drive, sound card, speakers or headphones, and media player software.

License Agreement for Delmar Learning, a division of Thomson Learning, Educational Software/Data

You, the customer, and Delmar Learning, a division of Thomson Learning, Inc., incur certain benefits, rights, and obligations to each other when you open this package and use the software/data it contains. BE SURE YOU READ THE LICENSE AGREEMENT CAREFULLY, SINCE BY USING THE SOFTWARE/DATA YOU INDICATE YOU HAVE READ, UNDERSTOOD, AND ACCEPTED THE TERMS OF THIS AGREEMENT.

Your rights:
1. You enjoy a non-exclusive license to use the software/data on a single microcomputer in consideration for payment of the required license fee, (which may be included in the purchase price of an accompanying print component), or receipt of this software/data, and your acceptance of the terms and conditions of this agreement.
2. You acknowledge that you do not own the aforesaid software/data. You also acknowledge that the software/data is furnished "as is," and contains copyrighted and/or proprietary and confidential information of Delmar Learning, a division of Thomson Learning, Inc. or its licensors.

There are limitations on your rights:
1. You may not copy or print the software/data for any reason whatsoever, except to install it on a hard drive on a single microcomputer and to make one archival copy, unless copying or printing is expressly permitted in writing or statements recorded on the diskette(s).
2. You may not revise, translate, convert, disassemble, or otherwise reverse engineer the software/data except that you may add to or rearrange any data recorded on the media as part of the normal use of the software/data.
3. You may not sell, license, lease, rent, loan, or otherwise distribute or network the software/data except that you may give the software/data to a student or and instructor for use at school or, temporarily at home.

Should you fail to abide by the Copyright Law of the United States as it applies to this software/data your license to use it will become invalid. You agree to erase or otherwise destroy the software/data immediately after receiving note of Delmar Learning, a division of Thomson Learning, Inc., termination of this agreement for violation of its provisions.

Delmar Learning, a division of Thomson Learning, Inc. gives you a LIMITED WARRANTY covering the enclosed software/data. The LIMITED WARRANTY follows this License.

This license is the entire agreement between you and Delmar Learning, a division of Thomson Learning, Inc., interpreted and enforced under New York law.

This warranty does not extend to the software or information recorded on the media. The software and information are provided "AS IS." Any statements made about the utility of the software or information are not to be considered as express or implied warranties. Delmar Learning, a division of Thomson Learning, Inc. will not be liable for incidental or consequential damages of any kind incurred by you, the consumer, or any other user.

Some states do not allow the exclusion or limitation of incidental or consequential damages, or limitations on the duration of implied warranties, so the above limitation or exclusion may not apply to you. This warranty gives you specific legal rights, and you may also have other rights which vary from state to state. Address all correspondence to Delmar Learning, Executive Woods, 5 Maxwell Drive, Clifton Park, NY 12065-2919. Attention: Technology Department

LIMITED WARRANTY
Delmar Learning, a division of Thomson Learning, Inc. warrants to the original licensee/purchaser of this copy of microcomputer software/data and the media on which it is recorded that the media will be free from defects in material and workmanship for ninety (90) days from the date of original purchase. All implied warranties are limited in duration to this ninety (90) day period. THEREAFTER, ANY IMPLIED WARRANTIES, INCLUDING IMPLIED WARRANTIES OF MERCHANTABILITY AND FITNESS FOR A PARTICULAR PURPOSE, ARE EXCLUDED. THIS WARRANTY IS IN LIEU OF ALL OTHER WARRANTIES, WHETHER ORAL OR WRITTEN, EXPRESS OR IMPLIED.

If you believe the media is defective please return it during the ninety-day period to the address shown below. Defective media will be replaced without charge provided that it has not been subjected to misuse or damage.

This warranty does not extend to the software or information recorded on the media. The software and information are provided "AS IS." Any statements made about the utility of the software or information are not to be considered as express or implied warranties.

Limitation of liability: Our liability to you for any losses shall be limited to direct damages, and shall not exceed the amount you paid for the software. In no event will we be liable to you for any indirect, special, incidental, or consequential damages (including loss of profits) even if we have been advised of the possibility of such damages.

Some states do not allow the exclusion or limitation of incidental or consequential damages, or limitations on the duration of implied warranties, so the above limitation or exclusion may not apply to you. This warranty gives you specific legal rights, and you may also have other rights which vary from state to state. Address all correspondence to Delmar Learning, Executive Woods, 5 Maxwell Drive, Clifton Park, NY 12065-2919. Attention: Technology Department.

Audio CD to Accompany
Basic Keyboarding for the Medical Office Assistant, 3e

Contents